INSIDE THE YOGA SUTRAS

INSIDE THE

YOGA SUTRAS

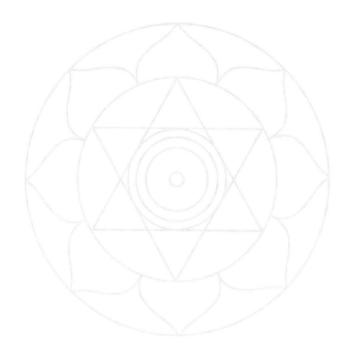

A COMPREHENSIVE SOURCEBOOK FOR

THE STUDY AND PRACTICE OF PATANJALI'S YOGA SUTRAS

REVEREND JAGANATH CARRERA

Integral Yoga® Publications
Yogaville, Virginia

Cover Art © 2006 Satchidananda Ashram–Yogaville, Inc.

Printed in the United States of America

Second Printing 2008
Third Printing 2011
Fourth Printing 2013

Library of Congress Control Number: 2005907687

ISBN - 13: 978-0-932040-57-2

Cover design by Tim Barrall
Layout by Kemper Conwell, Pixels of Charlottesville, Virginia.

Integral Yoga® Publications
Satchidananda Ashram-Yogaville, Inc.
108 Yogaville Way
Buckingham, Virginia 23921

Contents

Dedication. vi
Acknowledgments. vii
Preface. viii
Put Down This Book, Unless. ix
The Cosmic Drama:
   What You Perceive Is What You Believe. 1
Pada One:. 7
   Inside Pada One. 8
   Samadhi Pada: Portion on Absorption. 9
   Pada One Review. 92
   What to Do. 93
Pada Two:. 95
   Inside Pada Two. 96
   Sadhana Pada: Portion on Practice. 98
   Pada Two Review. 159
   What to Do. 161
Pada Three:. 163
   Inside Pada Three. 164
   Vibhuti Pada: Portion on Accomplishments. 166
   Pada Three Review. 201
   What to Do. 202
Pada Four:. 203
   Inside Pada Four. 204
   Kaivalya Pada: Portion on Absoluteness. 205
   Pada Four Review. 232
   What to Do. 233
Study Guide. 235
Appendix:
   The Yoga Sutras, the Dualism of Classical
   Sankhya, and the Nondualism of Advaita Vedanta. 239
Sutras-by-Subject Index. 245
Word-for-Word Sutra Dictionary. 293
Continuous Translation. 363
Glossary of Sanskrit Terms. 369
Resources. 401

Dedication

This book is dedicated to all who seek peace and understanding, both individual and universal. May you soon experience the unbounded peace and joy of your own Self.

It is also dedicated to that great light of Yoga, Sri Patanjali Maharaj. A compassionate and brilliant teacher, his universal teachings have informed and guided countless seekers to realize the Self and be free.

Above all, I offer this book with humility, love, and gratitude to my revered master, Rev. Sri Swami Satchidanandaji Maharaj, whose very life embodies and exemplifies the truths of Sri Patanjali's *Sutras*.

He is the root; this text, the fruit. His teachings, humor, vivid stories, and memorable analogies are for me the foundation for understanding the *Yoga Sutras* and permeate this publication. This, along with his admonition always to "look beyond the letter, to find the spirit of the law," encouraged me to express my own humble thoughts regarding this classic text.

I can never repay him for all he has done for me. To him, I offer my prostrations.

Acknowledgments

This text has been published through the dedicated and loving efforts of many. I can never repay them for their selfless efforts in bringing this text to light. They truly embody Yoga in action.

To my wife, Rev. Janaki Carrera, who patiently reviewed draft after draft, providing organization, commonsense guidance, and the title of this volume.

To Swami Karunananda Ma and Swami Sharadananda Ma, masterful teachers of Raja Yoga, whose countless hours of service provided both insights into these teachings and perceptive editing. They helped give clarity and depth to the text.

To Paraman Barsel, a great Raja yogi (and the teacher in the first Raja Yoga class I attended) whose editing skills helped elevate both the ideas and prose of this text. He was on call at all hours to serve.

To Rev. Prem Anjali for her unflagging support, Ganesh MacIsaac for his advice and help, Gill Kent for the clear editing that put the polish on the apple, and the many students and teachers of Yoga who encouraged and inspired me.

To Tim Barrall, a great artist and Karma Yogi, for his inspired cover design and to Kemper Conwell who did a masterful job with the layout of the text, making it clear and inviting.

To the countless wise teachers, authors, and commentators whose profound knowledge and insights into this holy text inspired and informed me. Thank you.

Preface

I love the *Yoga Sutras*. They have been a part of my life, as both a student and a teacher of Raja Yoga, for over thirty years. Yet to comment on a sacred text requires a particular inspiration or, failing that, a peculiar type of daring or arrogance. After all, every spiritual classic is surrounded by the wise words of great sages and scholars. Before adding another viewpoint, one must ask: Do I have anything worthwhile to add to the discussion? Will it be a useful service to others?

The book you hold in your hands began as a personal project: to organize notes that had been jotted down on receipts, envelopes, and notebooks over years of study and contemplation. At the urging of students, this straightforward task transformed into the formidable undertaking of writing a commentary. Their requests gave birth to a rumor that took on a life of its own. Soon I was being asked when my book would come out!

In spite of the interest, the project initially seemed unnecessary to me, especially since my own master, Sri Swami Satchidananda (Sri Gurudev) had authored a magnificent translation and commentary. That text has been a treasured bible for me as well as countless others for almost two decades. I thought it might be impertinent even to suggest that my small voice should be added alongside his and the other brilliant translators and commentators on the *Yoga Sutras* that are available. Still, students continued their requests. Finally I found it hard to ignore the realities of students' interest and my expanding compilation of notes.

One day, during a meeting I had with Sri Gurudev, I brought these developments to his attention. His response provided insightful guidance along with his blessings: *"If it's a good service to others, why not? I've been thinking that it is time for a new approach. Go. Do it."* On another occasion, in response to my lingering hesitancy, he added, *"Someone motivated by their ego would not even be asking these questions. It's a good idea to do this. Yes, let's do it."* His blessings instilled a special life and spirit to this project and initiated five years of joyfully consuming effort.

My prayer is that this publication fulfills my master's charge to provide a useful service to others.

Put Down This Book, Unless . . .

. . . you agree with this fundamental truth: everyone wants to be happy, peaceful, and fulfilled.

If you are completely at peace, if there is no lack in your life, if nothing has the power to make you sad, anxious, or unsure, then perhaps for you the study and practice of the *Yoga Sutras* is not necessary; you are already living the goal. If, on the other hand, you feel there is something missing in fleeting occasions of joy; if you yearn to experience an abiding peace, are searching for meaning and a vision of life that will help you make sense out of the unexpected twists and turns you face; or if you would like to bring your mind to a clear and focused stillness, then consider reading on.

The *Yoga Sutras* of Sri Patanjali is the science of joy and a blueprint for living a deeply satisfying life. It is a timeless spiritual classic whose appeal is founded on a profound and unerring understanding of the human condition. Not simply a philosophy, it presents a holistic system of practices that provide clear progressive steps towards the elimination of suffering and attainment of spiritual liberation. These teachings reach beyond age, occupation, gender, and faith tradition. They touch the heart of the struggle to find peace amidst a world of uncertainties and challenge. They boldly proclaim that the joy we seek is within us, as none other than our True Identity.

The Cosmic Drama: What You Perceive Is What You Believe

Everything begins in the mind. If you want to see
clearly, you need clear vision.
Sri Swami Satchidananda

"Perception is reality" is an adage understood by publicists and ad
executives. They understand that—accurate or not—what we perceive
to be true determines our responses. Imagine walking into a dimly lit
room. As we look around, we notice a coiled shape in a corner. A
snake! Our heart beats faster. Breathing becomes agitated. Adrenaline
pours into the bloodstream. Our mind frantically searches for the
proper course of action: Should we run, call 911, scream for help?
Fear-based thoughts repeatedly interrupt reason: What if it's
poisonous and I get bitten? Who will care for my children if I die! Then,
instinctively, we reach for the light switch. Light has the power to dis-
close the mysteries written by shadows. There is no snake; there never
was. What we thought was a snake was nothing but a coiled piece of
rope. Even though we were never in any danger, by falsely perceiving
the rope for a snake, we experienced the same thoughts, physiological
responses, and actions as if it were a snake. Our perception of the
coiled rope in the dim light became—for a while—our reality.

Perceptions become the basis of belief systems, and belief
systems, regardless of how subtle and sophisticated, are like filters
that allow certain bits of information to pass through while blocking
others. We might believe that a loving, merciful God exists, that
human nature is intrinsically good, that the purpose of life is to serve
others, that angels exist, that the policies of our own political party
are best for the country, that an apple a day keeps the doctor away,
that virtue is its own reward, and that a penny saved is a penny
earned. But what elements of truth might these beliefs be filtering?
Are these beliefs only partially true? Could they be completely false?
How many coiled ropes does our belief system contain?

Examine the "realities" that define your life. How have assumptions,
past experiences, hopes, and fears sculpted your universe? Do you *see* a
dog-eat-dog world, or does life resemble a bowl of cherries? A rat race
or a bed of roses? Is the world a dangerous place or a Garden of Eden?
If you wake up every morning to find that you are in the midst of a rat

race, large rushing rodents will populate your world. It follows that if you perceive the planet as choked with cutthroat activities, it will be necessary for you to "look out for Number One" and watch your back. Life will be a stressful experience. On the other hand, if you see a Garden of Eden outside your window, contentment and joy will surround you.

For most of us, life involves swinging from a measure of contentment and security to sadness, restlessness, and fear. Our experience of life depends on how we perceive the happenings of the moment. If everything seems to be proceeding according to our plans, we see sunshine and heaven; if our plans do not happen to match what life allows, existence can take on hellish hues.

Swinging back and forth from heavenly to hellish experiences is itself a source of suffering. We cling to pleasurable experiences while trying to escape painful ones. Those who tire of the relentless and unpredictable ups and downs of life comprise the majority of spiritual seekers. Others are drawn to spiritual life because they are dissatisfied or disillusioned with at least some aspect of life. Regardless of the specific reasons, the first steps toward spiritual life are often motivated by some measure of discontent, insecurity, or restlessness.

Thorny questions follow this agitation: Is there something more to life? Something deeper and more fulfilling? What is the true nature of life, and is there any purpose or meaning to it? Do we have to suffer? Why are we born? How and where does God fit into all of this? Does God even exist?

The answers to these questions—and more—can be found in the *Yoga Sutras*.

The teachings and practices of the *Yoga Sutras* are based on three principles:

- Suffering is not caused by forces outside of us but by a faulty and limited perception of life and of who we are. Our basic misperception gives rise to endless cravings for sense satisfaction. Since everything in the universe is constantly changing, nothing in Nature is capable of bringing lasting fulfillment.
- The unwavering peace we seek is realized by experiencing the unlimited and eternal Peace that is our True Identity. Though obscured by ignorance, it exists within us, waiting to be revealed. This experience is enlightenment—Self-realization.

- Self-realization is attained by mastering the mind. Just as only a clean, undistorted mirror can reflect our face as it truly is, only a one-pointed and tranquil mind can part the veils of ignorance to reveal and reflect the Self.

The effort to free the mind from the limitations of ignorance is a drama that has been repeated since time immemorial. The foundation of this drama is summarized in three basic precepts: *Purusha, Prakriti, and Avidya.*

Purusha: Pure Unbounded Consciousness, the Indwelling God; Self, Seer, Spirit

The experience of the Purusha as our True Identity is enlightenment or Self-realization. The direct experience of the Purusha provides the ultimate quest.

Much, although not all, of the *Yoga Sutras* is based on the Sankhya philosophy. Sankhya proposes that there are an infinite number of separate Purushas, all being omnipresent and omniscient. Yet during Sri Patanjali's time, there existed other philosophical schools that used the term Purusha to designate One Absolute Truth or Self. The *Yoga Sutras* part ways with Sankhya at several key points and the sutras themselves offer no direct reason to believe that Sri Patanjali held to the multi-Purusha principle. *(See the Appendix for more on this subject.)*

Prakriti: Undifferentiated Matter; Nature

Prakriti is the setting for this epic. Due to ignorance, Prakriti may sometimes seem to behave like an obstacle, obscuring our experience of the Purusha. In reality, it provides us with the challenges and lessons that lead to Self-realization. In doing so, Prakriti helps to uncover our hidden strengths and weaknesses.

Avidya: Spiritual Ignorance

Every hero has a weakness: Superman has kryptonite; Achilles, his heel. In this epic, Avidya, ignorance, obstructs the experience of our True Identity. It is the fundamental confusion of the Seer (Purusha) with the seen (Prakriti): regarding the impermanent as permanent, the impure as pure, the painful as pleasant, and the non-Self as the Self. Avidya is the cause of suffering. And the teachings of Yoga point the way to its removal.

The only element missing in this saga is a hero or heroine. That role belongs to you. And there is no better guidebook than the *Yoga Sutras*.

In Sri Patanjali's day, it was common for teachings, including sacred texts, to be preserved and transmitted orally. Those teachings, which for centuries have been passed down from master to disciple, are the basis of the text you hold in your hands today. We do not know when or by whom the sutras first made the transition to written form. There are 196 sutras presented in four sections or *padas*, each emphasizing a different aspect of the science of Yoga.

"A picture is worth a thousand words." So is each sutra. The most useful strategy to employ when studying the *Yoga Sutras* is to approach them as you would a piece of art or poetry, where a literal, there-is-only-one-way-to-understand-this outlook can smother the nuances, beauty, and various levels of meaning. The *Yoga Sutras* can be examined and enjoyed from many angles, each facet exposing another aspect of truth. You will discover more levels of meaning for yourself as you continue your study and practice.

The *Yoga Sutras* are also commonly known as Raja Yoga, the Royal Yoga. They earned this noble status because they present spirituality as a holistic science, universally applicable to people of all faith traditions. These are teachings that are alive, that resonate at the level of our inner spirit, awakening memories of our True Identity. The guidelines and practices of Raja Yoga bring the attainment of spiritual enlightenment within the reach of anyone through a practical step-by-step process rooted in real life experience.

Sri Patanjali

Details regarding Sri Patanjali's life are scant. It is believed that he was born sometime between 5000 BCE and 300 CE, with many modern scholars placing his birth at sometime in the second century BCE. He may have been one person or several with the same name. Some say he was a physician, lawyer, or a grammarian. Maybe he was all three. Certainly, by examining the *Yoga Sutras*, we can glimpse the mind-set of a holistic physician, an insightful legal mind intent on closing the loopholes in his presentation, and a master of concise language. Though Sri Patanjali is called the "Father of Yoga," he did not create it. The essential teachings are so ancient that no one knows for certain when they started. Sri Patanjali is the "Father of Yoga" because he was a masterful teacher who clearly perceived the cause of suffering and was able to prescribe a practical step-by-step way out of it. Though the *Yoga Sutras* are filled with wonderful philosophical insights and revelations, his intent never strays from the practical. Sri Patanjali never forgets that theory without practice will never truly satisfy us—and it is in this that we can find evidence of his great compassion. Only someone who fully empathizes with the suffering that attends spiritual ignorance would be so unwaveringly determined in pointing out the path to freedom. Sri Patanjali does not want us to while away our time admiring dazzling philosophical insights. His intent is to help us out of ignorance as quickly as possible.

Several tales of Sri Patanjali's birth have survived the centuries. According to one legend, Sri Patanjali was the grandson of Lord Brahma—creator of the universe. Another tale gives us the origin of his name. In this story, Sri Patanjali is the incarnation of Ananta, the thousand-headed serpent. Ananta (lit., the infinite) is the guardian of the hidden treasures—the sacred teachings—of the earth. Ananta also serves as the couch upon which Lord Vishnu—the form of God as preserver—rests before the beginning of creation. Ananta himself is also considered an incarnation of Lord Vishnu.

Ananta desired to bring the yogic teachings to earth, but he needed to take birth in the womb of a virtuous woman to do so. His search ended with Gonika, who was a great *yogini* (a female practitioner of Yoga) and who had been praying for a son worthy enough to receive the knowledge of Yoga. One morning, while engaged in worship, she offered to the Lord the only thing she had—a handful of water. She reverently lifted the water into her cupped palms. Just as she was about to make the offering, she noticed a tiny serpent swimming in the little pool of water in her hands. Her amazement increased as the tiny snake form of Ananta assumed full human form. He prostrated before her and asked if she would accept him as her son so that he could bring the great science of Yoga to humanity. Gonika joyously agreed and named her divine son Patanjali: an offering (*anjali*) who fell (*pat*) from heaven.

Sri Patanjali is often depicted as half human and half serpent, with his four-armed human torso emerging from the coils of his serpent lower half. Two of his hands are together in front of his chest in reverent greeting, a gesture that is referred to as an *anjali*. When given by a sage or God, this gesture reflects both a greeting and a blessing. One upraised hand holds the *chakra*, or discus, which symbolizes the turning wheel of time and the law of cause and effect. His other uplifted hand holds the conch, symbolic of the energy of the primordial sound, OM. This calls his students to practice and announces that the world as they know it will be transformed.

A note on the Sanskrit transliteration and translation used in this text.

We have decided not to use one of the standard methods for the transliteration of Sanskrit terms. Instead, we have used a simplified system meant to make the reading of the text more fluid. Also, while it is not strictly grammatically correct to add "s" to pluralize Sanskrit words, we have done so for certain key terms because it is in keeping with the trend of anglicizing Sanskrit. For example, it is now common to add an "s" to asana *and* mantra *to indicate their plural.*

In the commentary, Sanskrit terms are italicized when first translated.

The translation used in this text is based on The Yoga Sutras of Patanjali *by Sri Swami Satchidananda (Integral Yoga Publications, 1990).*

Pada One
Samadhi Pada: Portion on Absorption

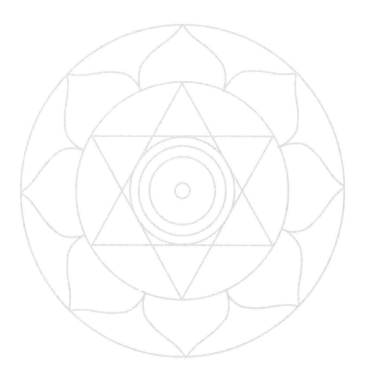

Inside Pada One

Pada One introduces you to key themes, terms, and practices that are expanded on in the rest of the text.

Sri Patanjali presents the goal of Yoga—our destination—in sutra two of this section. Where we are now—stuck in a misperception of our True Identity—is addressed by sutra three and several sutras scattered throughout the text. You will also find descriptions of the various mental modifications that color the mind, several meditation techniques, and practical hints for gaining and maintaining undisturbed calmness of mind.

Key Principles:
- Basic definition of Yoga
- Five categories of mental modifications (vrittis)
- Practice and nonattachment
- Obstacles and the ways to overcome and prevent them
- Various levels of samadhi: absorption or superconscious states

Key Practices:
- Several classic meditation techniques
- Nonattachment
- The four locks and four keys—a way to retain calmness of mind in any situation

Other Key Terms:
- *Nirodha*: cultivation of stillness of mind and the cessation of the misidentification with the mental modifications; it is both the goal of Yoga and the means to attain the goal
- *Chitta*: the mind-stuff
- *Yoga*: spiritual disciplines and effort; the experience of union between seeker and Purusha
- OM: the Cosmic Vibration; the source of all mantras (sound formulas used for meditation)
- *Samadhi*: the superconscious state, absorption into the object of contemplation
- *Ishwara*: the supreme cosmic soul; God

Pada One
Samadhi Pada: Portion on Absorption

1.1. Now, the exposition of Yoga.

Not later, not soon: now. If we wish to understand the principles of Yoga, our minds can't be bogged down in the past or fretting about the future. With all other concerns at least temporarily put aside, our minds are free to be completely in the moment. The ability to focus attention is an important requisite in all areas of learning but especially in spiritual matters, which contain subtle philosophical observations.

Atha, translated as "now," implies Sri Patanjali's fitness or authority to teach. He is calling the class to order, so to speak. Only a qualified teacher would do that. The word was also traditionally used to indicate the beginning of a course of study intended to remove doubts. With regards to Raja Yoga, the doubt to be addressed refers to students' uncertainties regarding the validity of the science of Yoga.

The word *anusasanam*, "exposition," was used to signal the beginning of the study of a subject that either was composed of commonly held concepts or had been previously taught on a more elementary level. Considering this, it is apparent that Sri Patanjali was not claiming that his was a new teaching but rather that it was an explanation of what had been taught before. It is also reasonable to assume that there were certain givens that Sri Patanjali didn't refer to when speaking to his students. It's like an instructor in a seminary who knows that it is not necessary to define the Golden Rule or list the Ten Commandments when speaking to his students.

We can now reexamine this sutra and imagine that Sri Patanjali's students might have understood it as, *"Be alert, stay focused, for any doubts you have concerning the timeless teaching of Yoga will now be erased."*

1.2. The restraint of the modifications of the mind-stuff is Yoga.

This is the heart of Raja Yoga. Each word is heavy with meaning. This sutra alone could form the basis of a lifetime of contemplation and practice.

The four words that comprise this sutra are, in Sanskrit: *Yogas chitta vritti nirodha.*

Yoga

The word "Yoga" has become so much a part of our everyday language that we take for granted that we understand its meaning. Derived from the root, *yuj*, it refers to the act of yoking. In common usage, it referred to the harnessing of animals to carts in order to make use of them. It is the root from which we derive the English word "yoke."

Later, the word was applied to the control of the senses and referred to harnessing the power of a concentrated mind toward an object of worship. It was then generalized to refer to any spiritual disciplines. "Yoga" is also used to refer to the essential union or Oneness of the individual with the Self. This last principle, common in the philosophical system of Vedanta, has influenced the understanding of this term in many schools of Yoga.

We don't have to limit our understanding of the word to any one definition. Why not include them all? Just as we value a gemstone for the way each facet reflects light, each meaning adds breadth and depth to our understanding of the term. All spiritual uses of the word "Yoga" can be considered when studying the word. In this spirit, let's look at a partial listing of definitions compiled from three Sanskrit dictionaries and then apply them to this sutra:

> Yoga: mental concentration, effort, application, practices leading to the state of Yoga (spiritual disciplines), conveyance, unity, opportunity, remedy, cure, religious abstract, undertaking, device, connection, relation, acquisition, gain, sum, fitness, endeavor, zeal, vehicle.

In the following example, the words in parentheses refer to the definitions listed above. Yoga could be defined as:

> The concentrated effort applied to the accomplishment of spiritual disciplines (mental concentration, effort, application, spiritual disciplines)...

> ...designed to bring the practitioner (conveyance, vehicle)...

...to a cessation of identification with the ego-sense, leading to the elimination of the false sense of separation from the Self (unity, union).

As such, know Yoga to be the means to remove the affliction of ignorance (remedy, cure)...

...and the essence of all spiritual paths (religious abstraction).

Chitta

Chitta comes from the root, *cit*, "to perceive, know, observe." Translated as "mind" or "mind-stuff" throughout this text, it refers to the mind in its totality: conscious, subconscious, and unconscious.

The chitta is not a separate component of Prakriti or an equivalent to the Purusha. It is the reflected consciousness of the Purusha *on* Prakriti. As such, chitta is a way of understanding the relationship between the Purusha (the Seer) and Prakriti (the seen) (*see sutra* 2.23). Since Purusha and Prakriti are omnipresent, the chitta is also all-pervading, though it appears to be limited through contact with the ego.

The chitta is composed of three functions: *manas, buddhi*, and *ahamkara*. Though these terms are not mentioned in the sutra, they were commonly known because of their use in Sankhya philosophy, which shares a number of principles with Sri Patanjali's Yoga.

Manas. The recording faculty of the chitta; that aspect of the mind-stuff through which impressions enter. Manas, mentioned three times in the sutras (1.35, 2.53, *and* 3.49), seems to be associated with the functioning of the senses. It is through manas that the individual comes into contact with external objects.

Buddhi. Buddhi has two meanings:

It is the discriminative faculty of the mind. Buddhi takes the impressions from manas and, through a process of comparison and discrimination, categorizes them, allowing the impressions to be stored for access at a later time.

Buddhi is the first, purest and most subtle product of the evolution of Prakriti. It is the liaison, so to speak, between Spirit (Purusha) and Nature (Prakriti). From buddhi evolves ahamkara, the three gunas (constituents of Nature), the senses, and the subtle and gross elements. When used in the context of the evolution of Prakriti, it is also sometimes called *mahat* (*see Glossary*).

Ahamkara. Ahamkara is the ego, the sense that we are individuals, separate from each other and our environment. Ahamkara claims the impressions from manas and buddhi as its own, bundling thoughts together to form the individual mind. Without ahamkara, there is no individual mind.

The ego is something like a dog marking its territory in a forest. Before the dog came along, the trees were simply there, belonging to no one. When the dog adds its scent to the trees, it feels that they're his. The pooch now has something to defend—property to worry over. Likewise, the ego stakes out the borders of self-identity and then exerts effort to maintain and strengthen it, while avoiding anything it regards as threatening or unpleasant.

It is at the level of ego that suffering arises. The ego prevents us from perceiving the Purusha as our True Identity. It harbors expectations and cravings, becomes frightened, insecure, angry, and envious. Yet it is the same ego that experiences love, caring, and compassion. So, in the name of Yoga, what will we be asked to do with the ego?

The yogi's first task is to eliminate not the ego but the selfishness that pollutes it. When this is accomplished, negative traits disappear, leaving the virtues intact. But even a clean ego has limitations—the ego, by definition, *is* limitation. It defines and maintains our most basic parameter: our sense of separateness. Enlightenment requires one more stage: the transcending of the ego, a shift from identifying oneself as the body-mind to the realization of oneself as Purusha.

Vritti

Vritti: literally to whirl, turn, revolve, to go on. It's a colorful term that suggests an incessant and maybe dizzying movement. It is the word that Sri Patanjali uses to describe the primary activity of the mind. A vritti is not simply a thought; it is the *activity* of forming conceptions from individual thoughts that arise in the mind. It takes place both on the conscious and subconscious levels of the mind. Vritti activity is the mind's attempt at making sense of the experiences it encounters. To a large extent, it determines our conceptions of who we are and the world we live in.

Let's examine how vrittis are born and the way they develop. Let's say, for example, that an outside stimulus rouses the senses, which brings the resulting impression into the mind. The mind takes that solitary thought (*pratyaya*) and begins a tornado-like dance, rapidly weaving together webs of thoughts in a frenetic search for other, related thoughts. Through a process of comparing, contrasting, and categorizing, individual thoughts cease their existence as isolated bits of information and become part of a complex web of ideas.

Right now your mind is attempting to find relationships between this new information regarding vrittis and any past experiences that seem to have a connection with it. The search for correlation and patterns is incessant and automatic. When we gaze at clouds, we don't have to force the mind to find foxes, dragons, and castles in their random shapes; the mind naturally seeks to make sense out of their billowy forms. This same process is how vritti activity creates our reality—our world, our family, our very self-identity. We are at the axis of a universe that we created; we are the weavers who spin the realities of our life. What this means is that our experience of life is largely determined by the nature of the webs we have woven. Hence vritti activity is the practice of constructing and deducing concepts of reality from mental impressions.

How does the apparently innocuous act of weaving thoughts create realities? Isn't there a real, tangible universe outside of the conceptions that our minds construct? Yes, there *is* a world of matter that exists independent of our perception of it (*see sutra* 2.22). Well then, we might wonder, shouldn't it seem more real than our mental constructs? In our daily experience, Reality, the unvarnished, unmodified truth of things, rarely pierces our mind's conceptions.

Vritti activity creates filters that can distort perception, selectively admitting and rejecting information. Our understanding of the world is limited and skewed by the biases and limitations that are built into and result from vritti activity. In other words, we project our conception of reality onto the screen that *is* Reality. However, the truth does peek through our mental constructs when vritti activity stops or winds down. And when vritti activity ceases, when all thought processes are stilled, then every filter is removed from our vision, and we perceive Reality in its entirety. In perhaps the most colossal "aha" moment a human being can have, we realize that we have been staring into the eyes and heart of Truth all along, almost assaulted by omniscience, omnipresence, and omnipotence, but have been allowing only bits and pieces of it into our minds.

Vrittis encourage identification. The obscuring power of whirling vrittis is only half the story; the real trouble comes when we identify with the "realities" our mind has woven. Identification with vritti activity obscures our experience of our True Self (*see sutras 1.3 and 1.4*). It takes us away from the objective truth of pure experience and involves us in the drama of the mind—the dance of light and shadows that is vritti activity.

In order for identification to take place, several factors are required:
- *Ignorance.* To be unaware or forget that our True Identity is the Purusha.
- *Egoism.* The belief that we are the body-mind.
- *Vritti activity.* The habitual behavior of the mind to form or find relationships. The mind identifies not so much with individual thoughts, but with patterns of thoughts. It is the way the mind deduces "reality" from mental impressions.

It is important to emphasize that vritti activity occurs under the influence of ignorance—forgetting our True Identity and then mistaking the body and mind for the Self (*see sutra 2.5*). The effects are much like being under the influence of alcohol. You are deprived of the ability to discriminate, to put ideas and experiences in the proper proportion. You lose mental clarity and judgment and suffer impaired reaction time. Under the influence of alcohol, inappropriate and even bizarre behavior passes for normal. Under the influence of ignorance, we cannot experience our True Identity.

Our identification with vritti activity superimposes fragmentation and limitations on the unity and harmony that is the Self. We lose our inner peace and any hope of finding Truth or the happiness we seek. That is why it is not an oversimplification to summarize spiritual life as stilling the persistent movement in the mind and the cessation of the habitual identification with vrittis.

The beguiling symphonies of vritti activity. A single note is not a song. It cannot inspire or move us. However, our attention is aroused when a note links to a few other compatible notes, generates a rhythmic pulse, and becomes a musical phrase. When that phrase joins other notes and phrases, it creates more propulsive rhythms and adds the dimension of harmonies. Our minds become even more entranced. Add counterpoint and a few related movements to create a symphony, and we will find ourselves beguiled. Each step engages us more deeply in the musical realities the mind has constructed. It is the same with vritti activity. The multilayered and multifaceted concepts formed from vritti activity are seductive, because a solitary thought offers little in the way of the understanding and meaning we seek.

Vritti's role in building self-identity. You are at a dinner party where you meet someone who asks you to say something about yourself. Your response, unhesitating and natural, is that you are an accountant, married, have three children, and love the opera. Unless prodded, you will not relate particulars such as: you routinely use a calculator, kiss your daughter good-bye every morning, and are especially moved by the first act of La Traviata, because these thoughts (although they contribute to your uniqueness) are not sufficiently comprehensive to define you. In short, when it comes to defining your sense of self, you more easily and strongly identify with broader categories or inclusive patterns of thought rather than the individual thoughts themselves.

The mess we are in. What is stunning is that the version of reality that we have created through vritti activity is based on whirls of largely nonsequential activity in which our attention constantly shifts (often rather wildly) among many different thoughts, beliefs (both true and untrue), and memories. You can confirm this for yourself after a few minutes of attempting quiet inner awareness.

For example, the act of planning a party for your uncle's eighty-eighth birthday is actually a ride on a disjointed roller-coaster of scattered thoughts. As you plan the menu, you recall that your uncle loves Italian food. Watch as the whirling begins:

eggplant is nice   it's a nightshade   I'm getting hungry aren't nightshades bad for arthritis   wasn't there something on the internet about arthritis what's that sound   my back hurts   I need a new computer   I can't afford one right now   my sister makes great sauce maybe I should get a new job   good, it's almost lunch the economy is not doing so well   we need a new

15

president   it's a little chilly in here   boy, summer is
almost over   I sure am hungry   I should ask my sister
if she can help   maybe pasta is better   I can't afford
a computer right now   yes, pasta is better

All this—and much more—happens over the span of only a few
moments. Just like some sci-fi, mutant, hyperactive superspider mad
on radioactive steroids, the mind's incessant whirling weaves webs of
conceptions from perceptions and memories. Is it possible to for us
to freely function among the many vritti webs—sticky with ignorance—and not get caught?

Yes, and Raja Yoga teaches us how. Back to the spider: since not
all the strands it weaves are sticky, it doesn't get caught in its own
web. In the same way, students of the *Yoga Sutras* learn that vrittis not
tainted by selfish attachment are free from stickiness.

How vritti activity affects perception. Let's examine what experience is like before vritti activity alters it. Imagine yourself as a baby,
having mashed banana as your first solid food. At that first taste, the
senses relayed the taste, color, texture, and aroma to your mind. At
that moment, there was no sweet fruity taste, no yellow, and no
banana aroma. Your eyes shone with wonder and curiosity when the
fruit touched your tongue. You simply experienced it for what it was.
You were in the moment, not influenced by biases, fears, or precon-
ceptions. In that moment, you truly knew the nature of a banana.

Great sages and saints of all times and traditions teach that to
experience enlightenment, we need to forget all we have learned
and become like a child. We need to regain the clarity and wonder of pure experience. This innocent awe is part of the greatness,
the holiness, we perceive in Self-realized masters. Their experiences of life, not colored by webs of thoughts, are direct, immediate, and complete.

The practical side of vritti activity. Vritti activity gives us shortcut
ways of dealing with the world of experiences. A cat sees a sparrow
perched on a branch overhead. In the cat's mind, the sparrow shape falls
into the category of potential dinner. She instinctively gets ready to
pounce. The same cat, upon seeing the mere shadow of a hawk flying overhead, hunkers down and scurries to safety. In both cases, there is no analysis needed. Each bird's shape fits into a category of the cat's reality: one

nutritional, the other a threat. It is easier to access information by category than by sifting though a multitude of individual, random thoughts.

Ultimately, the problem with vritti activity isn't the categories or correlations themselves. Instead, it is the identification with that activity, rooted in ignorance, that prevents us from seeing Reality as it truly is.

Vritti activity summarized:

- Vrittis are the mental activities through which the mind-stuff experiences and attempts to understand and organize the experiences of life.
- Vrittis are formed under the influence of ignorance.
- When individual thoughts (pratyaya) arise, they are contrasted and compared with other thoughts and then grouped into categories with similar impressions. This non-stop activity can take place on a conscious or unconscious level. The created thought-webs are also referred to as vrittis.
- The activity of vrittis generates and sustains a false sense of identity. Like cosmologists of the Dark Ages who believed that the earth was the center of the universe, vritti activity creates a counterfeit center of consciousness, a false limitation for that which is omnipresent. Through the process of identification, vritti activity creates the illusion of a self-identity separate from the Purusha.
- Vrittis provide only a limited perception of existence and are the means by which we project our conception of reality onto objects and events.

(See Vritti and Pratyaya in the Sutras-by-Subject Index. Then, by turning to the Sutra Dictionary, you can deepen your understanding of the relationship between vritti (mental modifications) and pratyaya (individual thoughts) by examining the sutras listed in the Index.)

This brings us to *nirodha*, the final word in the sutra which is the way out of the negative effects of vritti activity.

Nirodha

Nirodha is used to denote both a process and a state. It is often translated as restraint, cessation, restriction, suppression, prevention, control, and inhibition. The difficulty with these renderings is that they sometimes lead us to reduce its meaning to something like "a forceful, mechanical halting of thought processes." And since nirodha is usually associated with practices for stilling the mind—making it quiet, clear, and one-pointed—the difficulty in understanding it becomes compounded. However, nirodha's ability to still the activity of vrittis is not due to brute repression, but a process of selective focus: redirecting and holding attention on one object or idea. In this process, other vrittis are naturally restricted from consciousness, breaking the usual routine of vritti activity. This frees the mind from the habitual patterns of perception that obscure the true nature of life and self. The mind begins to perceive everything in a fresh new light, to see things as they are. That is why practices such as worship, prayer, selfless service, and study that also rely on selective focus lead to releasing the hold of the vrittis on the mind.

Since it is not the vrittis themselves but our identification with them that causes us stress and suffering, our understanding of nirodha should include any process that ends ignorance's hold over the mind-stuff. This understanding is reflected in Sri Patanjali's description of perfection in nirodha. Note the difference in a mind with and without nirodha:

> With nirodha:
> Then the Seer (Self) abides in Its own nature (Sutra 1.3)—a description of Self-realization.

> Without nirodha:
> At other times (the Self appears to) assume the forms of the mental modifications (Sutra 1.4)—a description of spiritual ignorance.

Practices, tenets, and lifestyle guidelines are valued because they foster nirodha. Nirodha ends the suffering that accompanies misidentification with the body and mind as well as ignorance's influence over mental functioning.

In the context of the *Yoga Sutras*, nirodha is best understood as a multifaceted approach to mental mastery, capable of transforming self-identity. It requires the cultivation of discipline, the redirection of attention, the attainment of discriminative discernment, the development of nonattachment, and is supported by clear moral and ethical principles.

Attainment of higher states of nirodha signals the end of the influence of subconscious impressions (samskaras) on behavior and perception. Ultimately, nirodha leads to the transcendence of all psychological limitations and the direct realization of the individual as Purusha. How does this occur?

Imagine that you have never seen your own face. You've heard that it is beautiful, and now you've developed a longing to see it for yourself. But you cannot see your face because it is the face that does the seeing. If you want to see your face, a mirror is needed to reflect the image back to you.

But to see yourself as you truly are, the mirror needs to be free of distortion and dirt. If you look at your reflection in a cracked, warped, or unclean mirror, you won't see your face as it is, you'll see a distorted image. Perceiving that you are deformed, you become disheartened. It should be obvious that you are fine and that the distorted image is due to a deformed mirror, but you persist in identifying with the reflected image.

Enter Sri Patanjali. He knows that your misery is caused by confusing the reflected image with the Self and begins gently to guide you out of ignorance. He doesn't spend much time talking about the nature of your face but instead suggests practices for gently but surely cleaning and straightening the mirror. As you persevere, the changes in the mirror cause the reflected image to change. Little by little a divine image emerges. When the mirror becomes perfectly straight, your face is revealed to you as it has always been.

The mind is the mirror in which we perceive ourselves. If it is distorted by vrittis, we often see ourselves as limited, frail beings, not one with the Self. We are fooled by the reflection in the mind-mirror again and again, missing the truth of who we really are. Vrittis swarm like locusts, clouding our discriminative faculty and reinforcing the faulty self-assessment that ignorance impresses on us. Nirodha is the means to regain the memory of who we truly are. We cease to identify with the vrittis. We realize that all of our turmoil, fears, doubts, anger, and depression are in the mind, not in our Self. The drama, conflict, humor, romance, adventure, horror, and comedy exist only on the level of the reflection. Though we might adore the image we behold, we really haven't gained anything we didn't already have; the mirror just revealed what has always been. We are not the reflection but the face. We are the Seer, the Purusha. This is enlightenment or Self-realization.

This is all good theory, but without direct experience of this truth, it doesn't help that much. Our minds are victims of habit, accustomed to restlessly running here and there. The mind's deeply ingrained restlessness can bring even the most robust seekers to despair, especially if the only image of nirodha they have is of sitting cross-legged, exerting Herculean efforts to prevent the mind from thinking. If this were all there was to Yoga practice, most of us would be doomed to brief careers as yogis. Fortunately, this scenario is not suggested in the name of Raja Yoga. Sri Patanjali presents an appealing, time-tested path that is clear, practical, and concise.

Nirodha is achieved through a holistic approach. To ensure success, we are encouraged to utilize and refine all our innate capacities: physical, social, psychological, and spiritual. In addition to stilling the mind through concentration and meditation, we are offered many other approaches that engage all of who we are in the search for Self-realization:

- The body: Yoga postures and breath control
- The intellect: study and self-analysis
- The heart: prayer and worship
- Social interaction: dedicated service to others
- Personal integrity: the cultivation of moral and ethical virtues

Related Sutra: 2.29: The eight limbs of Yoga.

By understanding the important facets and implications of nirodha, we can grasp the essence of Yoga and of all spiritual disciplines.

Nirodha is exercised by redirection. The real secret to making progress in Yoga lies in cultivating helpful habits while breaking harmful ones. The way to develop new habits is the purposeful redirection of attention. The roots that make up the word nirodha suggest this.

Derived from *rudh*, "to restrain, arrest, avert," and *ni*, "down or into," nirodha suggests "to avert into." Practitioners strive to restrain their attention from unyogic pathways by averting it toward endeavors that are consistent with the goal of Yoga. You could think of this process as retraining rather than restraining (*see sutras 2.33 and 2.34, on pratipaksha bhavana, the practice of replacing negative thoughts with positive ones*).

Training the mind is like training a puppy. Having a well-behaved and happy pet is accomplished by firm, loving redirection rather than harsh words or stern punishment. Good dog trainers know that this is the best way to create good habits.

Every time we disconnect our attention from an unwanted temptation or habit and redirect it to something beneficial to our growth, we will have gained a little more mastery over our minds.

How nirodha affects our understanding of the world. It is difficult to know an object, person, or event as it is, because biases affect perceptions. It is as though we are looking at life through a grimy camera lens that has been improperly focused.

Nirodha cleans and focuses our lens by stilling the vrittis that color our perceptions. Through a spotless, focused lens (a clear and steady mind) we come to know the nature of objects as they are. The mind naturally exercises its capacity to penetrate whatever is held steady within its focus.

Measuring progress in nirodha. Progress in Yoga is not necessarily characterized by daily mind-bending revelations. Instead the path is marked by small but significant changes in how we act and react. Perhaps we will be more patient when cut off in traffic. Or we may find ourselves a little less fearful or anxious when speaking in public. Attraction to violent movies may be replaced with more tranquil diversions. Next Christmas, we might decide to reduce our gift budget so that more can be given to charity. Sages and saints are born from these beginnings.

There is one infallible sign of growth: we will be more peaceful and happy. Maybe not everyday in every way, but if our happiness were marked on a chart, the trend over a period of time would definitely be upward.

Nirodha, repentance and the Bible. Repentance is an important recurring theme in the Bible. Though we usually consider repentance as an expression of remorse, it originally meant to undergo a radical change in values and behavior. It signified a turning away from the darkness of ignorance (sinful ways) and toward leading a life based on spiritual principles (turning toward God). Both nirodha and repentance represent turning points, fundamental changes in objectives. They form the nexus of life for those who seek to end the darkness of ignorance and the turn toward the Spirit.

Related Sutras: 3.9 and 3.10: A more technical description of the process of nirodha.

1.3. Then the Seer (Self) abides in Its own nature.

What or who is the Seer? In sutra 2.20, Sri Patanjali gives the definitive answer: *"The Seer is nothing but the power of seeing which, although pure, appears to see through the mind."* Seer is another way of referring to the Purusha: pure consciousness; unchanging, unconditioned awareness.

The word *abide* means to dwell or take permanent residence in. Because of the mind's constant fluctuations, the Seer, though always present as our True Identity, seems to appear and disappear. What *abide* suggests is that the Seer will no longer be a visitor, coming with periods of mental stillness and leaving when the mind becomes restless.

The last two sutras present the essential theoretical core of Raja Yoga; that in a perfectly still, clear mind, all traces of ignorance vanish and the individual experiences him or herself as pure, eternal, unbounded awareness: the Self. It is like a wave that experiences that it is now, was, and always will be one with the ocean.

(If you would like to look at a more detailed description of this experience, see sutra 4.34.)

This truth has been rediscovered by women and men of many cultures and times. When Lord Jesus taught, *"Blessed are the pure in heart, for they shall see God"* (Matthew 5.8), he was presenting the same principle. What does it mean to have a pure heart?

At some point in your grade-school years you were probably asked to memorize a poem to recite the next day. What did you say if you knew it perfectly? "I know it by heart." Not by head, mind, or brain, but by heart. Heart implies the totality of the mind, something deeper and more stable than the usual thinking apparatus. To have a pure heart is to have a clean, steady mind—a state of nirodha. The result of this purity is that we *shall* see God. There is no choice implied. If your heart is pure, you will see God; no ifs, ands, or buts.

The Old Testament contains a very similar idea. It appears in Psalm 46.10. This time it is God speaking: *"Be still and know that I am God."* Stillness is the requirement. Stillness; not simply refraining from motion, but absolute stillness, like the calm, clear surface of a lake which can reflect like a mirror.

All those who have achieved nirodha have the gift of dual vision. They see the unity that is God behind the diversity of names and forms. They never lose sight of the Cosmic One that is the ground of all creation. How do those of us who have not attained this lofty state view the world? What happens to our perception of the Self when the mind is colored by ignorance?

1.4. At other times (the Self appears to) assume the forms of the mental modifications.

This describes the habit of clinging to individuality: the ego identifying with mental activity. The whirl of mental modifications (vrittis) has a way of captivating our attention. It is a drama so captivating that we lose ourselves (and Self) in the theatrics. We forget that we are really witnesses to the play.

The process of misidentification is deceptively innocent. For example, if we look at our bodies in a mirror, we think we are the body. "I am tall." "I am thin." "I am male." "I am sick."

When we identify with the contents of the mind we make different statements. "I am a professor of physics." "I am a doctor." "I am happy." "I am sad."

Notice how language reveals that our "I" *appears* to undergo changes. Yet the Self hasn't changed. It's the *reflection* of the Self in the mind-mirror that changes. Our face, reflected in a distorted mirror, remains unaffected. In the same way, the Self remains unaffected and unlimited even though it is reflected on a mind that, under the influence of ignorance, is distorted by vrittis.

1.5. There are five kinds of mental modifications, which are either painful or painless.

Sri Patanjali describes vrittis in two ways: by category and by effect.

By Category

The categories consist of the five primary activities that the mind performs when engaging in daily life (*see sutra* 1.6 *for the list*).

By Effect

Fundamentally, mental activity is motivated by a dualistic principle. The mind's attention habitually flows in one of two directions: toward activities that are pleasurable or away from those that bring pain. In this sutra, we are being introduced to a deeper understanding.

Note the words used in this sutra: "painful or painless." Why not use the word pleasurable, the natural opposite of painful? We mistakenly think (sometimes subconsciously) that there is a philosophy or set of spiritual exercises that will put an end to suffering and *bring* pleasure. We believe this because we forget that the pleasure we seek is, in reality, who we already are. And although it is true that vritti activity does have only two effects, they are not pain and pleasure. The truth is that vritti activity can either obscure the happiness that is our true nature or leave that happiness undisturbed.

The flow toward the painless is characterized by clarity, discernment, and selflessness. This thought-stream leads to the disbanding of ignorance. On the other hand, mental activities that bring pain are influenced by ignorance and help maintain its power and influence. These two fundamental movements are like whirlpools, gaining or losing momentum according to the thoughts and actions of the individual.

We have become accustomed to the mind-flow that maintains ignorance and are habitually drawn into its currents much of the time. Through the practices of Raja Yoga, we increase the pull of the painless whirlpool. Each and every instance of meditation, prayer, selfless action, study of high ideals, or mantra repetition adds force to the momentum of painless vrittis, strengthening their influence in our lives. Over time, the pain-free whirlpool gains sufficient force to overcome the painful one. No yogic act, no matter how small, is ever wasted and contributes to Self-realization.

If we examine moments of joy and peace, we will discover that what they offer are veiled, fleeting glimpses of the Self. They are the instances when the mind, through a combination of factors (primarily the suspension of craving), has momentarily become steadier, enabling it to reflect a hint of the peace within.

Without self-motivated expectations, there is nothing to disturb the mind. As my master often said, *"Where there is no appointment made, there can be no disappointment."* The source of our pain is our own appointment or expectation. The mind, when no longer prodded by self-centered thought processes, gradually settles down, becoming clear and still. Operating the mind in a selfless mode does not directly bring pleasure; it simply leaves the mind alone so that the inner joy can shine forth.

(See the Sutra Dictionary to see the relationship between the painful vrittis of this sutra and the fundamental obstacles, the klesas of sutra 2.3.)

1.6. They are right knowledge, misperception, conceptualization, sleep, and memory.

This sutra tells us what vrittis "look like." If we wish to catch thieves, it is helpful to have a good description of how they look or act. If our goal is to attain nirodha over the vrittis in the mind, a description of them is very useful.

These five vrittis can be grouped into three categories. The first is concerned with the ways we gather information, whether valid or invalid. The second is the opposite of gathering data—the thought of nothing and its consequence, the state we call sleep. It is how the mind attains a state of deep rest. The third is memory, which makes learning possible by retaining experiences and giving continuity to life.

Sleep, memories, and knowledge—right or wrong—all this is in the realm of mental modifications and therefore, according to Sri Patanjali, should ultimately come under our mastery.

1.7. The sources of right knowledge are direct perception, inference, and authoritative testimony.

Our understanding of life is built on a foundation of knowledge we gain over a lifetime. But that knowledge can be trusted only if it is attained by valid means.

There are two ways of interpreting this sutra:
- There are three reliable means for attaining information regarding life and the Self.
- A piece of information is considered trustworthy after passing through this three-pronged process.

Direct Perception

Information gained through direct perception can be trusted as valid, meaning that it conforms to the actual facts. By placing direct perception first, Sri Patanjali implies that experience is the cornerstone of the learning process. Experience is not only the best teacher; it is the only teacher. Even to read a book or take a class is to benefit from someone else's experience. We may read of fire that it generates heat and can be put to either destructive or constructive uses. It could all make sense, but if our experience with fire has been confined to words on a page, it remains a reality outside of our experience. We cannot say that we *know* the nature of fire. But when we put our finger near the flame, we know that it can burn flesh; and after cooking food over a fire, we will understand its benefit. Assuming that our senses are working normally, direct perception is a source of knowledge that we can trust and use in our investigation of the world and our innermost Self.

Direct perception is the initial impact of a stimulus on individual consciousness. However, when the mental functions kick in, what was a pure direct experience can become colored by the limitations of the thought process itself. If there is a lack of focus during the act of perception, the knowledge gained can be incomplete. Then, when the ego, ahamkara, stamps its imprint on that experience, claiming it as unique to itself, the experience usually becomes colored by biases, desires, aversions, and fears. Finally, when recalling the experience, the mind becomes vulnerable to the corrupting influences of faulty or incomplete memory, causing vital facts to be lost or extraneous information added.

Since we can't directly experience everything ourselves, we need to be able to gain knowledge from other sources. For example, we routinely compile and process information through reading or listening. (If the source of the information is considered expert, we would then be using authoritative testimony, the third category for attaining right knowledge.) The data we gather forms an internal library of information: true, false, or mixed. This stored information, when used to augment direct perception, is what is called inference.

Inference

Inference, primarily a function of the discriminative faculty of the mind (buddhi), relies on previously gained knowledge. It requires that we know at least some of the characteristics of the object being inferred and can correctly relate those characteristics to the object. The classic example is that fire can be inferred when we see smoke, because it is known that one characteristic of fire is that it is accompanied by smoke.

Inference as a means for attaining knowledge is only as reliable as the analytical means employed. If I spot smoke rising on a distant mountaintop, I can infer the presence of fire, but only after I determine whether what I see is truly smoke, not a wispy cloud, steam escaping from a factory vent, or dust kicked up by a truck. Simply seeing a hazy, billowy shape in the air does not provide enough information to draw a valid inference. However, I may be able to correctly infer fire if I draw closer and detect the smell of smoke or hear the sound of a fire truck approaching. Any attempt to conclusively identify what I'm seeing before gathering sufficient information would be jumping to a conclusion.

The mind's tendency to jump to conclusions is probably one reason why Sri Patanjali would like us to consider the proper way to make inferences. Consider how much trouble is caused when the mind assumes facts not in evidence. False accusations and interpersonal strife are only part of the problem. Our minds can become littered with falsehoods and half-truths about life and the world we live in. In order to avoid this dangerous habit, it is helpful to be aware of the state of mind that makes it more likely.

The primary factor that marks jumping to conclusions is an interruption or corruption of the fact-gathering process due to:

• A loss of focus in the act of perception
• The impatience to experience something we think will bring us pleasure
• The anxiety to avoid that which we think will bring us pain

Ideally, how should the process of inference work?

The Sanskrit term for inference, *anumana*, holds important clues for the effective analysis of information. It comes from the roots, *anu*, "after," and *ma*, "to display, measure, prepare." "To display after" can be understood as the use of recollection; "to measure" suggests assessment; and "to prepare" implies the drawing of a conclusion. Therefore inference is the process of drawing a logical conclusion regarding an experience through accurate recall and assessment.

Accurate recollection. Unlike direct perception, in which the *object* itself is the stimulus for (and the focus of) perception, in inference, it is a *characteristic* of the object that catches our attention.

Example: I put a sweet potato casserole in the oven. Meanwhile, I busy myself with some intense housecleaning. Two hours later, I catch a whiff of something alarming. My memory, searching for similar smells, quickly reports that the aroma I am detecting is that of burning food. I have not directly observed the burning food but have perceived one of its characteristics. The unpleasant aroma then stirs another memory: I recall the casserole that I placed in the oven two hours earlier.

For inference to be of value, memory needs to be accurate and readily accessible. Accurate recollection is enhanced by having a clear, focused mind unhampered by bias or personal attachment.

Assessment. Since inference deals with characteristics, I need to be able to find relationships between the characteristic I am experiencing and its object. If my understanding of the relationships between what I am experiencing and that which is being inferred is correct, and if my mind follows a logical progression of reason and resists jumping to conclusions out of anxiety, fear, or some other stressor, my measure of the event is something I can rely on as accurate.

Example: Using the information I have at hand, I assess that my recollections of the smell of burned food and an overcooked casserole have a logical relationship.

Drawing a conclusion. This is the process of summarizing information into usable knowledge.

Example: I conclude that it is my sweet potato casserole that is burning. Direct visual perception of my casserole will verify my inference.

Drawing a reasonable and logical conclusion about an idea, object, or event allows us to find correspondences to other pieces of information and may also prompt us to form general principles or plans of action. In the above example, I quickly decide to remove the casserole from the oven and then later shop for an oven timer with a loud bell.

Authoritative Testimony

Agama, literally, "to go toward a source," is expert advice and guidance from scriptures and from spiritual adepts or enlightened individuals.

The direct experience of sages, saints, prophets, and spiritual masters is a valid source of knowledge, since it is knowledge that has proven its reliability to countless seekers over time. It should also be knowledge that has the potential to be verified by the individual through his or her own direct perception. We can verify the validity of our guidebook's road maps when we drive the roads for ourselves.

Now let's examine how direct perception, inference, and authoritative testimony work together to help ensure that any knowledge gained is accurate and therefore useful in contemplating spiritual teachings.

Assuming that the senses are in good working order, there is no delusion in direct perception. Therefore it is a valid source of gathering knowledge. Yet it does have practical limitations. The scope of learning is limited to personal experiences. Also, there are no concepts, words, value judgments—no way of communicating the experience to others or of assessing its purpose in life. Although the information is true, it is stark and isolated from other facts.

Inference allows us to work with information. We compare, contrast, and evaluate bits of information on many levels, refining them until they can be used in everyday life. Inference not only helps bring our experiences into the world but assists us in coordinating, organizing, and utilizing all the knowledge we acquire. But, as we noted above, the process of inference is susceptible to the distorting influence of the thought processes. This is where authoritative testimony comes in.

In order to prove that personal knowledge is sound, it is prudent to measure it against expert, objective testimony.

Let's look at a hypothetical example to demonstrate how the three sources of right knowledge balance each other. Suppose that you have recurring bouts of abdominal discomfort. The sensation of pain is direct experience. Your concern motivates you to refer to several medical texts, research on the Internet, and talk to a few friends who have had similar problems. Through inference you deduce that it is a case of acid reflux. You conclude that it is not serious and purchase over-the-counter drugs to treat it.

Of course, you may or may not be correct. If you wish to be certain, or if the attempts at self medication prove unsuccessful, you would naturally consult experts—doctors. Similarly, if we wish to confirm the validity of our understanding of spiritual matters, we would do well to consult authoritative texts and those who have experienced the truths of these teachings for themselves.

This three-limbed approach to gaining understanding—direct perception, inference, and authoritative testimony—helps keep the yogi's attention focused on endeavors that are conducive to their spiritual maturation.

1.8. Misperception occurs when knowledge of something is not based on its true form.

The word translated as misperception is *viparyaya*. The word's roots offer a clue into what it is and how it occurs.

Viparyaya is from *i*, "to go, flow," with *vi*, "asunder, away," and *pari*, "around," giving *Viparyaya*, "to flow away or around."

Misperception occurs when the mind misses the point and flows away from or around the truth when drawing conclusion about an occurrence.

Note how this definition of misperception is almost the direct opposite of nirodha—holding the mind's attention steady. The implication is that observations can be faulty when the mind lacks steady focus. Misperception is grounded in problems that occur during the act of perception or in the process of inference. It could be that the information relayed by the senses is incomplete, the logic is faulty, irrelevant information is added, or the memory does not contain facts pertinent to the object perceived. The consequence of misperception is that mental impressions (vrittis) that do not correspond to actual facts become stored and treated as true knowledge.

The classic example of misperception is mistaking a coiled rope for a snake in a dimly lit room. The mistaken perception produces the same impact as if the snake were actually present.

Misperceptions usually contain a kernel of truth. Continuing with our example, the senses correctly perceived a coiled shape and relayed that information to the discriminative faculty. Maybe because of a deep fear of snakes or because the memory of a documentary on rattlesnakes was fresh in our mind, the orderly process of inference was short-circuited. We jumped to a conclusion that did not correspond to reality. Without mental equanimity, we are easily sidetracked during acts of perception or inference. Our minds, thrown into an uncontrolled chain reaction of subconscious impressions, desires, and biases, falls prey to misperception.

It is interesting to note that Sankhya philosophy lists the causes of misperception as:
- Ignorance
- Egoism
- Attachment
- Aversion
- Clinging to bodily life/self-love

If you look ahead to sutra 2.3, you will see the same five factors listed as the five obstacles (klesas). In short, misperception rests on the fundamental ignorance of the True Self.

1.9. Knowledge that is based on language alone, independent of any external object, is conceptualization.

The mind constructs our understanding of life through various avenues. Knowledge born of conceptualization is based on language alone: on our familiarity with words and the knowledge symbolized by words. Conceptualization is the creating of subjective realities from the mind's incessant inner dialogues. It is perhaps the most prolific creator of our notions of reality. Consider for a moment how many of our ideas concerning existence are formed from or are based on what we hear in conversations and through novels, newspapers, movies, TV shows, and lyrics.

In conceptualization, the mind weaves realities by combining memory and language in various creative ways. It is important to note that knowledge gained through conceptualization may or may not be correct. For example, consider the adage, "Love is blind," a proposition with no perceptible object that we can connect to it. It is a reality constructed of words alone that may indeed reflect a reality. Next, we encounter the saying, "God is love." Once again, there is no object detectable by the senses, and once more—using only words—we treat these words as a truth. These two sayings echo, in a poetic way, personal feelings that are real and that can become building blocks of our worldview. However, until we experience the objects associated with these conceptualizations (*love* in one case, and *God* in the other) or have them confirmed by authoritative testimony, we can't treat these sayings as right knowledge. Here's one good reason: conceptualization can easily get out of hand and lead us into ignorance. Using a kind of equation-based thought process, we can arrive at a new "truth" by combining the two sayings above: If love is blind and God is love, therefore God is blind. With no external object to restrain our minds from fantasy or no acknowledged authority correcting us, we might indulge in flights of fancy. These mental excursions can take us from word-formulas that reflect a truth to fantastic images assembled from memories: a thirty-foot crab with a horse's head, for example. The fact that conceptualization can make us abandon proper inference, authoritative guidance, and direct perception in favor of word-constructed realities is nicely depicted in the Sanskrit for conceptualization, *vikalpa*. Its root translates as "to depart from the well-ordered or suitable."

Because conceptualizations have no external point of reference, they can obscure our perception of reality as it truly is. We can study exacting similes describing the taste of a banana, but until we actually taste one, it remains a conceptualization—a reality not experienced. For yogic students who are interested in direct perceptions of reality, the deeply ingrained habit of conceptualization:

- Forms blocks to direct perception
- Distracts the mind from the logic of inference
- Hinders us from benefiting from the wisdom that comes from authoritative testimony

Knowledge gained through conceptualization is not considered valid until and unless there is an actual object or event that is directly perceived or if it can be corroborated by an authoritative source. All genuine truths can be corroborated, at which point they are then considered authoritative testimony: a "source of right knowledge"(*see sutra* 1.7).

Conceptualization does have a positive side. It is how we form the metaphors and similes that help us make sense of data stored in the mind. Conceptualization also forms the basis of the creative process necessary to produce poetry and the other arts.

Misperception and Conceptualization Compared

In contrast to misperception, in which the mind alters the perception of an external object, conceptualization is devoid of any object, any corresponding reality. In misperception, we mistook a rope for a snake. Here there is nothing but the power of language to create vrittis.

One of the ways we fall into the pitfalls of conceptualization is when the search for truth is abandoned in favor of things feared or hoped for. In such cases, relying on conceptualization as a source of valid knowledge often nudges the mind to jump to conclusions.

There is a fictional story of a young man who was a high jumper of little ability. He was recounting to his classmates—and anyone else who would listen—the amazing events that transpired at the county championships.

He proudly told his friends that on his first jump he tied the school record. The crowd cheered wildly. But unfortunately, he emphasized, he could not prove that this happened because no one was there to see it. His classmates were amazed at his accomplishment. Was this the same boy who barely made the team?

His next jump broke the state record. The crowd jumped to its feet, cheering in thunderous acclaim.

"I know that this is hard to believe, but it's true. The only regret I have is that no one was there who can verify my story."

"Amazing!" exclaimed one of his friends. "What a shame that the media was not there."

On his final jump the crowd grew hushed as the bar was raised above the national record. He mustered his concentration, focused on the crossbar, and, in a mighty effort, broke the record. The crowd, again on its feet, cheered long and hard, chanting words of praise for their hometown hero. "But sadly," the young man said, "no one was there to see it."

Then one young girl said, "No one was there to see this?"

"No," replied our hero, "no one."

Another classmate chimed in, "But the crowd...the crowd cheered for you, didn't they?"

"Why, yes they did."

Suddenly, they understood. With loud sighs and rolling eyes, they began to walk away. Caught up in the drama of his story, they had fallen victims to conceptualization.

In our daily lives, when we learn of facts or events from words alone, it is beneficial to allow the mind time to examine the related circumstances and, when applicable, consult "experts." Often we can avoid the problems that follow from jumping to conclusions.

Related Sutra: 1.43: Describes nirvitarka samadhi, the state in which the mind is immune to the pitfalls of conceptualization.

1.10. That mental modification which depends on the thought of nothingness is sleep.

This refers to dreamless sleep. It is the state in which all other vrittis are suspended, except that of nothingness. The fact that we remember sleeping proves that sleep is not the mere absence of mental activity. We remember only that which we perceive.

Although deep sleep provides the body with much-needed healing rest, the deeper and more subtle function of sleep is the rejuvenation of the mind. The body, though it needs rest so it can regenerate, can get some recuperation in other ways. For the advanced yogi, deep states of meditation provide profound rest and rejuvenation for both the body and mind.

1.11. Memory is the recollection of experienced objects.

All experiences impact the mind as vrittis. After a time, the vrittis become subtler and sink to the bottom of the mental lake, where they become samskaras: subconscious impressions. Samskaras can lie dormant and not affect us, become active on a subconscious level and influence our conscious mental states, or get stimulated and return to the surface of the mental lake as a memory (*see Samskara in Sutras-by-Subject Index*).

This sutra has a link to the previous one. Dreams are memories that assert themselves in sleep. These memories may present themselves in symbolic form and so are often not recognized as such.

Memory is the only one of the five thought waves that concerns the past. Without it, we could not learn from experience.

1.12. These mental modifications are restrained by practice and nonattachment.

This two-pronged approach typifies a principle used by holistic health care practitioners. While appropriate treatment for the current complaint is prescribed, measures that strengthen resistance to future occurrences are also suggested. Practice is analogous to treatment, and nonattachment, to prevention. Both practice and nonattachment are necessary for success in Yoga. They are complementary approaches that help the mind become clearer, calmer, and stronger.

Practice without nonattachment can lead to a superinflated ego that relishes using power to satisfy self-interest regardless of consequences. Many demons in Hindu mythology were advanced yogis who fell from the path of righteousness when they succumbed to a tragic flaw, usually a burning craving. On the other hand, without the strength and mental clarity gained from practice, true nonattachment may never really dawn. Instead, the mind can slip into apathy. This faux nonattachment can provide a temporary haven for the fearful—a spiritual facade where they can hide in order to avoid challenges and responsibilities. When fears remain untouched, innate capacities remain undiscovered. We become Clark Kent, never knowing that Superman lies within. It is *practice* that mines our untapped inner resources.

The combination of practice and nonattachment leads to becoming an individual who develops his or her capacities to the fullest and who is guided by a clear, selfless mind.

1.13. Of these two, effort toward steadiness is practice.

"Effort toward steadiness" refers to focusing and stilling the mind in meditation, to the cultivation of regularity, and to developing an unwavering awareness of the mind's activities (especially the ego's limiting and harmful impact). In the most general sense, practice is the continued effort to stay within the flow (the habit) of mental activity that leads to the dissolution of ignorance.

The practices presented in the *Yoga Sutras* fall into the following categories:

- The physical practices of *asana* and *pranayama*
- Meditation (*dharana, dhyana, samadhi*)
- Devotion to God or self-surrender (*Ishwara Pranidhana*)
- Understanding and accepting suffering as a help for purification (*tapas*)
- Discriminative discernment (*viveka*)
- Study (*svadhyaya*)

In all these practices, good results can be obtained only when the mind attains steady attentiveness to the task at hand.

But Yoga practice is not limited to formal meditation or prayer. Daily life is the stage upon which vrittis perform their dance. Therefore our lives—every act—should reflect a clear and steady focus of mind. We won't make satisfactory progress if we practice control of the mind for an hour a day and then let it restlessly wander during the other twenty-three. Our lifestyle and environment should support our goals. That is why we need to live fully in the moment and to develop attentive focus on whatever task is at hand. That is also Yoga practice.

By using the word "effort," this sutra reminds us that Yoga is not for the lazy. Nothing great was ever achieved without effort. Take, for example, the great dancer Fred Astaire. We see him gracefully gliding and leaping—seemingly immune to the law of gravity—and are amazed. How effortless his movements seem. Yet many people don't know how hard he worked to achieve that mastery. Many times, the cast and crew would go home after a hard day's filming only to return the next morning to find that he had never left the studio. He continued rehearsing through the night, striving to perfect every subtle nuance of the dance. His story is not unique. It is shared by many women and men who achieved greatness.

It is significant that this sutra does not make any reference to sectarian traditions. Sri Patanjali doesn't mention anything specific to Hinduism, Buddhism, Islam, or any other religion. He doesn't mention God, Truth, or Cosmic Consciousness. When it comes time to define practice, Sri Patanjali demonstrates the universality of his understanding by simply presenting steadiness of mind as the foundation of spiritual practice.

That is why it is not a stretch to say that when a Catholic prays the rosary, it is essentially what the *Yoga Sutras* define as Yoga practice. It is the same with a Buddhist monk engaged in walking meditation in the jungles of Thailand and the Jew who reverently prays in front of the Western Wall in Jerusalem or the Muslim facing Mecca in prayer. They may or may not know the name "Yoga," but according to the authority on the subject, they are engaged in Yoga practice.

Experience It

If you haven't done so already, now is a good time to begin a daily routine of Yoga practices. It's a good idea to include practices that help make the body stronger and more relaxed, meditation and/or prayer to help steady the mind, and at least a little study to help keep inspired and on track.

Consider starting a spiritual diary. Make a daily chart listing all the practices you intend to perform, and note how long you spend with each practice. You can also track your progress in other areas that need improvement, such as dietary changes, virtues to cultivate, and negative habits to eliminate. You could also devise a system of reinforcements to help you if and when you slip from your commitments. You could add an extra sitting of meditation or do a few extra rounds of breathing practices, for example.

Note how lapses in your commitments affect the quality of your practices and the way you experience your day. A late night today may make tomorrow's meditation dull and unfocused. Missing meditation altogether may bring an increase in irritability during the day.

Review your resolves every month or so and revise them as you progress. A spiritual diary can serve as a good reminder of your objectives.

Be practical in structuring your program. Estimate how much time you need for your other duties and realistically calculate how much time you can spend with your Yoga practices. Students are often very enthusiastic in the beginning and bite off more than they can chew. It is better to spend less time and be regular than a great deal of time occasionally.

Don't be obsessed with your progress. Even a trip to a vacation destination can seem interminable when we all we care about is arriving. The anxiety will make us miss many beautiful and worthwhile sights along the way. Learn to appreciate and enjoy the process.

1.14. Practice becomes firmly grounded when well attended to for a long time, without break, and with enthusiasm.

What is a "firmly grounded" practice and why is it a desirable state? A firmly grounded practice is one that occurs daily without strain or grudging participation. It is meaningful, inspired, and focused. It is a joyful habit that accompanies practitioners throughout their lives and becomes the unbroken thread that guides them to Self-realization.

A firmly grounded practice is not simply an ingrained routine of spiritual exercises but an anticipated time of connection to deeper levels of self. It is a time of growing acquaintance with our True Identity, of spiritual discovery and nurturance. Times in practice are times of integration and increasing wholeness. This vision of practice is the ideal and is achievable by anyone who follows the advice presented in this sutra.

The attainment of a firmly grounded practice marks an important stage in spiritual pursuits: it is the shift from "doing Yoga" to having Yoga practice become a natural expression of who we are. Practices are no longer activities outside us—techniques or observances that have been added to our daily life. Practices become as integral to our life experience as eating and sleeping.

Yet most practitioners know that there are times when practice is not a pleasant experience. Initial enthusiasm—the anticipation and zeal to experience the peace and joy of higher spiritual states—can gradually give way to complacency and carelessness. These are times when much of our energy is spent on cajoling, persuading, and sometimes even intimidating ourselves to practice. When practice is irregular, the hoped-for benefits are not realized, leading to a downward spiral of even less frequent, less focused practice. To avoid this pitfall, Sri Patanjali offers a simple, effective formula for cultivating a firmly grounded practice.

Long Time

Success in any worthwhile endeavor requires time, and with regard to achieving nirodha, a long time. How much time depends on variables such as past activities, temperament, and current environment. But chief among these is how much effort and focus we put into our practices (*see sutras 1.21 and 1.22, which discuss the relationship between enthusiasm and strength of effort and success*).

We are not told how long we will need to wait for our practices to be firmly grounded, but clearly we need to have a measure of patience. What can be said is that success in spiritual endeavors requires persistence.

There is a story in which Lord Buddha was asked how long it takes to reach nirvana.

"Do you really wish to know the answer?" the Compassionate One asked his enthusiastic student.

"Oh yes, Master. I am eager to know how long I will have to practice before I reach enlightenment."

"Very well, my son. Can you imagine a cube of solid granite one hundred by one hundred feet?"

"Yes, sir, I can do that."

"Very good. Now, also imagine that a bird carrying a silk scarf in its beak flies close enough to the granite block so that the scarf brushes the top of it. Are you still with me?"

"Yes, sir, but what does this have to do with my enlightenment?"

"You will soon understand. Can you further imagine that this bird flies over the granite cube only once very one hundred years?"

"Yes, sir, I am able to think of that, though it is a bit difficult."

"Good. If you wish to know how long it takes to attain nirvana, understand that it is the same length of time it takes that scarf to wear the granite to the ground."

The eager student's jaw must have dropped. There may be many reasons why Lord Buddha relayed the message of this story to his disciple. Regardless, we can rest assured that enlightenment probably doesn't come after a month or two of practice for most of us.

This story can be disheartening, especially to those new to the practice of Yoga. But don't fret. Keep reading. A little further on in the commentary on this sutra is another story that balances this one.

Without Break

Any student would love her or his practice to be as ingrained a habit as toothbrushing. If you decide tonight to skip tomorrow morning's dental routine, there is a good chance that tomorrow you will find yourself in front of the bathroom mirror with a mouth full of foam, having completely forgotten the previous day's resolve. Such is the power of habit. Yoga practice can also become that habitual.

To attain an easy, flowing regularity in practice, a considerable length of time is not enough. The practice has to be regular. There is no lack of Yoga practitioners who complain that they are not much better off now than ten years ago when they began. If you question them, you will often find that though they have been practicing for ten years, their practice has been an on-and-off affair. Progress cannot be made without regularity—not just in Yoga but in any worthwhile endeavor.

However, no effort in Yoga is wasted. Every mantra repeated, every asana, each occasion of dedicated service to others, every prayer, act of worship, or bit of sacred knowledge learned adds to the momentum and depth of practice.

With Enthusiasm

Years of regular practice still might not produce the expected results if it is not done with the proper attitude. Enthusiasm means to have faith and love for the practices and what they will bring. It is the key that enables us to practice for a long time and without break.

In the beginning, enthusiasm is inspired by the promise of benefits to come. As we progress, the peace and joy of the Self dawning on the mind becomes the great motivator.

Remember the story of Lord Buddha and the block of granite? Here is a story that demonstrates a complementary principle. It features the sage Narada, who was well-known for his travels to and from heaven.

One day, while Narada was walking through a forest, he came across a yogi who had been sitting in meditation for so long that ants had built an anthill around his body, covering it totally. Only his face was sticking out.

This meditator, of obvious resolve and stamina, saw Narada and called out, "Revered sir, where are you traveling to?"

"Oh, I'm soon off to visit Lord Siva in heaven." Lord Siva is known as Lord of the Yogis. Our ardent practitioner recognized an opportunity.

"When you are there, could you ask the Lord a question for me?"

"I'll be happy to. What is it you wish to know?"

"I have been here such a long time. How much longer will I need to be meditating like this until I reach enlightenment?"

"I'll be certain to ask the Lord for you. When I come back this way, I'll let you know His response."

Narada resumed his journey. After a few more miles, he came to a clearing and spotted another man. In contrast to the motionless, anthill-covered yogi, this fellow was dancing and chanting with joy. After a moment, he noticed Narada.

"Narada, what brings you here? Where are you going?"

"I'm going to heaven for a visit."

"Wonderful. If it is not too much trouble, I have this question. Could you kindly present it to the Lord?"

"Yes, I'm happy to do so."

"How much longer will I need to practice before I get final liberation?"

"Okay. I'll be sure to ask Him for you."

After some time, Narada returned to the forest and encountered the first man, still covered by the anthill.

"Namaste, Narada, did you see the Lord? What did he say about me?"

"Yes, I saw Him and asked your question. He said that you will have to be meditating like this for four more lifetimes."

"FOUR? FOUR!!! I can't believe it! Haven't I done enough?" He cried and moaned over the news.

After consoling the great meditator, Narada walked on and found the second man, still dancing and chanting the name of God.

"Greetings Narada. Did you receive an answer to my question?"

"Yes. Do you see that tree over there, the very large one?"

"Yes, sir."

"Can you count the leaves on it?"

"Yes, I'll start right away if you wish."

"Oh no, you don't have to count the leaves for me. But, Lord Siva said that you will need to take as many births as there are leaves on that tree before you get liberation."

"At least the time is finite. I'm so happy to hear the answer, Narada. Thank you."

Suddenly, a magnificent chariot descended from heaven. The driver looked at the young man and said, "Please come. Lord Siva has sent for you."

"I don't understand. I'm going to meet the Lord now? I thought I must wait until I took so many births."

"Yes, but the Lord has been watching you and He is pleased with your joyful patience and perseverance. So there is no need to wait. Come."

Patience, perseverance, joy, and dedication combine to shorten our journey. Even a one-hundred-foot cube of granite can quickly disintegrate under this pressure.

Yoga is a science. If you practice diligently, you'll get the results. There is no doubt about it. We develop into better people, seeking within ourselves to find the place where devotion lives, where consistency is the natural state, and where the roots of love are hidden. We could replace, "long time, without break, and in all earnestness" with "devotion, consistency, and love." These qualities will serve us well in any endeavor.

How can we tell if our practice has become firmly grounded? One simple answer is: when it is harder *not* to practice than to practice. Another touchstone is: when, for reasons beyond your control, practices are missed. Does skipping a day or two or a change of schedule initiate a cascade of irregularity? If so, the practice is not yet firmly grounded. Those who have firmly established their practice are not thrown off by changes in schedule, place, or time. For them, the joy and benefits of the practices are stronger than worldly distractions.

Dedicated practice generates a flow of mental energy toward Self-realization so strong and vital that no other result can follow. If we persist in promoting that flow, we will someday experience help (grace) in the form of the pull of the Absolute (*see sutra 4.26, "Then the mind-stuff is inclined toward discrimination and gravitates toward Absoluteness"*).

1.15. Nonattachment is the manifestation of self-mastery in one who is free from craving for objects seen or heard about.

Nonattachment, *vairagya*, literally means "without color." It is the ability to keep the distortions of selfish motives and intents out of every relationship, action, and process of learning.

Selfish desires are the typical motivating forces of the mind, pulling it toward hoped for pleasure or away from the dread of pain. However, for those interested in Self-realization, selfish desires are not the appropriate mode of functioning, since they are based on relieving the discomfort of craving and not on what is physically, mentally, socially, or spiritually beneficial. Seekers are called on to cultivate a different foundation for their actions: nonattachment.

Nonattachment emerges when the mind voluntarily changes its underlying motivations from selfish to selfless, from seeking sense satisfaction to seeking an experience of peace that transcends external circumstances. Selfless desires gradually release the mind from the sway of sense-motivated activity and open it to the powerful influence of the Purusha.

Relating nonattachment to self-mastery might lead us to confuse it with fanatical exercises in repression and self-deprivation. That path often leads to failure and an unbalanced view of the world as a dangerous and evil place. Instead, the self-mastery that expresses as nonattachment is a process of reeducating the mind through:

- The careful observation of the limitations of sense satisfaction; it is the cultivation of realistic, healthy relationships with objects and attainments based on understanding what the world can and cannot offer.
- Assessing life's experiences in regard to their ability to decrease or increase ignorance
- The effort to live according to principles that foster spiritual growth rather than what feels good at the moment
- Cultivating an inner awareness: an introspective mind-set that is aware of the motives for actions
- The redirection of the will when making choices; not by repression of desires but by directing the attention away from selfish actions and toward those that are selfless

But these explanations are probably not enough to inspire confident, enthusiastic practice. It is hard to drop the feeling that nonattachment is somehow unnatural; that it rejects human emotions and promotes a dour view of life. That is why success in nonattachment requires a deeper understanding of the nature of attachments and of why we are being asked to avoid them.

Attachments are attractions we feel toward objects or people that we believe have brought us pleasure (*see sutra* 2.7). Aversion, the feeling of repulsion for certain objects or events that we believe bring discomfort, is attachment in reverse (*see sutra* 2.8).

As seekers, we sometimes find ourselves caught in a contradiction. We believe that it is unreasonable to expect the world to provide permanent fulfillment. Meanwhile, even as we strive to experience the unbounded Peace that is our True Identity, we cling to a list of things we think we need to be happy. This contradiction occurs because we habitually attribute the power to confer happiness onto objects and attainments.

We catch a whiff of warm apple pie. Immediately, without any apparent thought, a craving develops. Craving, never a comfortable state, nudges us into action. We expend the time, energy, and funds necessary to get some nice apple pie. After enjoying a slice, a thought arises. It may seem harmless, yet it exemplifies a way of thinking that leads to suffering: "*That* made me happy." Our beliefs seemed to have switched from "Happiness is my True Nature," to "I can't be happy without apple pie." What happened?

We expended effort to get the pie, driven by the discomfort of the craving and the anticipation of experiencing pleasure from satisfying that craving. After eating the pie, we felt a release and, *mistaking* it for happiness, attributed our happiness to the pie. Actually, we just returned to the state we were in before the craving took hold of the mind, albeit with more calories and sugar in our bloodstream.

This is not to say that apple pie is bad—or good. It is neutral. Things in Nature are neutral. It is our approach that determines whether sense objects are experienced as sources of pain or pleasure. As my master often said, "*Electricity is good when you plug in a radio but bad when your plug in your finger.*" If we are interested in knowing the true nature of electricity, the mind must be kept neutral. To maintain a clear, balanced mind; to perceive things as they are, without bias; and to act without prejudging, constitute the core of nonattachment.

Your own experience with transitory sense pleasures will tell you that they are often mingled with guilt or the pain of seeing them slowly vanish. Rarely, if ever, are we perfectly satisfied. Most often we are left wanting a little more or better food, movies, shoes, money, or relationships. This lack of real satisfaction is inherent in the mistaken notion that something outside us can make us happy. The more we rely on the outside world for happiness, the more we experience dissatisfaction and craving. We forget that an undisturbed state of mind reflects the essence of our being, the Self, which is happiness itself. The paradox is that the only way *not to* experience perfect happiness is to be seeking it outside the Self.

One might wonder: Does the practice of nonattachment require staying away from things we love, those things that bring enjoyment? Isn't it natural, even good, to want a meaningful job or a loving partner; aren't they, at least, exceptions to this principle? Didn't God create the universe for us to appreciate?

Nonattachment is not a negation of the world but the cultivation of the appropriate relationship to the transitory pleasures and pains of the world. It isn't sense objects that cause grief but our inappropriate relationship to them based on unrealistic, often selfish, expectations. This principle is illustrated by an answer Sri Swami Satchidananda gave in response to a student's question at a public program years ago.

"Is it okay for a yogi to have chocolate ice cream from Maygolds?" Maygolds was a dairy farm and restaurant about twenty minutes from the ashram. It was popular with ashram residents who enjoyed dipping into one of the restaurant's homemade desserts on warm summer evenings.

"That is a very good question. Allow me to answer it in this way. Everyone please imagine that tonight's program has ended. It is very warm outside and you decide to go to Maygolds for some chocolate ice cream. Is everybody with me so far?"

"Yes."

"So you drive over to Maygolds, order an extra large chocolate sundae. Can you taste it? Is it good?"

"Yes, Gurudev." I suspect that a few ashramites were ready to turn this exercise of imagination into a reality once the program was over.

"Are you feeling happy?"

"Yes."

"Okay. Fine. Now let's try it again, but with one small change. After the program, you drive to Maygolds, but find it is closed. How do you feel now? Are you still happy? If the answer is yes, then it's okay for you to occasionally have some ice cream. If the answer is no, it is better for you to stay away from it for awhile and analyze your attachment to it."

We have to ask ourselves if we are really enjoying life or if we are simply on a roller-coaster ride of cravings, the efforts to fulfill them, and temporary satisfaction. Scratching an itch does not bring happiness, only temporary relief, followed by more itchiness and irritation.

Change is the nature of life. Even when something or someone makes us happy, the situation is bound to change. We change, the thing changes, or the external conditions change. One day or another, everything we counted on to bring us comfort and joy slips away, along with the hopes for happiness that we linked to it.

Nonattachment is a difficult subject because it speaks to our fundamental motivations and beliefs regarding life. In the name of nonattachment, we examine what we hold dear and question if it is necessary to happiness. Do I need a certain sized paycheck to be happy? Is it necessary to have children to be complete? Can I still be happy even if I lose my health? Is it even possible to live without desires? To help clarify the reason nonattachment plays such a vital role in spiritual growth, we will briefly look at seven key manifestations.

Nonattachment Brings Fearlessness

Fear is founded on concern over potential loss. We are anxious over losing that which we perceive brings us happiness or security. These fears are based on attachments and the resulting anxiety over not attaining what we desire or losing what we have gained. As attachments decrease in number and intensity, fear naturally begins to evaporate. Those who are free from selfish attachments know freedom from fear (*see sutra 2.15, which among other things, shows the relationship between fear and attachment*).

Nonattachment Expresses as Service

The inclination to live for the sake of others exists within us. Sacrifice is the law of Nature. The cherry tree happily lets go of its fruit after years of laboring to grow from seed to maturity. It also provides shade, oxygen, and a home to many creatures. Finally, when it becomes too aged to produce fruit, it offers its body to become firewood to give us warmth.

The same principle holds true for those who harbor no selfish desires. Their actions naturally bring benefit to all. They experience joy *in* every act and not as a result of gain from their actions. From Sri Swami Satchidananda's commentary on this sutra:

> Try to remove the suffering of other people. Once you are
> unattached in your personal life, you can serve others,

and by doing that you will find more and more joy. (By nonattachment) you become the happiest man or woman. The more you serve the more happiness you enjoy. Such a person knows the secret of life.

Dedication, devotion, and love are expressions of nonattachment.

Nonattachment Frees Us to Love Purely

I can care and love only to the extent that I am nonattached. If I am 100 percent concerned with what's in it for me, how much love is left for you? Zero. If I am 75 percent attached, there will 25 percent remaining for your welfare. Only when I am 100 percent nonattached am I free to love and care without reservation. Nonattachment is the polar opposite of being indifferent, aloof, and uncaring.

The objective in any relationship should be to continually reduce selfishness so that more love can be brought forth. Nonattached love seeks to increase the welfare and well-being of everyone.

Nonattachment Includes Taking Care of Ourselves

If we are interested in being useful, we should take good care of ourselves. But it should be done with the proper understanding. Our own heart serves as a good example. It tirelessly fulfills its responsibility for decades. Yet the first blood it pumps is not to the body it is working to serve, but to itself. The heart knows that without first partaking in a little life-giving blood, it would not be able to serve the body. Rest, recreation, and rejuvenation can all be part of service to others.

Nonattachment Brings Skill

It is mainly a person with a nonattached mind who can do a job perfectly. Freed from the anxiety born of selfish expectations, the full power of the mind is available to engage in the project at hand. As the Bhagavad Gita states: *"Yoga is skill (or perfection) in action"* (2.50).

Nonattachment Cultivates Nirodha

Attachments comprise the major source of distractions that prevent steady mental focus. Even when we are determined to direct our full attention to the task at hand, the mind *wants* to think about other things. That wanting is an expression of attachment. Without attachment, we could make the mind focused at will.

In a way, we could think of meditation as the concentrated practice of nonattachment. Success in meditation requires not only the ability to direct and keep the awareness on the object of attention but the skill of letting go of distracting thoughts as well. This skill can be beneficial in daily life. If we can learn to let go of our "to do list" while we meditate, we can someday let go of the thought of impatience over getting caught in a traffic jam or the anger we feel toward our spouse or employer.

Nonattachment Opens the Door to Wisdom

Wisdom is the ability to rise above perceptions that are clouded by biased self-interest to discern the meaning concealed in a fact or event.

Nonattachment lifts us over the trees so that we can see the forest. If our attention is captivated by the disappointment we feel for a tree that has fallen, life in the forest can seem cruel and senseless. But if we expand our vision, we will see that this same fallen tree is returning needed nutrients for the forest floor as well as continuing to provide a home for countless creatures. Nonattachment frees the mind to rise above self-centered notions of the way of life so that we can glimpse the Divine Plan.

Understanding and working with nonattachment is a challenge but it is also highly rewarding. One day we will discover nonattachment's character as inner strength, objectivity, loving and caring, and the best way to enjoy life. Even a little success in nonattachment brings great benefit.

Experience It

This exercise should be done over at least three weeks.

Week 1: Keep a diary listing all the times you become anxious, sad, angry, fearful, shy, and so on. Any disturbing experience will do.

Week 2: Review the incidents in your list. Ask yourself: What is it that I wanted but didn't get? Don't automatically accept the first response as final. Keep asking why. Let's say, for example, that you become upset because you couldn't find your heirloom punch bowl for a dinner party. At first, you think your anger stemmed from failing to provide the best for your guests. After some self-analysis, it seems more likely that it was your faulty memory that provoked you. Continuing with your soul-searching, you come to realize that what you really wanted was to impress your guests. Your subconscious hope had been that by garnering raves over the punch bowl, you would be happy. The next task is to discover why you need your guests' appreciation to be happy. It could be a lack of self-worth, for example.

Week 3: Now that you have seen directly how selfish attachments cause your woes, you can ask: Do I really need this to be happy? Is it possible for me to be happy without it? Start simply: Can I be happy without [fill in the blank: coffee, a hair dryer, TV, a punch bowl]? Over time, the questions become more personal: Can I have this crooked nose and still be happy? Can I be happy without getting the appreciation of others?

1.16. When there is nonthirst for even the gunas (constituents of Nature) due to realization of the Purusha, that is supreme nonattachment.

There are three gunas or qualities in Nature: *sattwa*, illumination or balance; *rajas*, restlessness or activity; and *tamas*, dullness or inertia. Every object in creation (including the mind) is composed of these three qualities. The mix of the gunas in a given object differs and is not stable, their interactions accounting for changes in matter. By using the gunas to describe the highest nonattachment, Sri Patanjali is underscoring the utter lack of craving that attends this state. There is absolutely nothing in Nature that the advanced yogi craves (*see sutras* 2.18 *and* 2.19 *for more on the gunas*).

This stage of nonattachment is the natural outcome of the process begun in the previous sutra, which explained vairagya as a "manifestation of self-mastery," a state that requires effort and analysis. When the mind desires something inappropriate, you tell the mind, "No," and it stays away. Although you may be able to free yourself of new temptations, there are still subtle impressions stored in the mind—memories that will tempt you. The cravings that result from subtle impressions are not easily erased. But on this higher level of nonattachment, you don't even think of attaching. Supreme nonattachment is based on having an inner experience so sweet, satisfying, and compelling that there is nothing on the outside that can compete with it. The yogi is completely free from cravings for anything in creation.

Before reaching this state, you are in-between, perhaps having experienced something nice from the Yoga practices but still susceptible to the objects of the senses and past samskaras.

Experience It

Methods for strengthening nonattachment:

Pratyahara. The events that lead to attachment usually begin with the mind being attracted to experiences through the sense organs. *Pratyahara* is the ability to neutralize the attraction we feel towards sense objects by disconnecting our attention from them.

Think of something you are attached to and try to "fast" from it for awhile. Maybe you are attached to having four teaspoons of sugar in your tea. Resolve to have only three teaspoons every Monday. When you become comfortable with this, expand it to three teaspoons everyday. After a while, three will become your habit. Now reduce it to two on Mondays, and so forth. In this way, you exercise your will, gradually making it stronger. At some point, you will have eliminated sugar from your tea completely. When you have achieved that mastery and discover that you could not only still be happy without sugar but be happier due to the joy of mastery, you will have made a great stride forward in attaining vairagya. You no longer *need* sugar in your tea to be happy (*see sutras 2.54 and 2.55 for more on pratyahara*).

Prayer and worship. Through devotional practices, selfish attachments naturally fall away. Until we can grasp onto something more fulfilling, we hesitate to let go of our attachments. In this we are like monkeys who swing from branch to branch, not letting go of one until they grasp another. We can use a higher attachment to help us let go of all others. Nonattachment flourishes when we focus our love, dedication, and devotion on God. The difference with attachment to God-realization is that when we fulfill it, when we realize oneness with God, all other desires naturally fall away.

Learn the nonattachment motto. Avaiyar was a renowned saint who lived many years ago in India. Her sayings are used to help children memorize the alphabet, much in the same way our children learn the "A, B, C" song. One of her sayings would be useful to memorize: *"Kita dayin, vetana mara"* (If you can't get it, immediately forget it). Once you realize that something cannot be attained, then forget it.

It's not for you, at least at this point in time. Repeat this saying often; it will help.

God's fail-safe plan. Attachments bring pain either now or in the future. If and when all else fails, pain will teach us very well. No philosophy or Yoga technique is needed to drop a hot pot that burns our hands. When the pain is enough, we drop it. Likewise, when the pain of selfish attachments increases sufficiently, we will drop them.

Pain points out where our attachments were hidden. It is a perfect indicator of the limitations that are our selfish expectations. That is why, to the yogi, pain is a teacher—a stern one, yet one that has nothing but the liberation of its students at heart (*see sutras 2.1, 2.32, and 2.43, on tapasya [austerity]*).

The "Sweet Sixteen" Sutras

If you are looking to gain a firm grasp on the fundamentals of the *Yoga Sutras*, become familiar with the first sixteen sutras. Here they are, summarized and paraphrased:

- The fundamental definition: the restraint (nirodha) of the modifications of the mind-stuff. Through nirodha, habitual misidentification with the mental modifications is ended.
- The yogi realizes her/his True Identity as the Self: Purusha.
- Mental modifications are experienced as being painful or painless depending on whether our motivations are selfish or selfless. (In fact, these two categories represent the basic "operating systems" of the mind-stuff. Selfishness sustains the influence of ignorance, while selflessness leads to Self-realization.)
- Nirodha is achieved by practice and nonattachment.
- Practice is the effort to still the mind and to remain steadfast on the path.
- Practice becomes firmly grounded when well attended for a long time, without break and with enthusiasm.
- Nonattachment (vairagya) is based on the realization that peace, happiness, and fulfillment come from within. It is

the establishment of proper, healthy relationships with sense objects.

• Nonattachment is perfected with the experience of Self-realization.

1.17. Cognitive (samprajnata) samadhi (is associated with forms and) is attended by examination, insight, joy, and pure I-am-ness.

In Yoga, higher states of awareness are generally referred to by the term *samadhi*, a word commonly translated as contemplation, super-conscious state, or absorption. Before going on to the commentary for this sutra, let's take a brief overview of the state of samadhi, since it is central to understanding Yoga philosophy and practice.

In a general sense, samadhi is a way of attaining knowledge that is supra (above)-rational. Samadhi differs radically from our usual method of gaining understanding in that there are no steps of logic and no comparing or contrasting of bits of information in order to arrive at an understanding of the object being contemplated. Instead, knowledge gained from samadhi is direct, spontaneous, and intuitive, the product of achieving at least some significant measure of unity with the object being contemplated.

Although the insights revealed in samadhi are not the product of a rational thought process, they do not contradict rationality, but transcend it. Samadhi (and Yoga theory and practice in general) is not a journey into an irrational mental landscape where flights of fancy rule the day. Recall that Sri Patanjali designated inference as one of three valid means of attaining "right knowledge" (*see sutra* 1.7). But since samadhi has the power to go beyond the confines of the physical senses, personal biases, and the inherent limitations of relativistic thought processes, it completes and verifies knowledge gained through direct perception, inference, and authoritative testimony.

Samadhi is a journey of exploration that begins by learning to hold steady attention on an "effect," a perceivable aspect of Prakriti— for practical purposes, whatever the practitioner has chosen as the object for meditation. The mind then naturally probes that object in order to discover its immediate cause, such as a more subtle element (*see Tanmatra in the Glossary*). The discovery of the immediate cause doesn't end the journey, since it too was brought into being by other, even more subtle factors. The journey continues as layer after layer of matter is stripped away until we reach the mother of all objects: pure undifferentiated Prakriti.

But another fundamental aspect of samadhi should be understood if we are to make sense of the various categories of it discussed in the *Yoga Sutras*: we need to understand what happens to the mind in states of samadhi. Here too, samadhi is a process of evolution in reverse in which the factors that formed our individual mind—our very sense and experience of self—are revealed. This voyage to Self-discovery occurs as we trace back the act of perception to its most subtle and fundamental root, the ego-sense. We then transcend even *that* to experience our True Identity as the pure, eternal, unbounded consciousness that yogis call Purusha.

Keeping in mind what we have discussed thus far regarding samadhi, we can understand that the levels or categories of samadhi that are found in the *Yoga Sutras* are essentially based on two factors:

- The relative subtlety of matter the mind is perceiving
- The degree to which the individual mind (manas, buddhi, ahamkara) and subconscious impressions continue to be active in the process of perception

Now we are ready to consider the samadhis of this sutra.

The first category of samadhi presented in the *Yoga Sutras* is referred to as cognitive (acquiring information or understanding) because it is marked by the attainment of knowledge regarding the object of contemplation. It is a suprarational mode of functioning that brings insights regarding aspects of Creation.

In samprajnata samadhi, the mind focuses on some aspect of Creation in order to uncover its inner truths, the causes behind the effects. It identifies with (by becoming united with) the object of contemplation. Familiar, day-to-day thought processes are replaced by a new way of perceiving and gaining knowledge. Rather than the acquisition of information that is categorized, compared, and contrasted with other bits of data (fundamental vritti activity), knowledge gained in samprajnata samadhi is spontaneous and intuitive.

The samprajnata samadhis listed in this sutra correspond to the four stages of Prakriti's evolution: gross matter, subtle elements, sattwa (pure mind), and the ego-sense.

- Gross elements (bhutas)
  Individual objects or aspects of creation perceivable by the sense organs. Gross elements include material objects perceivable by the senses. Samprajnata samadhi at this level is said to be attended by "examination."
- Subtle elements (tanmatras)
  Sound, touch, sight, taste, and smell. They are the cause of the gross elements. At this level of samprajnata samadhi, the mind gains intuitive knowledge of the subtle nature of the object of meditation and is said to be attended by "insight."
- The mind (composed of pure sattwa)
  Samprajnata samadhi at this level is attended by "joy," the experience of the still, pure, sattwic mind.
- Pure Ego-Sense (asmita)
  Sense of individuality; the immediate cause of the mind. Samprajnata samadhi at this level is attended by "pure I-am-ness."

In essence, the four stages of samprajnata samadhi describe a mind that is probing the phenomenon of perception, of what constitutes experience.

Our daily experiences are comprised of two factors that change and one that doesn't. The object and action change, but the subject always remains the same. I throw the ball. I eat the raisins. I enjoy sunsets. I sleep in the guest room. The "I" can throw, eat, enjoy, or sleep. "I" can do much more: skip, read, build, sneeze, or drive, for instance. The objects of these actions can be almost limitless, too. But the ego, the sense of "I," stays the same. In short, samprajnata samadhi can also be understood as a process in which the act of perception is gradually reduced to its most elemental aspect: ego-sense.

Let's examine each level of samprajnata samadhi in more detail.

Examination

Vitarka, the word translated as examination, can also be interpreted as debate, reasoning, or question. It accompanies samadhi, in which the focus is on objects or elements that are tangible to the senses.

Learning is a natural impulse. It is the nature of the focused mind to continually probe more deeply into the object of attention. It wants to know more, to discover and explore.

In vitarka samadhi, the process of examination is powered by a mind that has achieved a measure of union with the object being contemplated. It is examination in its freest, most creative expression. The focused mind naturally uncovers increasingly deeper and subtler levels of the object of attention. It pierces through layers of gross matter, revealing the object's inner structure, the *tanmatras* or subtle elements.

The knowledge gained through vitarka samadhi stops at the level of the tanmatras. In order to behold the subtle elements, the mind needs to be even more focused. This brings us to *vichara*.

Insight

Vichara, insight, can also be translated as reflection, inquiry, introspection, or investigation. It is a more refined form of inquiry than vitarka and is performed on the tanmatras.

Like vitarka, there is no asking of questions. It is a matter of the mind attuning itself to the level of the subtle elements. Knowledge—intuitive insight—comes through attaining resonance or identification with the object of contemplation.

Imagine what it would be like to meditate on taste. Not the taste *of* something, but just taste or sight, hearing or touch. How about movement, time, or space? These are very difficult to imagine without tangible objects to relate them to. Yet in the vichara samadhis, this is done. These subtle objects may be specifically chosen by the practitioner or can come as a natural product of the vitarka samadhis.

(*See sutras 1.42 and 1.43 for detailed descriptions of the two "tarka" samadhis, and 1.44 for the two "chara" samadhis.*)

Joy

Ananda is Sanskrit for bliss or joy. This samadhi is the experience of the pure (*sattwic*) aspect of the mind which is beyond the subtle elements. It is the bliss of a mind free of worries, stress, fears, and burdens. The joy of ananda samadhi is infinitely more satisfying than our usual experiences of happiness, since the mind reflects the unbounded joy that is the Self.

As wonderful as the experience of ananda samadhi is, we shouldn't mistake it for the highest enlightenment. *"Although the sattwic guna is pure, luminous and without obstructions, still it binds you by giving rise to happiness and knowledge to which the mind readily becomes attached"* (Bhagavad Gita, 14.6).

Happiness is seductive. After all, for many of us, our interest in Raja Yoga was motivated by the wish to be happy. With ananda samadhi, we seem to have attained our goal. We might be tempted to discontinue our efforts toward Self-realization. This samadhi does not make us immune to ignorance. We are not yet completely free.

Pure I-am-ness

Asmita is the ego-sense. In this samadhi, the ego-sense itself is the object. This is the highest samprajnata samadhi. There is only awareness of individuality, just the feeling or thought of "I," or "I-ness." It is simply awareness of one's existence.

The samprajnata samadhis are a process of tracing the manifestations of Prakriti back to their source. By going inward, we turn back the pages of evolution. The ego creates the mind. The mind is the cause of the subtle elements, which in turn are the basis for the gross elements.

1.18. Noncognitive (asamprajnata) samadhi occurs with the cessation of all conscious thought; only the subconscious impressions remain.

Asamprajnata: asam, "without," and *prajna,* "knowledge," giving "without knowledge," or *a,* "not," and *samprajnata,* giving "not samprajnata" samadhi (the "other" samadhi).

Asamprajnata samadhi is noncognitive because there are no objects in the conscious mind to discern; even the ego is temporarily transcended. Though the conscious mind becomes completely still, the subconscious impressions (samskaras) remain. Asamprajnata samadhi is the experience of the reflection of the Purusha on a perfectly still, clear mind.

The steps from samprajnata to asamprajnata samadhis are:

- First you understand Nature (gross and subtle elements; the mind and ego)
- Then bring it under your control
- Finally, you transcend it by freeing the mind of all mental activity. Only subconscious impressions remain

The yogi cannot be freed from the ego until the samskaras are transcended. Samskaras are remnants of past experiences that help perpetuate vritti activity by maintaining the structure of the ego. To reach the highest samadhi, nirbija samadhi, even the samskaras need to be wiped out. Sri Patanjali addresses nirbija samadhi in the last sutra of this pada (*see sutra* 1.51).

(*Also see* Samadhi *in the* Sutras-by-Subject *Index.*)

1.19. Yogis who have not attained asamprajnata samadhi remain attached to Prakriti at the time of death due to the continued existence of thoughts of becoming.

This sparsely worded sutra (the original Sanskrit is only five words) can be interpreted in several valid and useful ways, all of which demonstrate the same underlying principle: the continued existence of ignorance is what prevents the seeker from advancing to asamprajnata samadhi.

In samprajnata samadhi, the mind has penetrated to the foundation of matter, to the pure mind, and finally, to the ego, the sense of "I" itself. Yet the influence of ignorance over mental functioning remains. The "thought of becoming" is the persistent desire to experience sense objects manifested from Prakriti. This desire, if not transcended in life, persists even after passing from the physical body. The "thought of becoming" ceases with the attainment of asamprajnata samadhi, the state in which "all conscious thought comes to a standstill and only the subconscious impressions remain "

1.20. To the others, asamprajnata samadhi is preceded by faith, strength, mindfulness, (cognitive) samadhi, and discriminative insight.

"To the others" refers to those seekers whose progress is not stalled by the "thought of becoming."

Faith

We look to faith to sustain us through difficulties and to provide meaning even in trying situations. Faith is not simply a higher form of belief. It is not a powerful wish for something to be true. Faith is a state of certainty; of knowing. It is related to direct perception (*see sutra* 1.7).

Putting our finger in ice water produces sensations of cold. We say with full faith that the water is cold. Looking out my window, I see that it is raining, and I have faith in what my senses report to me. But consider this example: I wake up, take a mental inventory of my health, and conclude that I am fine. I have abundant energy and no aches or pains. Yet, later that day, I am surprised when my doctor finds that my blood pressure is so high that I need to take medication to control it. What went wrong with my direct perception?

My mind was not steady or clear enough to make the proper assessment; it was insufficient to the task. My mind's assessment was tested and proved incorrect by an instrument capable of detecting subtle physiological states, a blood pressure gauge.

Seekers look to experience the source of life, the essence of all things: God. They may encounter sensations or thoughts in prayer, worship, and meditation that lead them to believe that what is happening is holy, that their belief in God is being confirmed. But how can they be sure? In the above example, our perceptive powers could not detect hypertension, even though it existed. Our mind can be fooled in many ways.

Many years ago, there lived a simple, illiterate man whose job was to ring the temple bells before sunrise as a call to worship. He had unfailingly dispatched this responsibility since he was a young boy.

It so happened that one day he became too ill to go to work. He was at home recuperating in bed when suddenly he became agitated. His wife rushed to his bedside.

"What is it, dear husband, what disturbs you so?"

"This is terrible, what are we to do? I am too sick to ring the temple bells tomorrow morning."

"Yes, this is so, my husband. But the doctor said that in a few days you will be well enough to continue with your duties."

"Don't you understand? If I cannot ring the bells, the sun will not rise."

He had linked the bell ringing with the rising of the sun. He had no recollection of a sunrise that was not preceded by his bell-ringing. He had faith, but it was based on an error (*see sutra* 1.8, *on misperception*). That type of error is easy to make: we act, experience a reaction, and believe that the action and reaction are linked. No doubt all reactions are linked to a previous action, but the difficulty lies in deciphering which cause(s) generated which effect. Beliefs need to be challenged by the rigors of everyday life. The bell-ringer was able to cling to an erroneous belief for many years because it had never been challenged. His illness was an opportunity for him to test his faith.

Most items of faith begin as conditional and need to be confirmed through the tests that life brings. The word *convinced* gives a clue to this truth. It means to be "well won." Spiritually, to be convinced is to measure our beliefs and inner experiences against the events, challenges, and sufferings that come our way (*see sutra* 2.1, *on accepting pain as a help for purification*).

As faith grows, it brings steadiness of mind. It provides the psychological "room" for life's lessons to be learned. Faith becomes the context in which we experience events. The result is that life is not experienced as a series of events without rhyme or reason but as a profoundly rich, subtle, and complex field for learning and growth.

Faith is cultivated when we think of all the blessings we have already received in our lives. This helps to develop gratitude, gratitude ripens into devotion, and devotion culminates in faith.

Strength

The goal of Yoga is not easy to attain. It requires dedication, resolve, and perseverance to master the mind.

Strength is a foundation of all vows and commitments and is needed for success in any significant undertaking.

Whenever we make resolutions, it seems we are tested. Temptations, distractions, and old habits spring up from every side. We need to find the inner strength to persevere and to discover ways to succeed. If we pass the tests, we will be living heroic lives, demonstrating strength and integrity in our undertakings.

Strength is also what sees us through the dry periods of our practices. It is easy to meditate, pray, and do pranayama when sweet benefits are experienced. But what keeps us going when we pray and feel no one is listening or meditate and spend the time half asleep or wondering what we should eat for breakfast?

Every seeker goes through difficult times. What once seemed rational now seems foolish. "Why should I be nonattached? I don't seem to be getting any benefits or having any fun. And why should I spend a couple of hours a day meditating? I seem to be missing out on a lot of enjoyment in life."

In times of trials we continue simply because we said we would. Our practice is not based on how we feel but on adhering to principles. That is strength, and it is beautiful.

(*See sutra 1.32 for one good way to build spiritual strength.*)

Mindfulness

Mindfulness (*smriti*) includes remembering our mistakes, their consequences, and the lessons learned. It also implies being vigilant—maintaining alertness and focus in everything we do.

Mindfulness helps cultivate strength and faith.

Cognitive Samadhi

Samprajnata samadhi is a preparation for asamprajnata samadhi.

Discriminative Insight

Discriminative insight (*prajna*) is the intuitive knowledge necessary to reach higher states of samadhi through continuous self awareness.

(*See Viveka in the Sutras-by-Subject Index.*)

1.21. To the keen and intent practitioner this samadhi comes very quickly.

Success in Yoga comes more easily to those who have the exuberance of youth. Adolescents have a fearlessness—a willingness to explore and experience unknown areas of life. They believe that if they try hard enough, they can achieve any goal. As we get older, we learn that we cannot have everything we strive for—and that is part of maturing. But in that process, we sometimes lose the willing energy of youth. Certainly we should look before we leap, but once the decision to leap is made, it should be done wholeheartedly. Seekers who dive within themselves with vigor and zeal attain results sooner. Success breeds even greater inspiration and enthusiasm. If we are focused, inspired, dedicated, unafraid of setbacks, and always seeking to grow and learn, we will make progress quickly.

A sincere student once approached his guru with a question: "Master, I have been meditating and practicing all sorts of disciplines for many years. Still, I have not seen God. What is necessary for me to do? What am I missing?"

Instead of speaking, the master escorted his young student to the banks of a nearby river. He asked him to bend over. Suddenly he grasped the young man by the back of the neck and thrust his head underwater.

Soon the man was squirming, struggling to break free. A few long moments passed before he was released.

Gasping for air, he asked, "Master, why did you do this to me?"

"When your head was underwater, what were you thinking?"

"I was only thinking of breathing. Nothing else."

"You didn't think of your wife, your job, your finances?"

"No, only getting air to breathe."

"When you think of God with the same one-pointed fervor, know that the experience of Him is very close at hand."

Practitioners who place the highest value on activities that promote their spiritual progress realize samadhi more quickly than students with a tepid attitude.

1.22. The time necessary for success also depends on whether the practice is mild, moderate, or intense.

The previous sutra spoke of the zeal of the practitioner. This sutra expands on the idea of the intensity, the number of practices performed and the degree to which they are integrated into daily life. The more practices that are incorporated into daily life, the sooner the influence of ignorance diminishes.

A mild practice describes one that lacks steady enthusiasm and is most likely irregular. For these students, practice is minimal and regarded as a necessary chore. Practitioners in the middle category usually find at least some time everyday to fit in Yoga practices. They enjoy benefits, but much of their practice remains disconnected from the rest of their lives. Zealous practitioners make sadhana their priority. They keep inspired and focused and look forward to periods of practice. They also tend to see every aspect of their lives as an opportunity for growth. For them, practice becomes a character trait.

Although success in Yoga requires full application of our resources, we should be on guard against fanaticism. Any practice or lifestyle that abandons balance and harmony can lead to lopsided development, rigidity of outlook, and interpersonal strife. Practice should be balanced by nonattachment.

1.23. Or samadhi is attained by devotion with total dedication to God (Ishwara).

Up to this point, the focus has been on practices that work directly with the modifications in the mind by redirecting or holding attention. Here we find another path to Self-realization. Devotion (pranidhana), translated literally, means "to place or hold in front." It means giving prime importance to the dedication of our time, capabilities, and energy to God. In short, this sutra presents selfless love of God as a legitimate path to Self-realization. Our minds naturally dwell on that which we love. In worldly relationships, when we love someone we can't stop thinking about them. We look forward to seeing them, talking to them, pleasing and serving them. There is nothing we would rather do more than be with our sweetheart. It is the same with love of God. Those who have a loving, devoted attitude toward God find that the selective focus of nirodha is easier to attain, and because loving is fun, it is more enjoyable. Regularity and enthusiasm are also more easily attained (*see sutra* 1.14, *on firmly grounded practice*). Obviously there are advantages that attend devotion to Ishwara. But who or what is Ishwara?

Ishwara is derived from *ish*, "to rule or own," and can be thought of as the Supreme Ruler of Creation. It is the Purusha as experienced from within the confines of Prakriti and perceived through the limitations of the ego. Ishwara is not separate from Purusha (Self), but is a way of externalizing It.

The externalization of the Self is natural tendency. It is part of a learning process. When grappling with subtle truths, we look for symbols that help us understand the nuances of those truths. In Christianity, for example, a three-leafed clover is used to symbolize the mystery of the trinity: how the one God could also be three separate personalities, Father, Son, and Holy Spirit. Instead of contemplating complex theological arguments that attempt to reconcile this principle, we could draw analogies with the three leaves on one stem. Similarly, it is difficult to grasp surrendering to the indefinable, infinite Self. Externalizing the Self as Ishwara offers something for the mind to grasp onto. A one-pointed, devoted relationship with Ishwara allows reverence and affection to grow. From this, surrender follows.

This sutra speaks to countless devotees who are devoted to their faith and who sincerely worship, pray, and attend church, synagogue, or temple. They do not need to learn about mantras, Prakriti, buddhi, or vrittis to achieve liberation. What they are doing is sufficient. To love and be devoted to God in any form is a valid path in Raja Yoga. The catalyst for growth is the complete giving of oneself to worship, devotion, and service. One of the reasons that loving devotion is highly valued as a spiritual practice is because it is the best way to overcome fear.

Fear is one of the most entrenched obstacles that Yoga practitioners encounter. Fear is how the ego responds when it perceives its existence is threatened. The ego calls itself "I," so its dissolution is experienced as "I am dying." Whenever it is in a vulnerable position, the "I" reasserts itself because of the fear of extinction. Since the ego stands between the seeker and Self-realization, ignorance continues.

Fear can be overcome by the will, but for most of us, it is more easily accomplished through love, which naturally evaporates fear. For the lover, nothing is more natural or desirable than union with the beloved. What begins as the reverent devotion of the seeker to Ishwara gradually grows to a love so consuming that the fear of self-extinction is overcome.

Overcoming the fear of self-extinction is daunting enough, but the dread is aggravated when we attempt to surrender to a Reality without name, form, or quality. It is like leaping into a vast unknown. We have nothing familiar or inspiring on which we can pour our attention. We have to overcome a deep-seated fear when attempting to submit to an Infinite Cosmic Principle whose face cannot be seen and who is devoid of any recognizable characteristics.

On the other hand, it is much easier to imagine giving ourselves to the One:

- Who is the supreme Purusha, unaffected by any afflictions, actions, or fruits of actions or by any inner impressions

- Who is unconditioned by time and the teacher of the most ancient teachers
- In whom there is the complete manifestation of the seed of omniscience (*see sutras* 1.24—1.26)
- Who is changeless (*see sutras* 4.18 *and* 4.22)
- Who, when experienced, brings the seeker spiritual independence and complete rest (*see sutras* 1.3 *and* 4.34)

These characteristics of Ishwara are ways of describing some of the experiences seekers can expect as they move closer to realization of the Self.

Raja Yoga does not require choosing between the will or loving surrender. For most, it is better to exercise both capacities, though the emphasis will vary according to the individual.

Experience It

Surrender is the active side of faith. Opportunities to cultivate it occur when our beliefs meet realties that differ from our conceptions or expectations. Surrender can't be forced; it is the outcome of a vision of life based on trusting that there is divine wisdom behind all events. But it is a mind-set that can be cultivated through dedicating the fruits of actions to God and by the practice of acceptance.

Dedication. We know from studying nonattachment that actions motivated by selfish expectations bring pain (see sutra 2.15). One way of overcoming selfish expectations is to engage in actions but dedicate the fruits of those actions to God. Dedication transforms ordinary actions into powerful spiritual practices.

Acceptance. The entire creation exists to give the experiences necessary for the liberation of the Purusha (see sutra 2.18). Our common experience tells us that our intents and actions cannot necessarily change the course of history—personal, familial, societal, or global. We develop acceptance every time we remind ourselves that no matter what occurs, it ultimately brings about our spiritual unfoldment.

With acceptance, there are no expectations or demands placed on anything to change or to conform to our personal conception of how life should be. Acceptance is trust in Ishwara (the Supreme Ruler) to oversee the universe wisely.

(*See* Ishwara in the Glossary. *Also see* Purusha, Ishwara, and True Identity in the Sutras-by-Subject Index.)

1.24. Ishwara is the supreme Purusha, unaffected by any afflictions, actions, fruits of actions, or any inner impressions of desires.

How are we to relate to God?

The sutra refers to Ishwara as the "supreme Purusha." Meanings for "purusha" include spirit, individual soul, or person. It is a word that is commonly used when referring to any individual. We are all purushas, but Ishwara is the supreme one, since He/She/It is free of subconscious impressions and not affected by any afflictions or karma. In other words, Ishwara is just like us, but without ignorance and its consequences. Of course, the equation read from the other side is that we are Ishwara, limited (apparently) by ignorance.

1.25. In Ishwara is the complete manifestation of the seed of omniscience.

This emphasizes the worthiness of Ishwara as an object of worship.

This sutra can also teach us something of the relationship between finite and infinite and serve as a proof for the existence of the Infinite. There can't be finite without infinite. Close your eyes and picture a circle. What do you see around it? Blackness. Where does the blackness end? It doesn't. Make the circle bigger. What is there around it? More blackness. Where does this blackness end? It doesn't end. And so on. All thoughts, facts, conjectures, and aspirations are finite realities projected upon the infinite omniscient screen that is Ishwara. The limited self can be known because it appears against an omniscient backdrop.

1.26. Unconditioned by time, Ishwara is the teacher of even the most ancient teachers.

In the previous sutra, we learned that Ishwara knows everything there is to know. Now we discover something of the nature of Divine knowledge. This precious knowledge is not to be saved, like valuables in a safe deposit box. It fulfills its destiny only when communicated to those who lack it. Just as it is our nature to seek knowledge, it is Ishwara's nature to share it.

"Unconditioned by time" implies that Ishwara's infinite store-house of knowledge and wisdom is eternally present and always accessible. The knowledge that was available to the yogis of yesterday continues to be available today and will continue to be available for an infinite number of tomorrows.

The wording of this sutra is noteworthy for another reason. We are not told that Ishwara is the source of knowledge. Instead, Ishwara is characterized as the teacher (literally, *guru*) of teachers. The word "guru" likely held significance for students who lived in a culture with a long-established tradition of receiving spiritual knowledge through the guidance of a qualified teacher. For them, seeking direction from a master was probably as natural as getting the weather report from the TV is for us.

The following quote predates the *Yoga Sutras* by perhaps two thousand years:

> To know the Eternal, let the seeker humbly approach a Guru devoted to Brahman and well-versed in the scriptures. To a disciple who approaches reverently, who is tranquil and self-controlled, the wise teacher gives that knowledge faithfully and without stint, by which is known the truly existing, the changeless Self.
>
> Mundaka Upanishad, 2.12–2.13

Only a lit candle can light an unlit one. Since time immemorial, the same spark of knowledge continues to be passed from teacher to student.

We live in times when many Yoga students question the necessity of studying under a master. Our culture places a high value on self-reliance and prizes the ability of the individual to reason through problems on his or her own. Our fascination with self-reliance is demonstrated by bookstore shelves that are crowded with self-help books and the many TV and radio talk shows that regularly include self-help segments. Though we seek to be self-reliant, we also seem to always be looking for someone to show us how to be so.

In such an environment, Yoga students might conclude that they can successfully practice Yoga without a teacher. Though this might be possible with the physical practices of Hatha Yoga or to begin practicing meditation, the path of self-help is not well suited to the subtle, difficult, and delicate task of cleaning the ego of ignorance. In this area, our objectivity will often be skewed. A competent third party to guide and instruct us is invaluable. After all, great ballet dancers attend master classes (the more advanced they are, the more important this is). Accomplished athletes appreciate their coaches' daily observation and corrections. Thousands go to health clubs to exercise under the knowledgeable eyes of a trainer. The basic principle is simple and sound: make use of those who have traveled the road before us. They correct our mistakes and help us to avoid wrong turns.

Even though knowledge of the Self is within us, it needs to be called forth. To some extent, we can experience this calling forth of knowledge through books, tapes, and classes. But it is more quickly and completely awakened within the context of a master/disciple relationship. The disciple finds in the master the fulfillment of spiritual potential. Enlightenment becomes real—a possibility within reach that fills the disciple with inspiration, hope, and challenge.

The inner environment necessary for good discipleship is described in the following quote from the Bhagavad Gita:

> If you seek enlightenment from those who have real-
> ized the truth, prostrate before them, question them,
> and serve them. Only then are you open to receive
> their teachings of sacred knowledge.
>
> Bhagavad Gita, 4.34

This attitude can be characterized as receptivity. A good disciple should be not only open to learning something new but ready to let go of or change former conceptions. Receptivity is based on humility, accepting that we do not know everything and that there is much to learn that would benefit us.

There is another important principle at work in the master/disciple relationship that we should explore: emulation.

Every Little League coach knows the power of emulation. By the time young children come to their first practice, they already have many of the skills they will carry with them throughout their playing years, even to the major league level. They attained this high degree of skill at such a young age by watching their heroes on TV and emulating them.

They bat, throw, and run like their favorite player, learning exquisitely subtle techniques that would take a coach years to teach. Of course, they pick up some habits that though not necessarily harmful, are not vital for success. Maybe they will imitate their heroes' facial expressions or the way they touch their helmet before stepping into the batter's box. Many of these unnecessary habits fall away, and the students will develop refinements and advancements on their own or with the help of their coaches. Emulation is natural, simple, and incredibly powerful. Yoga students emulate their master and, in that emulation, learn more than words alone can convey.

Emulation is one of the principles behind apprenticeship. It is the method of study most valued by those who are advanced in their field. Where do advanced pianists go to refine their skills further? They study under the watchful eye of someone they feel has accomplished what they seek. The same is true in spiritual matters. Find someone in whom you have faith, who you feel has experienced the goal of Yoga. If that is not possible, it is still worthwhile to study under someone who is at least a few steps ahead of you. Wisdom passing from one human being to another is like being kissed by the Truth. It is beautiful and powerful.

1.27. The expression of Ishwara is the mystic sound OM.

This sutra introduces us to the mantra OM, which denotes Ishwara. In the Sanskrit, the word "OM" isn't mentioned. Instead, we find the term, *pranavah*, the humming of prana. OM is the hum of the business of Creation: the making, evolving, and dissolving of beings and objects. You can hear it in the roar of a fire, the deep rumble of the ocean, or the ground-shaking rush of a tornado's winds. Since the pranavah is not something we can easily chant, the name is given as OM. It is always vibrating within us, replaying the drama of creation, evolution, and dissolution on many levels. This hum can be heard in deep meditation, when external sound is transcended and internal chatter stilled.

The identity of primordial sound with God as the creative force of the universe is not limited to Raja Yoga. It is a principle found in many spiritual traditions. The Bible declares, *"In the beginning was the*

Word, and the Word was with God and the Word was God" (John 1.1). The Rig Veda, one of the most ancient scriptures in the world, contains a similar passage: *"In the beginning was Brahman (God) and with Brahman was sabda (primordial sound) and sabda was truly the Supreme Brahman."*

Since the use of mantras is a central practice in many schools of Yoga, it will be useful to examine them in a little detail.

Mantras

Mantras (literally, to protect the mind) are sound syllables representing aspects of the Divine. They are not just fabricated words used as labels for objects. They are not part of the language as such. They are the subtle vibratory essence of things, presented as sounds that can be repeated. Concentrated repetition of a mantra forms the basis of an entire branch of Yoga: Japa Yoga, the Yoga of Repetition.

Sounds have the ability to soothe or agitate us. Many people shudder when they hear a metal utensil scrape the bottom of a metal pan. At the same time, countless vacationers seek out the shoreline in order to lie back and let the sound of the waves soothe their tattered nerves. Mantras are sounds that calm and strengthen the mind, and for this reason they are ideally suited to serve as objects of meditation. The vibratory power of the mantra enhances the meditative experience.

Once a mantra has been chosen, practitioners generally make the best progress if they stick to it for life. Students may choose a mantra themselves based on trial and error or because it is associated with a particular deity with whom they feel a strong connection. For example, OM *Namah Sivaya* is a mantra connected with Lord Siva. However, since the word *siva* represents auspiciousness, the repetition of this mantra is not restricted to devotees of Lord Siva. Mantras transcend these designations. They are sound formulas whose fundamental benefit derives from their vibration, not associated ideas or images.

Some students receive a mantra from a master or adept in whom they have faith. In this case, they put their faith in the teacher to choose for them. The student is still making the essential choice in both scenarios. The difference is that in the former, the student chooses the mantra; in the latter, the student chooses the teacher who selects the mantra.

Japa Yoga is not limited to Sanskrit and Raja Yoga. Repetition of powerful sounds and prayers—*Shalom*, *Maranatha*, and *Ave Maria*, for example—is used in many spiritual traditions.

OM

The word used to denote Ishwara needs to be special; it should be free from the limitations of time, circumstance, or faith tradition. Not only should this designation be universal, it must also bring the experience of Ishwara to the practitioner. Sri Patanjali states that the name that accomplishes this is OM.

OM is the origin of all sounds. It comprises three letters: A, U, and M (OM rhymes with "home" since the A and U, when combined, become a long O sound). A is the first sound. You simply open your mouth and make a sound. All audible sound begins with this action. It represents creation. The U is formed when the sound rolls forward toward the lips with the help of the tongue and cheeks. This represents evolution. Finally, to make the M sound the lips come together. This last sound represents dissolution. So together A, U, and M signify creation, evolution, and dissolution. The entire cycle of life is represented in these three letters.

According to the philosophy of Advaita Vedanta (the philosophical school of nondualism), A is outer consciousness, U is inner consciousness, and M is superconsciousness. The same three letters also signify the waking, dreaming, and deep dreamless sleep states. Beyond these three states is a fourth state, the Absolute, the silence that transcends all limitations.

Although there are many mantras, the source of all mantras is OM. Some of the more widely known mantras include OM *Shanti*, *Hari* OM, OM *Namah Sivaya*, and OM *Mani Padme Hum*. Most but not all mantras used for meditation contain OM.

Considering its symbolism and power, it is understandable why Sri Patanjali identifies OM as the "name" for Ishwara.

Universality of OM

Sri Swami Satchidananda's commentary on this sutra says:

We should understand that OM was not invented by anybody. Some people didn't come together, hold nominations, take a vote, and the majority decided, "All right, let God have the name OM." No. He Himself manifested as OM. Any seeker who really wants to see God face to face will ultimately see Him as OM. That is why it transcends all geographical, political, or theological limitations. It doesn't belong to one country or one religion; it belongs to the entire universe.

It is a variation of this OM that we see as the "Amen" or "Ameen," which the Christians, Muslims, and Jews say. That doesn't mean someone changed it. Truth is always the same. Wherever you sit for meditation, you will ultimately end in experiencing OM or the hum. But when you want to express what you experienced, you may use different words according to your capacity or the language you know.

1.28. To repeat it in a meditative way reveals its meaning.
The two key words in this sutra are *artha* and *bhavanam*.
- *Artha* signifies meaning, purpose, or aim; from the root *"arth,"* to point out.
- *Bhavanam's* meanings include meditation, consideration, disposition, feeling, and mental discipline. Some branches of Hindu philosophy understand bhavana as a particular disposition of mind—one in which things are constantly practiced or remembered.

Mantra repetition is not the mindless parroting of a sound but an attentive and informed act set against a background of enthusiasm. Steady mental focus and an understanding of the significance of the mantra are needed. In this way the meaning (or purpose) of the mantra will gradually unfold. This understanding is in harmony with one of Raja Yoga's basic tenets: focused attention results in deeper and subtler perceptions

For keen seekers, each and every repetition is a moment of connection with the Self, an affirmation of the Truth of their own spiritual identity, and a reminder of their intentions.

1.29. From this practice, the awareness turns inward, and the distracting obstacles vanish.

When the mind "tunes in" to the vibration of OM, it becomes introspective and begins to awaken to Self-knowledge. Meanwhile, the distracting obstacles (*see sutra* 1.30), which are the product of a scattered mind, naturally dissolve.

By extension, we could claim a similar benefit for the repetition of any mantra and for the practice of meditation in general (*see sutra* 2.11, "*In the active state, they [obstacles] can be destroyed by meditation*").

This sutra introduces a key theme in Raja Yoga: the practices do not directly bring spiritual progress; they simply remove obstacles that prevent it. The evolution of the individual naturally occurs when that which retards its progress is removed. This principle is also found in sutras 2.2, 2.28, and 4.3:

- They [accepting pain as help for purification, study, and surrender] help us minimize obstacles and attain samadhi.
- By the practice of the limbs of Yoga, the impurities dwindle away and there dawns the light of wisdom, leading to discriminative discernment.
- Incidental events do not directly cause natural evolution; they just remove the obstacles as a farmer [removes obstacles in a water course running to his field].

1.30. Disease, dullness, doubt, carelessness, laziness, sensuality, false perception, failure to reach firm ground, and slipping from the ground gained—these distractions of the mind-stuff are the obstacles.

This list of obstacles will be familiar to those who have been practicing Yoga for any length of time. Every seeker faces them at various points on their spiritual journey.

Vikshepa, translated as "distraction," means false projection, scattering, dispersing, and shaking (of the mind-stuff). Vikshepa suggests that the obstacles are symptoms of a lack or loss of focus. It is interesting to note that misperception is also born of lack of steady mental focus (*see sutra* 1.8). Again and again, we see why nirodha—the ability to attain a clear focused mind—is the cornerstone of spiritual life.

The obstacles form a kind of chain reaction, one leading to the next.

Disease

This stands for dis-ease, any physical discomfort or disorder that prevents us from fully engaging in Yoga practices. It can present as any number of diverse problems, such as fatigue, aching lower back when sitting for meditation, nagging allergies, or frequent headaches. Whatever the reason, the student's practice becomes irregular due to the challenge of physical distress.

Dullness

What is the result of irregular practice? Not much progress is made. It's hard to be keen and intent if you don't experience anything nice in your practices. The mind begins to have a hard time focusing. Nirodha begins to seem like an impossible dream. The end result is dullness of mind.

When the mind can't focus, it can't penetrate into the deeper meaning of things. This being so, the next stage naturally follows....

Doubt

"I don't know. These teachings are awfully intense. And they seem too idealistic. Or maybe I don't have the talent for this. I'm also starting to wonder if maybe my teacher doesn't know what's really best for me."

We doubt the veracity or practicality of the teachings or, even more troublesome, we doubt ourselves. We have not made the progress we thought we would. We feel a bit let down. Our hearts are not in our practice like before. Our regular practice now includes a new factor: uncertainty.

Doubt can be a serious impediment to progress. When our practice has stalled due to doubt, our first duty is to have the doubts cleared. Ask questions of adepts and masters; read and study more; do whatever it takes to remove the uncertainties from your heart.

Of course doubt, in addition to being its own difficult obstacle, adds fuel to dullness.

Carelessness

Even though the first three obstacles are working their spell, being a good student, you persevere. But there's not much enthusiasm.

Your practices become mechanical and lack conviction and intensity (*see sutras* 1.21 *and* 1.22: *"To the keen and intent practitioner this samadhi comes very quickly"*; *"The time necessary for success also depends on whether the practice is mild, moderate, or intense"*).

The energy of the mind is torn by doubt and dissipated by disease and dullness. It is natural that such a practice be marked by carelessness. You barely pay attention to your practices.

"Did I just inhale or hold my breath? What round am I doing?"

The end of your meditation session comes, and you have no idea what you've been doing for the past thirty minutes—probably *not* repeating your mantra.

Not only do you cease experiencing progress, but whatever momentum and depth your practice had are slipping away.

Laziness

Yoga practice now becomes nothing more than a chore. Do you feel like practicing anymore? Not likely. You become lazy with regard to your practices.

Lord Buddha taught that the only sin was laziness. If we do not even attempt to better ourselves, how can there be hope for success in Yoga?

Sensuality

The mind is bored, and a bored mind always looks for a distraction—a new amusement or something to do. It gets mischievous. If it cannot find anything satisfying within the practices, it will look to gratify the senses.

The Sanskrit word for sensuality, *avirati*, also means "to dissipate" and refers to the dissipation of our energy that comes when the mind loses its focus and resolve and seeks to satisfy sensual cravings. The decrease in the energy exacerbates all the other obstacles.

False Perception

"Yes, I used to practice Raja Yoga. Don't get me wrong, some aspects of Yoga are good, but these Eastern philosophies miss the point. After all, shouldn't I live life with gusto, wringing out every drop of fun I can? And those yogis lived so long ago! Patanjali could not have anticipated today's world. Or maybe he just didn't face life as it is. It seems that Yoga is really about the suppression of natural impulses and emotions. I wonder how different these sutras would be if Patanjali were alive today."

What seemed so clearly true in the beginning now seems out of touch. We may begin to believe that our assessment of Yoga as meaningful for our lives was a mistake. Most practices are abandoned, with the exception of perhaps a few stress-relieving techniques.

False perception is noteworthy among the obstacles because it most resembles ignorance

(See sutra 2.5, which defines ignorance.)

Failure to Reach Firm Ground

It is difficult to make progress when the practices and attainments have not become firmly grounded, an integral part of how we experience life. Another way to understand this obstacle is that it is the inability to attain or maintain focused attention.

Related Sutra: 1.14: Describes the factors needed to make a practice firmly grounded.

Slipping from the Ground Gained

Slipping from the ground gained can happen because we fall back into to harmful habits, or due to extended periods of physical or emotional stress, or even because after making a little progress, we get a little complacent and "rest on our laurels." Whatever the reason, it is a common experience to lose, at least temporarily, some of the spiritual progress we have made.

It is very discouraging to work hard, make some progress, and then slip back. It can feel like Dante's vision of hell, where poor souls expend tremendous energy to crawl out of an immense, burning pit, only to fall back into the flames at the brink of escape.

If these obstacles are left unchecked, we will lose much of what we have gained. The guarantee of never falling back arrives only with the highest samadhi. Yet for those of us who have done our share of slipping, it is reassuring that Sri Patanjali understands our plight. He knows that this happens and has given us two powerful remedies

75

(see sutra 1.29, regarding the way to overcome obstacles, and sutra 1.32, which explains the best method to prevent obstacles).

It is easy to become discouraged when we experience these obstacles. We should remind ourselves that encountering obstacles is natural. Instead of becoming discouraged or worried, we can take the opportunity to look within and see what lessons the obstacles can teach us.

There is a story that demonstrates the sneaky way obstacles can slip into our lives and distract us from our intentions. Not all the obstacles are represented in this tale, but you will recognize a few of the key ones and the slippery slope they present.

There once was a young yogi who had lived at his guru's ashram for a number of years. He was a dedicated disciple who practiced with great fervor. One day, he noticed his master looking at him in a curious way.

"Master, is there something wrong? You are looking at me in the most peculiar way."

"No, nothing is wrong. But as I was watching you, it occurred to me that it would be good for you to experience a period of seclusion to focus on deepening your meditation."

"Fine, master. I'm happy to do as you say."

"Good. A few miles from here there is a nice forest with a small village nearby where you can go and beg for your daily food. Stay there until I come for you."

"It sounds perfect. I'll go at once."

Following his master's instructions, he took only a begging bowl and two loincloths. Arriving at the bank of a stream, he found an elevated spot where he built his hut.

He then began a routine that was repeated faithfully for many weeks; after morning meditation, he would take one loincloth, wash it, drape it on the roof of his hut to dry, and then walk to the village to beg for food.

Then one day, when he came back to the hut he noticed that a rat had eaten a hole in his loincloth. What to do? The next day, he begged for food and another loincloth. The villagers were only too happy to help him. Unfortunately, the rat would not go away and continued ruining one loincloth after another. One villager took pity on him.

"Son, look how much trouble that rat is causing you. Everyday you have to beg for food and also for a new loincloth. What you need is a cat to keep away the rat."

The young man was stunned at the simple logic of the answer. That very day he begged for food, a loincloth, and a cat. He obtained a nice kitten.

But things did not go as he anticipated. Although the cat did keep away the rat, it, too, needed food. Now he had to beg for a bowl of milk for his cat as well as food for himself. This went on for several weeks, until. . .

"Young man, I noticed you begging for food for yourself and milk for your cat. Why don't you get a cow? Not only can you feed the cat, you'll even have milk left over for yourself!"

He thought this was brilliant. It took a little time, but he was able to find a villager to give him a cow. By now, you may have guessed what happens next. While the milk from the cow fed his cat and provided some milk for him, it too needed to eat. Now, when he begged for food, he also had to ask for hay for the cow. After some time....

"Dear boy, what a burden it is to beg for food and hay for your cow, too! Just do one simple thing and all your problems will be over. You are living on very fertile soil. Beg for hayseed and plant hay to feed the cow. You will certainly have enough hay left over to sell in town. With the extra money you could buy whatever you need."

The young disciple wondered how he could have missed such a simple solution. He found hayseed to sow and soon harvested a rich crop of hay. But, one day a villager spotted him, looking haggard.

"Son, you are working too hard. You have a growing business to look after. What you need is a wife to share responsibilities with you. Later on, your children will also be able to help.

Of course, he thought. So simple. He did find a nice woman to marry. His business and family grew by leaps and bounds. In fact, his hut was soon replaced by a mansion staffed with servants.

One day there was a knock at the door.

The young man walked to the door and looked into the eyes of his master. A sudden rush of recognition brought back memories of long forgotten and neglected commitments. Looking heavenward, he raised his arms high and shouted. . .

"All for the want of a loincloth!"

The moral is *not*: don't have pets, a business, or a spouse; it's: always keep your eye on your goal. It is too easy to slip from the ground gained.

1.31. Accompaniments to the mental distractions include distress, despair, trembling of the body, and disturbed breathing.

In life, the obstacles don't necessarily appear to us as presented in the previous sutra. Not many practitioners have felt, "I am experiencing false perception these days." The obstacles are like viruses. We can't directly perceive their presence in our systems. We need to learn to recognize the symptoms. This sutra presents the main symptoms of the obstacles.

1.32. The concentration on a single subject (or the use of one technique) is the best way to prevent the obstacles and their accompaniments.

In sutra 1.29, meditation is presented as the way to overcome obstacles; here we learn that commitment is the preventive against future occurrences. Steadiness of mind is the basis for both remedies, manifesting as focused attention in meditation and perseverance in life.

There is a story that demonstrates the power of sticking to one thing. It begins with a young boy's first day of school.

The teacher welcomed the class warmly.

"Today is a special day: your very first day of school. We will treat this day as a holiday. I will send you home early, but only after teaching you something that you can show your parents."

At least in the beginning, most students look forward to going home to demonstrate what they learned in school that day.

"Class, today we will learn to write the number one."

The class was thrilled. The teacher turned to the blackboard and with the chalk traced the single stroke for all the class to see.

"Now you all try it."

One by one, she checked all the students' papers.

"Good. Good. Fine. Very nice. Class, you have all done very well, you are dismissed for today."

The next day, the teacher gave a new assignment.

"Boys and girls, you did so well yesterday that we can proceed to number two." She drew the sample on the board for all to see. Again, she strolled up and down the isles checking the papers.

"Good, Good. Fine. O, son, you must have misunderstood." She was talking to our young hero.

"You are still writing number one, and today we are practicing number two. Your number ones are fine, please move on."

"Teacher, I know we are doing number two, but somehow I don't think I have understood the number one yet."

"Well . . . okay. I'll let you continue with number one today, but you must catch up with the class by tomorrow, or you will fall too far behind."

The next day the teacher wrote the number three on the board for the class to copy.

"Good. Good. Fine...O, son, you are still practicing number one. Take it from me. I'm a college-educated teacher. Your number one is perfectly acceptable. There is no reason for you to continue practicing it."

"I understand, teacher. I don't want to cause any trouble; it's just that I don't feel like I *understand* the number one."

The teacher was not sure what to do. The boy was otherwise well-behaved and intelligent. Days passed and the class continued to advance, while our young man insisted on practicing number one. Finally, in a moment of exasperation, the teacher lost her temper.

"Get out. Go home. Maybe your parents can do something with you."

"Okay, teacher. I'm sorry to have been a problem for you."

The boy went home and explained what had happened to his parents. They were shaken. He had never exhibited any willful behavior before. They discussed the situation and hoped that maybe with their love and patience they could guide him through this perplexing problem.

Unfortunately, the boy continued the same behavior with his parents. Everyday they gave their best effort and everyday he replied, "I am so sorry to hurt you, Mom and Dad. I don't mean to disobey; it is just that I don't understand the number one."

After a few weeks of this, even the parents lost their temper.

"Get out of our sight. Just leave this house."

Quietly the boy left, eventually entering the large forest at the edge of their village. Moments later, the parents, regretting their outburst, searched for their son but could not find him.

Then one day, the boy appeared at the classroom. The teacher, excited yet restrained by the boy's past behavior, simply welcomed him and then added, "Is there anything we can do for you son? Is there anything you want to say?"

"Yes, teacher, I now know the number one."

"Would you like to come up to the front of the room and show everyone your number one?"

"Certainly, if you like."

The little boy calmly walked to the front of the room. Picking up the chalk and turning to the blackboard, he made the simple straight line of the number one...and the blackboard *split in half.*

The boy's attentive repetition of the number one resulted in an extraordinary demonstration of the power of a one-pointed mind. When he undertook the simple act of tracing a straight line on the board, it took on miraculous dimensions.

We need that kind of one-pointed perseverance to overcome obstacles and pierce the veneer of ignorance. We should never give up. Many people quit when they are on the brink of success. Determination always pays off. Ants, daily walking the same path across a stone wall, will wear a groove in it one day. Likewise, our practices will eventually eradicate ignorance.

Related Sutra: 1.14: Teaches that regular practice, done over a long period of time and with enthusiasm, results in the steadiness of practice discussed in this sutra.

1.33. By cultivating attitudes of friendliness toward the happy, compassion for the unhappy, delight in the virtuous, and equanimity toward the nonvirtuous, the mind-stuff retains its undisturbed calmness.

This sutra demonstrates how the mind can retain its peace in any situation. It has been referred to as the "four locks and four keys" by Sri Swami Satchidananda.

Sri Patanjali divides interactions into four categories. These are the "locks;" the puzzles or challenges we face daily. The "keys" that are applied to these situations help the mind retain undisturbed calmness. The locks and keys are not prescriptions for specific actions: we are not told what to *do* but how to *be*; how to cultivate attitudes that ensure that the instrument of perception (the mind) is in the best condition to make the proper assessments and choices.

Lock 1: Happiness; Key: Friendliness

We might think it is natural to be friendly toward someone who is happy. Unfortunately, this is not always true. There are times when another's happiness (or success) reminds us of our failures or unfulfilled desires. Though we may not become overtly angry or depressed, our well-wishing could be mixed with envy or jealousy. For example, this might happen if a friend receives the promotion we hoped for. Our good thoughts could be diminished by regret or envy.

Sri Patanjali recommends cultivating friendliness toward the happy as the key to undisturbed calmness. We should make friends with happiness, get to know it, give it proper attention and respect. If we dwell on happiness, looking for it like a miner's eye seeks gold, we will cultivate it in our lives.

Lock 2: Unhappiness; Key: Compassion

Sometimes the unhappiness of others feels like a burden. We may become impatient, wondering how our brother can make the same mistake over and over again. Perhaps we think that he should just get over his grief and get on with life. There are times when the suffering of others can make us uneasy or frightened. In our discomfort, we turn away from them.

Instead, whenever we see unhappiness we should use the compassion key. To be compassionate doesn't necessarily mean that we cry when our brother cries or become angry in order to support our sister's frustration. In the name of compassion there are times when the appropriate response is to deliver a strong piece of advice that is difficult to hear. However, behind our actions, we should cherish one overriding motive: the welfare of others. All actions should proceed from a place of caring and loving.

A compassionate heart is a comfort and support to many. We develop compassion by recalling acts of kindness that have benefited us while remembering the pain, alienation, despair, and confusion caused by suffering.

Compassion requires courage and strength: the courage to move beyond our own concerns to connect to the suffering of others, and the strength to help bear their suffering.

(Note: The word translated as unhappy is duhkha, variously translated as pain, suffering, sorrow, or grief. It is a central theme in the sutras, being mentioned seven times. Refer to sutra 1.31 in the Sutra Dictionary for a more complete explanation of duhkha.)

Lock 3: Virtuous; Key: Delight

Virtues are moral traits—such as patience, courage, reliability—that bring benefit to others and harm to no one. They are signs of spiritual maturity and serve as reliable compasses with which we can navigate the uncertainties of life's choices.

Virtues can be developed through study and contemplation or, as this sutra suggests, through recognizing their presence in others. In other words, we should cultivate the habit of celebrating virtues wherever we recognize them. The more we rejoice in them, the sooner they will be ours.

This practice is especially useful in encounters with people who make us uncomfortable or whom we do not like. Everyone has at least some virtues. Are we perceptive enough to recognize any in our enemies? We might find that behavior we once understood as obnoxious might reveal perseverance. What we once regarded as pushy now gives us a glimpse into the benefits of firm convictions.

Lock 4: Nonvirtuous; Key: Equanimity

Upeksha, translated as "equanimity," comes from upa, "to go near or toward," and iksha, "to look at or on." In the context of this sutra, we can understand it as the ability to clearly perceive the nature of the nonvirtuous act through close and unbiased examination.

Sad to say, we all too often witness or are victims of injustices. This sutra is not promoting aloofness or praising an uncaring attitude. Even though anger often feels justifiable and sometimes seems like the best way to correct an injustice, Sri Patanjali doesn't find it an acceptable attitude for a yogi to have. Instead, we are challenged to do something that may seem counterintuitive when we face a nonvirtuous act: keep our equanimity.

Though it's natural to feel like striking back when we are victims of someone's wrongdoing, anger causes great harm:

- It deprives us of peace and neutrality of mind.
- Our bodies become shaky and disturbed. Anger weakens us physically
- Anger destroys reason and stifles creativity. The loss of reason and creativity means that better approaches to resolving conflicts are often missed.
- Every act of anger predisposes us to further instances. Repeated actions create habits; and habits continued form character: we are in danger of becoming bitter people.
- Even if it brings benefit to others, our anger hurts us first.

While anger sometimes motivates people to correct an injustice, there is a state of mind better suited for dealing with the nonvirtuous. The mind possessed of equanimity is in the best position to find solutions. It is strong, clear, and free of bias.

We don't need anger to motivate us to do what is right. We can act from higher motives: compassion, the clear knowledge of what is right, and the strong wish to bring about harmony. With clarity of mind we will understand the wicked act and its implications, increasing the chances of finding creative and effective solutions.

This brings us to a related topic: how, when, and whether we should attempt to correct another who is engaged in nonvirtuous actions. There are occasions when taking corrective action is not the best course. It could even be counterproductive. For example, someone you care for may not be ready to hear your helpful advice concerning some careless habit. They may react in anger to your suggestions and then hold a grudge, making it even harder for you to serve them in the future. Although you may be able to point out your concern gently and tactfully and mention your availability to serve them, sometimes the most beneficial and compassionate act is to allow them to face the consequences of their actions. There are also times when you simply have to wait until the one you care for demonstrates readiness to change by approaching you or someone else over the matter.

Finally, it is interesting to note one result of practicing this key: it opens the door to compassion for the unhappy. We realize that nonvirtuous acts are based on misdirected attempts to find fulfillment.

In studying the locks and keys, we should remember to apply them to ourselves.

We need to cultivate:

- Friendliness toward our own happiness. This is one instance in life when a little indulgence is good, especially when our happiness has its roots in spiritual acts or values.
- Loving compassion for our own sorrow. Be kind to yourself.
- Joy when we manifest virtues.
- Strength, patience, and equanimity when working to eliminate our weaknesses. Forgiveness plays an important role with this.

The next six sutras give various techniques and suggested objects of meditation that help steady the mind. All these sutras begin with the word "or." They are the "oars" that help us row to the shore of peace.

1.34. Or that calm is retained by the controlled exhalation or retention of the breath.

The mind and breath are related. When the mind is calm, so is the breath. When the breath becomes agitated, the mind follows. When we regulate the breath, the mind will become more clear and calm. By gently extending the duration of exhalations and gradually increasing the retention of the breath, we exert a powerful calming influence on the mind.

(A note of caution: breath retention is a very powerful practice. To avoid any potential physical harm, it should be attempted only under the guidance of a qualified teacher.)

1.35. Or that (undisturbed calmness) is attained when the perception of a subtle sense object arises and holds the mind steady.

For some seekers, the experience of something out of the ordinary acts as an encouragement to persevere in their practices.

Tradition suggests several ways to gain the experience of subtle sense perceptions: steady focus on the tip of the nose or tongue, for example. If your concentration is sufficiently deep and stable, you will experience a nice fragrance with the first technique and a wonderful taste with the second.

1.36. Or by concentrating on the supreme, ever-blissful Light within.

This sutra refers to meditation using a visualization technique. From this we can infer that any inspiring visualization, religious symbol, or form of God that points to the Self can be part of a Yoga practice.

We are asked to focus our minds on a truth that we have not yet experienced (that there is a Divine Light within). It requires a certain amount of faith even to try this. Eventually, the visualized Light will disappear and be replaced with the true experience.

1.37. Or by concentrating on a great soul's mind which is totally freed from attachment to sense objects.

This can be regarded as an alternative to the above sutra. If you cannot imagine or believe in your own Inner Light, then look to the heart of a great saint, prophet, or yogi in whom you have faith. Perhaps you can perceive the Light there.

1.38. Or by concentrating on an insight had during dream or deep sleep.

This sutra is referring to a particular type of dream: those that are spiritually uplifting, that in some way influence us for the better or teach us a helpful lesson.

With regard to deep sleep, Sri Patanjali is not asking us to meditate on sleep itself but on the peace of dreamless sleep.

1.39. Or by meditating on anything one chooses that is elevating.

Sri Patanjali knows human nature. There will always be someone who will find a reason not to take his suggestions. "It doesn't matter," he reassures us. "As long as you find it spiritually inspiring, go ahead. It will work."

The teachings of Raja Yoga are useful for everyone, regardless of background, era, or faith tradition. If the chosen object captures our interest, inspires and points us in the direction of the Self, it has Sri Patanjali's seal of approval.

1.40. Gradually one's mastery in concentration extends from the smallest particle to the greatest magnitude.

Through faithful practice, the yogi can focus the mind on any aspect of creation, from the most subtle to the almost unthinkably immense. A mind with this degree of focus and clarity is fit for meditating on the Infinite.

The next sutra begins a series of four on the topic of samadhi.

1.41. Just as the naturally pure crystal assumes shapes and colors of objects placed near it, so the yogi's mind, with its totally weakened modifications, becomes clear and balanced and attains the state devoid of differentiation between knower, knowable, and knowledge. This culmination of meditation is samadhi.

Why would we wish to experience a "state devoid of differentiation between knower, knowable, and knowledge?"

As was mentioned in the commentary on sutra 1.17, perception requires three factors: the knower; an object to perceive; and the act of knowing. This threefold process is useful for obtaining ordinary knowledge but is insufficient for experiencing subtle aspects of Prakriti and for attaining of Self-realization.

Samadhi is the zenith of the meditative process in which the "differentiation between knower, knowable, and knowledge" dissolves. It is state in which insight is gained through union with the object of contemplation. The mind, steady and clear as a crystal, temporarily gives up its self-identity and seems to vanish as it allows the object of meditation alone to shine forth.

In the next three sutras, Sri Patanjali expands the discussion of samadhi by examining two of the four samprajnata samadhis presented in sutra 1.17: vitarka and vichara. Vitarka samadhi is divided into two categories: with (*sa*) and beyond (*nir*) examination. In the same way, vichara can be either with or beyond insight.

Related Sutras: 1.17: On samprajnata samadhi; and 1.18: On asamprajnata samadhi.
(Also see Samadhi in the Sutras-by-Subject Index.)

1.42. The samadhi in which an object, its name, and conceptual knowledge of it are mixed is called savitarka samadhi, the samadhi with examination.

Savitarka samadhi is absorption on a gross object; one that can be perceived by the ordinary senses. This absorption initiates a spontaneous and intuitive examination of the qualities of the object contemplated. There is union with the object of contemplation, but it is mixed or interspersed with the word used to designate the object along with our learned knowledge of that object.

Savitarka samadhi also brings an intuitive understanding of the phenomenon of sense perception. What we experience as the simple perception of any object is a mixture of three distinct components: name, form, and knowledge:

- Name (sabda): the "handle" that we use to grasp outside objects
- Object (artha): the original object of perception as it exists
- Knowledge (jnana): the reaction in the chitta to the object

We usually do not perceive an external object directly. Knowledge obtained in the ordinary way is the result of the senses relaying the vibrations of an object into the mind-stuff, which reacts by forming vrittis. What we perceive is not the external object but the risen modifications in the mind. In addition, past impressions related to that object pop up. The sum total of this reaction in the chitta is "conceptual" knowledge. Conceptual knowledge can be a mix of accurate and erroneous ideas regarding the object under examination. Usually, this threefold process happens so quickly that the steps blur into what seems to be the single event we call perception.

For example, there is the external reality of a cow, the word "cow" that we use to think about matters bovine, and ideas about cows—that they moo, give milk, and chew their cud. We are not normally aware of the three distinct factors. We just "see" a cow, and all sorts of related ideas appear in the mind.

In savitarka samadhi, the mind gradually learns to isolate and focus on the object itself, leaving behind the relativities of our knowledge of it and its name. This prepares the mind for the next step in samadhi: nirvitarka.

Examples of objects of meditation in this category are the form of a deity, a candle flame, or the repeated sound of a mantra (rather than its subtle essential vibration).

1.43. When the subconscious is well purified of memories (regarding the object of contemplation), the mind appears to lose its own identity, and the object alone shines forth. This is nirvitarka samadhi, the samadhi beyond examination.

This is the second of the two *tarka* samadhis. The prefix, *nir*, means "without," but in the context of the *Yoga Sutras*, it may be best understood as "beyond."

As with savitarka samadhi, the object of contemplation is an object perceptible by the senses. Nirvitarka samadhi differs in that the object is now fully known, so the process of "examination" is complete and hence comes to a halt.

In nirvitarka samadhi, the name of the object and any perceptual knowledge of it that was filtered (and therefore skewed or limited) through ordinary thought processes cease to be influential factors in cognition. We are left with just the object as it exists, uncolored by any past impressions we have of it. The subjective experience of nirvitarka samadhi is that the mind gives up its own identity for the sake of union of the individual with the object of contemplation.

1.44. In the same way, savichara (with insight) and nirvichara (beyond insight) samadhis, which are practiced upon subtle objects, are explained.

The two *chara* samadhis parallel the *tarka* samadhis except that the objects of contemplation are subtle elements (*tanmatras*), such as the energies or potentials that make sound, touch, taste, color, and sight possible, rather than objects perceivable by the senses (*see Tanmatra in the Glossary*).

Specifically, savichara samadhi begins the process of understanding the causes that brought the object into being: the subtle elements and the factors of space and time.

Nirvichara samadhi is said to be "beyond insight," meaning that there are no further insights into the nature of the object to be had. There is complete knowledge of the object of contemplation down to its subtle essence.

1.45. The subtlety of possible objects of concentration ends only at the undifferentiated.

The mind gains the ability to focus and merge with every object in creation, down to undifferentiated Prakriti.

1.46. All these samadhis are sabija [with seed].

The "seeds" are the subconscious impressions remaining in the mind. They can sprout at any time, given the proper time, place, circumstance, and karma. When they do sprout, they can deprive the mind of the intuitive knowledge of samadhi and reopen the door to the influence of ignorance and egoism.

1.47. In the pure clarity of nirvichara samadhi, the supreme Self shines.

Although not conferring liberation, nirvichara samadhi, by virtue of its purifying action on the subconscious mind, allows the Self to reflect undistorted on the mind. A unique and subtle wisdom emerges from nirvichara samadhi…

1.48. This is ritambhara prajna [the truth-bearing wisdom].

Ritambhara prajna: ritam, "truth," bhara, "bearing," and prajna, "wisdom, knowledge," hence ritambhara prajna, the intuitive wisdom that is truth-bearing.

Sri Patanjali goes on to expand our understanding of this special state of knowing.

1.49. The purpose of this special wisdom is different from the insights gained by study of sacred tradition and inference.

Nirvichara samadhi unlocks the door to Self-realization. In this samadhi, the Self clearly reflects on the mind and confers a truth-bearing wisdom: the discernment of Purusha from Prakriti. This discernment cannot be achieved through study and inference. Its source is the intuitive insight of nirvichara samadhi.

Related Sutra: 1.7: "The sources of right knowledge are direct perception, inference, and scriptural testimony."

1.50. Other impressions are overcome by the impression produced by this samadhi.

This samadhi generates powerful subconscious impressions that incline the mind toward uninterrupted stillness, mastery, and ultimately spiritual union. The "other impressions" mentioned in this sutra, the ones that are overcome, are those that maintain the mind's deeply ingrained habit of externally oriented behavior. The reason that nirvichara samadhi has this overpowering impact on lifetimes of latent subconscious impressions is because the impressions it generates are "truth-bearing," supercharged with the reality and immediacy of the Self.

As wonderful as this samadhi is, there is still one more step to climb. Nirvichara samadhi is a dualistic state. Even the feeling "I have realized the Absolute" needs to be left behind. Though the image of the Absolute we see is totally engrossing, it is a reflection, a copy, not the original. We have not yet realized that we *are* that which we behold. The final step is the transcendence of the mind and the realization of our True Identity as the Self. This realization is described in the next sutra.

1.51. With the stilling of even this impression, every impression is wiped out, and there is nirbija [seedless] samadhi.

The finite mind cannot grasp the Infinite. The mind needs to be transcended to reach the final stage, *nirbija* samadhi. Even the impression left by nirvichara samadhi needs to be transcended. With both conscious mental activity and subconscious impressions (samskaras) completely stilled, the mind achieves (more correctly, realizes) perfect union with the Self. The universe and self melt into the experience of Oneness.

In the Vedas, this truth is expressed as: "Brahman [God or the Absolute] is One without a second." That means, all that there is, is God. Normally, we cannot think of a single unit of something without comparing it to at least one more. For example, it is impossible even to understand *one* apple (the oneness or singularity of it) unless we can compare it to two or more apples. Even to understand the concept of *nothing*, we also need to compare it to *something*. Similarly, we cannot understand the oneness of the Absolute through the use of the mind, which operates only with dualities and relativities.

Nirbija samadhi is the experience of complete oneness with the Absolute. You realize that the real you was never born and will never die. You are the Self.

Pada One Review

1. The goal of Yoga is stated:

When the mind becomes completely clear and focused (nirodha), the changeless Self is realized as one's True Identity.

2. The basic obstacle (ignorance):

The Self gets confused with the body and mind due to the ego's identification with modifications in the mind-stuff and the resulting impressions they leave in the mind.

3. Achieving nirodha:

We are introduced to the modifications (vrittis) that we are asked to restrain. There are five types (right knowledge, misperception, conceptualization, sleep, and memory) that either bring pain or are painless.

A two-pronged approach to achieving nirodha is presented: practice (abhyasa) and nonattachment (vairagya):

- Practice is the effort to steady the mind. It becomes second nature (firmly grounded) when engaged in for a long time, without break, and with enthusiasm. Several options for calming the mind are given.
- Nonattachment is presented on two levels: the effort to maintain the proper relationship with sense objects by not depending on them for happiness, and the highest nonattachment which comes with Self-realization.

Several levels of samadhi are explained, culminating in the complete cessation of all conscious and subconscious mental activity: nirbija samadhi. It is at this point that unity with the Self is realized.

4. Samadhi can also be attained by devotion to Ishwara (the supreme Purusha, unaffected by limitations).

What to Do

The practice of mantra japa is a gateway to experiencing Ishwara, an aid to overcoming obstacles and attaining samadhi (*sutras* 1.27–1.29). Anyone from any background can participate in this powerful practice. If you are an adherent of a particular spiritual tradition, you will most likely find mantras, short prayers, or names of God that can be used in your practice. There are a host of well-known and powerful mantras you can choose from, including OM Shanti, Hari OM, OM Namah Sivaya, Maranatha, Ameen, and Shalom.

Hatha Yoga makes a good foundation for a daily routine. It will help you gain some control over the mind as well as enhance your health and well-being. Be careful not to bite off more than you can chew. A little practice every day is better than occasional dramatic efforts. Moderation is a key to success.

Begin applying the Four Locks and Four Keys (sutra 1.33). Observe the challenges they present as well as the benefits they bring. You could choose one lock and key per day or week to practice. It will also be helpful to record your experiences in a daily diary.

Start a regular practice of meditation (*see sutras* 1.34—1.39). In the beginning stages, it is good to experiment with a few different approaches that appeal to you. But remember that the best results will be attained when you settle on one approach. If you are attracted to Mantra Japa, it can certainly serve as your meditation practice.

Some meditation hints for beginners include:

- Find a seated position in which your back can remain comfortably upright.
- Start with prayers or affirmations that remind you of your goal. Then add some easy deep breathing to continue the process of calming the mind. After a few minutes, turn your attention to the object of meditation you have chosen. Give it your gentle, unwavering focus. Just be aware of it.
- It's common for the mind to wander. When it does, gently let go of the distracting thought and refocus on your object of meditation. This refocusing of the mind will occur a number of times during your session. Over time, the mind begins to learn steady focus.

- After about fifteen minutes, begin to deepen the breathing and then end your session with more affirmations, remembering to send thoughts of peace and well-being to those in need.
- Try to have at least two sittings of twenty minutes each that include affirmations, breathing, and meditation. This routine insures proper preparation and helps you to bring the peace of meditation into your daily life.

Regardless of which meditation technique you use, it is beneficial to practice the mindful performance of daily tasks. See how you can make your everyday actions more efficient; when cutting carrots, do it with a focused mind and make every cut uniform. If painting a room, do it in an orderly manner, trying to not waste energy and resources. Mindfulness should extend to cultivating a greater awareness of the impact of your decisions and actions on others. This will not only benefit your Yoga practices but make you a better friend and neighbor as well.

Pada Two
Sadhana Pada: Portion on Practice

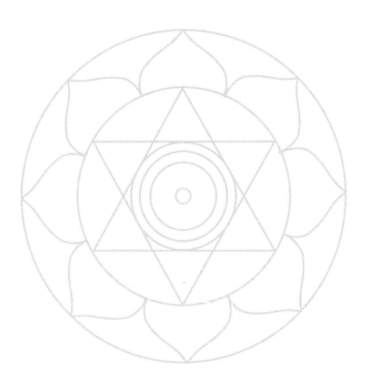

Inside Pada Two

Sadhana, the term used to designate spiritual practices, is derived from the root sadh, "to go straight to the goal," and is generally translated as "the means to liberation."

Pada One presented the theoretical foundation of Raja Yoga; the focus now shifts to providing the motivation for regular sadhana and presenting clear, comprehensive instructions for practice.

The motivation is achieved through sutras that discuss the nature of pleasure and pain, the length of life, and the circumstances of our birth. Sutra 2.15 confirms the experience of wise women and men of all times: that pain is inevitable in life. But we are not left feeling burdened by this uncomfortable observation. Subsequent sutras state that suffering can be avoided and that the cause of our suffering is ignorance, which can be removed by the practice of the eight limbs of Raja Yoga.

Speaking of practice, we are introduced to Kriya Yoga, a three-pronged approach that weakens the obstacles that impede progress. Then, in sutra 2.29, we encounter the heart of Raja Yoga practice, the eight limbs of Yoga. In a mere eight words we discover the fullness and harmony of Yoga sadhana.

Pada Two also begins the investigation of discriminative discernment (viveka), with a discussion on the distinctions between the Seer (Spirit) and the seen (Prakriti or Nature), a topic that will be resumed in greater detail in Pada Four.

Key Principles:
- The five klesas or obstacles: ignorance, egoism, attachment, aversion, and clinging to bodily life
- Karma: the law of action and reaction
- The Seer (Purusha) as:
  The power of seeing
  The "owner" of Prakriti
- The seen (Prakriti) as:
  Necessary to bring experiences and liberation
  Existing only for the sake of the Purusha
  Consisting of the gunas: sattwa, rajas, and tamas

Key Practices:
- Kriya Yoga:
  Accepting pain as help for purification
  Study
  Surrender to the Supreme Being
- Uninterrupted discriminative discernment (viveka)
- The eight limbs of Raja Yoga

Other Key Terms:
- *Avidya*: ignorance
- *Yama*: restraints
- *Niyama*: observances
- *Asana*: posture
- *Pranayama*: breath control
- *Pratyahara*: withdrawal of the senses
- *Dharana*: concentration
- *Dhyana*: meditation
- *Samadhi*: absorption, superconscious state

Pada Two
Sadhana Pada: Portion on Practice

2.1. Accepting pain as help for purification, study, and surrender to the Supreme Being constitute Yoga in practice.

The practices listed in this sutra, called Kriya Yoga, constitute the context in which all other Yoga practices are placed. They are the foundation of spiritual life in general and serve as a preparation for the eight limbs of Yoga (*see sutra* 2.29).

The three aspects of Kriya Yoga are a synergistic combination of:
- *Tapas*: the acceptance of challenges as a help for purification
- *Svadhyaya*: refinement of the intellect through introspection and the acquisition of knowledge (study)
- *Ishwara Pranidhana*: leading a life dedicated to God (self-surrender)

Related Sutra: 2.32: Lists these three observances as part of the niyamas.

Accepting Pain as Help for Purification: Tapas

No one wants to suffer, yet the first word from Sri Patanjali in the section on Yoga practice is *tapas*, "accepting pain." He gives prominent position to an attitude, a way of perceiving and responding to the experiences of life. We are challenged to engage life actively with an outlook that may seem far-fetched: that anything that happens—no matter how painful—can be used for spiritual growth. In some way, although not always readily apparent, everything truly is for the good—*our* good. Tapas is not resignation, a passive submission to the sorrows of life; it is the embracing of pain as friend and teacher.

Tapas begins to make sense only when we understand that pain—psychological or physical—is a sign that we have encountered a limitation in ourselves. Stretch a muscle beyond the limits of its tissues, and we feel pain. Push the mind beyond the limits of what it perceives to be just and proper, and we experience suffering. But to be free, we need to overcome our limitations. They need to be exposed, examined, and uprooted (a process, by the way, that is greatly aided by study and surrender to God). However, while some of our shortcomings are apparent, many others remain hidden in the subconscious, where they do their mischievous work. Tapas helps uncover hidden shortcomings by forcing them to surface in the conscious mind. Taken with the right understanding, suffering can bring forth the effort to overcome limitations. It also stimulates introspection and inspires creativity. For example, it can help us find fresh, meaningful ways to convince and entice ourselves to sit for daily meditation or to uncover a lesson hidden in our chronic disease that will bring us peace of mind.

Of course, adhering to the "no pain, no gain" philosophy is difficult while we are hurting.

Day after day, opportunities arise to practice acceptance, but instead we find ourselves caught up in resistance, anger, or depression. In the name of tapas, seekers expend great energy struggling to reconcile their beliefs with their own shortcomings and the disappointing realities of life. But the struggle is not fruitless; it brings us to a deeper self-knowledge and a truer understanding of life.

Tapas is not simply a patient, if unsettling, wait for painful events to come along so that they can be accepted. It can also be a voluntary act of will, a choice to embark knowingly on a path that might bring discomfort and challenge before producing its benefits. Fasting is an example of a voluntary practice of tapas. Some yogis willingly accept the discomfort of hunger one day a week as a help in purifying the body and strengthening the mind. The practice of tapas might also take the form of a shy person studying public speaking, someone who fears heights taking a ride on a Ferris wheel, or an individual who feels clumsy signing up for a class in tap dance.

Tapas also refers to the effort to be regular in the Yoga practices and to live a yogic lifestyle. For example, a comfy bed can beckon us to continue sleeping when the alarm signals the dawn of a new day. The effort—the inner voice coaxing us to get up, the exercise of the will, the mind's reminder that meditation promises great benefits to us, the prayer to God to help us leave the bed—all this is part of the practice of tapas.

We've talked about tapas as the struggle to understand and accept that life's trials have value for us. What can we expect from perfection in this practice? What does the practice of tapas ultimately bring the seeker? Obviously, the ability to endure and overcome problems strengthens the will. But that's not the whole story. Far from being a pessimistic resignation to suffering, tapas is the embrace of the

PADA TWO

entirety of life. Tapas is the foundation of an intimate relationship with the Intelligence that animates life. This relationship gives birth to wisdom, the certain knowledge—a steadfast faith—that the peace and joy of the inner Self is stronger and more enduring than any pain that life may bring. Through perfection in tapas, the fear that life is devoid of wisdom vanishes. Wisdom, faith, and fearlessness—these are the fruits of tapas.

Study: Svadhyaya

Ultimately, all study in Yoga is aimed at helping practitioners achieve Self-realization. Yogis have long recognized that this goal is more easily attained by including practices that prepare the mind for deeper insights, practices that inform intellect (the study of sacred tradition) and that clear and steady the mind.

Yogis should not be blind followers. Study enlists the cooperation of the mind by keeping it inspired and focused on the goal. The field of study is the nature of Spirit and the factors that obscure our experience of it. The primary source of information is scripture. We can also include the study of other authoritative works that teach accepted paths for spiritual liberation (*see sutra 1.7, in which authoritative testimony is given as a source of right knowledge*).

Hindu philosophy traditionally speaks of two avenues for attaining scriptural knowledge: the argumentative (*vada*) and the decisive (*siddhanta*).

The argumentative approach is taken up by those who are new to spiritual life—when the student appropriately engages in debate and the weighing of the pros and cons of any given point of theory. This period of debate and questioning is not argument for argument's sake; it is valid only if it increases knowledge and removes any doubts that prevent practice.

Questioning is a necessary stage for the student; there is no shortcut around it.

> If you seek enlightenment from those who have real-
> ized the truth, prostrate before them, question them,
> and serve them. Only then are you open to receive
> their teachings of sacred knowledge.
>
> Bhagavad Gita, 4.34

While we need to be honest about our doubts and reservations, dismissing teachings because we are uncomfortable with them is not a productive approach. We may deprive ourselves of some really useful gems. In reality, sometimes we are not ready to understand the truth. At other times, we may not have found someone who can explain it in a way we can relate to and understand. Regardless of the reason, we risk losing something of value if we dismiss precepts out of hand. To weigh our doubts against the evidence of countless thousands who have transformed their lives by following these teachings is central to a healthy practice of Yoga.

Seekers who have arrived at conclusions about spiritual life are ready for the decisive approach. Inner controversies have ceased. All fundamental questions have been satisfactorily answered. At this point, study primarily intensifies and refines convictions. This is why repetition is important. The advanced student of Yoga seeks not so much to gather new principles but to experience more profound depths of the truths already learned.

Traditionally, the repetition of mantras (or any other practice given by one's master) has also been considered an important aspect of study. The one-pointed repetition of a mantra strengthens the mind and brings the awareness within, taking the practitioner on a journey of self-discovery. It gradually reveals subtler levels of understanding, culminating with the realization of the Self.

Study informs and gives a balanced context for the practice of tapas. We understand and anticipate the benefits of forbearance. We know *why* we should turn the other cheek, accept our aches and pains—*why* it's okay when something doesn't go according to our personal plan.

Surrender: Ishwara Pranidhana

Surrender is the voluntary letting go of limited, personal desires for the sake of a greater and more fulfilling experience. It often takes the form of dedicating the fruits of our actions to God or humanity.

Normally, we try to keep the fruits of our efforts for ourselves. After all, it was *our* thought and energy that brought the rewards. We did the work; we deserve to be paid. Spiritual life takes a different view, one that can be observed in Nature: the law of life is sacrifice. The tree never eats its own fruits. The fruits have been produced *through* it, not *by* it. The air, sunshine, rain, and fertilizer were not created by the tree, but by God. Even the power of the tree to make baby trees came in seed form, which was given to it by its mama tree. And the mama got it from her mama, who got it from God.

Like the trees, nothing is ours—even our bodies and intellects were given to us. The strength we need to learn, grow, and accomplish are not ours either; they are provided by the food and air, which are given by Nature.

Most bodily functions that are essential to life are involuntary. We eat an apple and digest it without being burdened by having to direct the stomach and intestines to do their job. It is involuntary to us, but not to God, who makes it happen. God gives us the gift of life because we still have a part in the Divine plan. Since everything we have is the result of gifts, it is logical that we give—not take—credit for what we have accomplished.

The appropriate response when receiving a gift is gratitude. We give back to the Giver through our prayers of gratitude, when we sacrifice our selfish attachments, and by working for the welfare of others. To live for the sake of others is our highest calling and aligns us with God's will.

Another area that cultivates surrender is worship, which expresses as practices such as prayer and ritual. Although the sutras don't offer instructions on the way to worship, it is in keeping with the spirit of the teachings to choose whatever form of worship is meaningful to the seeker. However, if we look back to Pada One, we see that there are sutras that do provide guidance in how a yogi might understand and relate to Ishwara.

- We are told that Ishwara is unaffected by afflictions, actions, fruits of actions, or desires. It is a description that inspires us with thoughts of perfect freedom. It also gives us a role model to emulate. (*See sutra* 1.24.)
- Ishwara is the complete manifestation of omniscience, the source of all knowledge. Therefore we can attribute everything we know or will know to a Divine source. Every piece of knowledge can become a calling card from God. (*See sutra* 1.25)
- Ishwara is the teacher of even the most ancient of teachers. Ishwara is not only the source of all knowledge, but the guide for attaining it. Good students know what they don't know and

approach a teacher with deference. The humility that is central to any form of worship is suggested here. (*See sutra* 1.26.)

- We find that there is a link to God that is very intimate—a mantra—that represents an aspect of the Divine. Repetition of that mantra will bring us closer to experiencing God by removing obstacles and impurities. (*See sutras* 1.27 *and* 1.29.)

So, according to Raja Yoga, what is the description of God that we might surrender to? God is our guide, eternally free from all limitations, beyond all suffering, and the source of all knowledge.

Surrender can be found at the heart of meditation, obedience, and love: all three require giving up short-term personal wishes for a greater, more satisfying reality.

Meditation. Strenuous exertion to still the mind creates more mental modifications that need to be restrained. These forceful efforts are like attempts at calming the surface of water by using our hands to smooth out the waves. Instead, in the name of meditation, learn to surrender the distracting thoughts to the act (or object) of meditation. In other words, meditation is as much a process of letting go as of directing attention.

Obedience. We usually understand obedience to mean that we do what we are told. There certainly is some basis for this. But simply carrying out the orders of another is not obedience in the spiritual sense. A grumbling, resentful obedience is not really going to enhance spiritual maturity.

Obedience is more concerned with the inner attitude. The Latin verb *oboedire*, from which the word obedience is derived, means to listen intently and implies an open, receptive attitude. It is the attentiveness of a lover to the beloved or a mother to her infant rather than a slave to his master. It is the appropriate surrender of personal desires whenever they are in conflict with the Divine Will.

A Muslim immediately halting all worldly activity when the call to worship is sounded, the student of Zen following the advice of the Roshi, a yogi devotedly arising before dawn for meditation are all examples of obedience.

Love. There can be no love without surrender of self-interest. The very essence of what we recognize as love is giving and caring. It is the act of surrendering oneself to something greater (not necessarily simply to the other in the relationship but to the relationship itself) with the knowledge that a new, more vital reality will be created.

As you examine these three expressions of surrender, assess their presence or absence in your life. Are you now or are you becoming the kind of person whose nature is to accept, forbear, serve, and be self-aware, focused, and humble?

Related Sutras: 1.23, 2.32, and 2.45: All pertain to Ishwara Pranidhana.

2.2. They help us minimize the obstacles and attain samadhi.

The goal of Yoga is not to obtain something that is lacking; it is the realization of an already present reality. Yoga practice does not bring about samadhi directly—it removes the obstacles that obstruct its experience.

Related Sutra: 1.29: Describes the way to overcome the obstacles described as "distractions of the mind-stuff."
(Also see Obstacles in the Sutras-by-Subject Index.)

2.3. Ignorance, egoism, attachment, aversion, and clinging to bodily life are the five obstacles.

If our true nature is peace and joy, then what else but ignorance can be the cause of all our suffering?

This sutra again addresses the topic of obstacles (*see sutra* 1.30), but on a deeper level. Here, they are designated by the word *klesa*, which means affliction, suffering, and pain. Affliction is an appropriate term for the klesas. They are like a genetic disorder that torments us throughout our lives.

Like the earlier list of obstacles, the klesas are a chain reaction:
- Ignorance begins the process. Ignorance is the lack of awareness of the Self, which leads to identity with the self (body-mind).
- Egoism is the first result of ignorance. The peace and fulfillment of the Self now lost, the mind becomes restless.
- The ego begins to form attachments to things or circumstances, looking to them to bring happiness. The mind becomes accustomed to searching for externals for happiness.
- The brother of attachment is aversion: the avoidance of anything we perceive will bring pain or discomfort.

We cling to life in the body, since it is the medium through which the mind (through the sense organs) experiences the pleasure we seek.

The klesas are reminiscent of the notion of original sin in Christianity. Adam and Eve were enjoying communion with God and an idyllic life in the Garden of Eden. God's only instructions were that the land be cultivated and that Adam should not eat of the fruit of the Tree of Knowledge of Good and Evil, *"for in that day that you eat from it you will surely die"* (Genesis 2.17). Let's compare the biblical teachings with the klesas point-by –point.

Ignorance

The knowledge referred to in the Bible is the same as the ignorance spoken of in Raja Yoga. They are two ways to refer to the same experience. Adam and Eve gained knowledge of their individuality, but lost—or became ignorant of—knowledge of God.

Attachment/Aversion

"Good and evil" are analogous to attachment (we perceive as good that which brings pleasure) and aversion (we perceive as bad that which brings pain).

Clinging to Bodily Life

In the Bible, God tells Adam if he eats this particular fruit, he will die. In other words, he will identify himself with his finite body-mind, forget the reality of his immortal nature, and experience fear of death. This is comparable to clinging to bodily life.

Just as all humans become heir to ignorance, the sin of Adam and Eve is considered the inheritance for all humanity. Whether we call it ignorance or original sin, we are talking about that which alienates us from the experience of the Self.

2.4. Ignorance is the field for the others mentioned after it, whether they be dormant, feeble, intercepted, or sustained.

Our daily experience of life suggests that there is a truckload of causes for suffering, but ultimately they are grounded in only one cause—*avidya*, "ignorance." All the other klesas are born from ignorance of our True Identity.

Dormant

A dormant klesa has not yet found circumstances favorable for its manifestation. We see an example of this in a baby whose environment (including its young age) is not conducive to the expression of the foibles we see manifest in adults. The klesas are still there but not yet fully active. Another form of dormant klesas can be seen in advanced yogis, in whom the force of years of dedicated practice (in some cases, along with a controlled yogic environment) can submerge a klesa into dormancy.

Feeble

After years of sadhana, the klesas' hold on the advanced yogi is weakened.

Intercepted

This level represents the effort to control the klesas by Yoga practices.

Sustained

In this state, all the klesas are operating unhindered. This is what we see in people whose approach to life is centered on distraction and diversion rather than introspection.

This sutra is a reminder of the importance of environment. There is a wise adage: "Environment is stronger than will." Seeds will only sprout when all the needed conditions exist. The proper environment exerts a powerful influence that will help move the klesas from sustained, to intercepted, to feeble, and then to dormant.

2.5. Ignorance is regarding the impermanent as permanent, the impure as pure, the painful as pleasant, and the non-Self as the Self.

Spiritual ignorance is the result of projecting attributes of the infinite Self onto that which is finite in nature.

Magicians use misdirection to fool our senses and amaze us. In life, misdirection comes in such forms as name, fame, romance, beauty, youth, and financial security. These goals are harmless if we remember they are limited and cannot bring permanent joy. They become harmful when we treat them as sources of unshakable happiness.

In order to rid ourselves of ignorance, we need to be able to recognize its manifestations. With this sutra to guide us, we will be able to identify the signs of ignorance as they appear in our lives.

The Impermanent as Permanent

Though we know that everything in Nature changes due to passage of time and the influence of circumstance, we tend to feel that good situations will continue and that painful ones will never end. The boring lecture, the difficult financial times, or the budding romance can all seem as if they will last forever. When we catch ourselves with these thoughts, we know we have slipped into the grasp of ignorance. The impermanence of worldly experiences quietly waits to sting us, often when we least expect it. The only permanent, unchanging reality is the Purusha.

The Impure as Pure

The second manifestation of ignorance is mistaking the impure as pure. "Pure" here does not imply a moral judgment. The word is used in the sense of "not mixed or adulterated with any substance." The Purusha is not composed of, limited, or affected by any elements and does not evolve. Only compounded elements change; therefore, whatever undergoes change cannot be the Purusha.

This sutra can also remind us to beware of the pitfall of worshipping "false gods." It is reminiscent of the "idols" mentioned in the Bible: *"Do not make or worship idols, for I am the Lord your God"* (Leviticus 19.3). Time and again people deify fame, power, and money, looking to them for solace and peace. Yet all these attainments are destined to change. When we find ourselves idolizing limited goals, we can be sure that ignorance is expressing itself.

The Painful as Pleasant

We often mistake painful experiences for pleasant ones. In order to discern the difference, we need to remember the lessons of experience. Many painful experiences begin pleasantly, only to cause us pain later. We forget that the pleasure we get from them is not permanent. We may not be able to detect at what point the secure job, supportive relationship, or rich, tasty supper began its metamorphosis into unemployment, divorce, or indigestion. We are set up to repeat the same unsettling experiences. We forget that some questionable choices contributed to the unwelcome changes, or we fail to notice that we have depended on transitory circumstances to be unwavering and inexhaustible sources of satisfaction.

How can we avoid mistaking the painful for pleasurable? The first time we saw a flame, we got burned, because the flame intrigued and attracted us. The finger went in and was quickly withdrawn, carrying pain with it. The next time we saw a flame, maybe it looked a little different, perhaps calmly flickering atop a nice candle. So quiet and pretty. But it still burned our finger. In an effort to avoid future pain, we begin to practice Yoga. But a little spiritual knowledge does not make us immune to being fooled. This time the flame attains holy status in our eyes by being enthroned on an altar. The flame now represents God. But a flame is still a flame, and we get burned if our finger wanders over to it. How many times do we need to get burned before we know the nature of fire? The answer can be a little discomforting: only when we have suffered enough. We drop a hot pot when the pain of the heat is greater than our desire to hold the pot—not a moment before. However, this sutra suggests that we can use our intellect to help shorten this painful process by remembering and examining both the short- and long-term effects of our experiences.

This sutra is not meant to imply that painful experiences invariably bring benefit or that pleasurable ones are gateways to suffering. It is a reminder that the true and lasting impact of any occurrence cannot necessarily be assessed from our initial reaction to it. Experiences are not, therefore, valued because of their initial pleasurable or painful impacts but by whether or not they lead to the lessening of ignorance and the revelation of the Self.

The Non-Self as the Self

This not only sums up the characteristics of ignorance but serves as a call to return to our spiritual home. What word is more personal than "self?" Our mistaken perceptions cause us to live estranged from our own Self. We wander through lifetimes, searching for that which will bring us permanent peace, forgetting that the Self is *"nearer to us than anything else, is indeed dearer than a son, dearer than wealth, dearer than all beside"* (Brihadaranyaka Upanishad).

This sutra can also serve as a reminder that experiencing the changeless, eternal, unborn, and undying Absolute is our ultimate destiny. No spiritual philosophy or theology is fulfilled until the individual realizes the Absolute Self as her/his True Identity.

Ignorance may seem like an unassailable fortress imprisoning the Self. Yet, as the above quotes from the Upanishads suggest, the Self is really the most immediate of all realities. Whenever you perceive something as beautiful, remind yourself that on some intuitive level you are recognizing the presence of the Self. The perception of something as beautiful requires the recognition of unity or harmony in an object, person, or action. Inherent in the appreciation or enjoyment of a painting, piece of music, sunset, poem, a kind act, or the physical appearance of another is the perception that the various aspects of the object are connected, have relationship, and work together for a purpose. No one perceives beauty where he or she sees dissonance or chaos. To see beauty is to see unity. To perceive unity is to sense the presence of the Absolute.

The Self is the unifying reality behind all manifestations in creation. It is the ultimate point of harmony where all things converge and come to rest.

A sign that ignorance is losing its influence on us is when our habitual identification with externals—possessions and attainments—begins to diminish. We begin to realize that we are not greater if we have them or less if we lose them. Our True Identity, the Self, is beyond all these conditions.

2.6. Egoism is the identification, as it were, of the power of the Seer (Purusha) with that of the instrument of seeing.

Egoism, the firstborn of ignorance, is a case of mistaken identity. It is the confusion of the instrument of seeing, the chitta (individual consciousness) and the sense organs, with awareness itself. As an analogy, think what might happen if we, the driver, identified with the instrument of driving, our car; if we actually thought we were our car. When the car was new, we would believe ourselves to be young and beautiful. And when it aged, becoming a cantankerous unreliable jalopy, we would believe that we were becoming frail and crabby. Of course, we don't make that mistake; it's not difficult to discern that the car is not us but an instrument we use. However, the confusion between the instrument of perception and the Seer presents a difficult test, because this misidentification is deeply hypnotic, persistent, and pervasive.

> The Self will always be falsely represented by the ego until our ignorance is removed. I often refer to these two "I"s as the little "i" and the capital "I." What is the difference? Just a small dot, a little blemish of ego. The capital "I" is just one pure stroke, just as the highest truth is always simple and pure. . . . Without the dot we are always great, always the capital "I." All the practices of Yoga are just to remove that dot.
>
> Sri Swami Satchidananda

Related Sutra: 2.20: "The Seer is nothing but the power of seeing which, although pure, appears to see through the mind."

2.7. Attachment is that which follows identification with pleasurable experiences.

The "that" in this sutra is craving.

Attachments are limitations that always result in deepening or maintaining ignorance (avidya). They are cravings that deny the peace and joy of our Self by insisting that outside experiences are the root of happiness.

The series of events that leads to attachment begins innocently: we engage in an activity or obtain an object and find pleasure in it. Identifying that activity or object as a source of happiness, we crave to repeat it. In fact, we often reason that if a little of the experience is nice, more would be better. Having conferred on pleasurable experiences the power to bring happiness, we expend time, energy, and resources looking to gain and retain happiness through them. It takes a long time to realize that this approach doesn't really lead to anything permanently satisfying.

Related Sutras: 1.15 and 1.16: The sutras that define nonattachment.

2.8. Aversion is that which follows identification with painful experiences.

Aversion is attachment in reverse. It is the effort to avoid objects or events that we perceive—or fear—will make us unhappy.

We experience some of life's occurrences as relatively neutral; they usually slip from our conscious memory. Other experiences are either sufficiently pleasurable or painful to be prominently placed in our storehouse of past impressions. Since our overriding motivation is to be happy, we tend to run after that which feels good and avoid that which is unpleasant. This two-sided coin of motivation lies behind most all our decisions in life.

On some level, it doesn't really sound like a bad strategy for living life. Who wants to be in pain? Who relishes suffering? It may sound reasonable, but there are a couple of problems with this approach to living life.

It overlooks or underestimates the value of principles. Just because something feels good doesn't mean it is right. It could be harmful to others or us—either now or later.

> The good is one thing; the pleasant another. These two, differing in their ends, both prompt to action.... The wise, having examined both, distinguish one from the other. The wise prefer the good to the pleasant.
>
> Katha Upanishad, 2.1

It's dangerous to adhere to a philosophy of life based on what *feels* right at the moment. This belief system contains the seed of disregard for others' welfare. This nasty seed could sprout at any moment, given the appropriate circumstances. Under the influence of an "if it feels good, it must be right" philosophy we may avoid situations that foster the welfare and well-being of others because they seem too challenging or hold the potential for personal loss.

Also, living life based on the "run *to* pleasure and *from* pain" principle doesn't take into account the vast number of factors that cannot be controlled or anticipated. In order for me to make choices that will unerringly steer me away from discomfort, I need to know the outcome of all actions and all the implications for everyone involved. It requires an absolute certainty about the future and the implications of all facets of an act or event. No one can sanely live in this way.

2.9. Clinging to life, flowing by its own potency (due to past experience), exists even in the wise.

"Clinging to life" conjures images of hanging on the edge of a cliff by our fingertips or a child desperately clutching its mother for safety.

Clinging to life, *abhinivesah*, is the desire for continuity of bodily existence. In examining this obstacle, let's begin by looking at the body's biological instinct to preserve itself.

Our bodies have built-in protective instincts: broken bones mend, our immune system fights infections, our eyes snap shut when dust blows their way, and our hands instinctively reach out to break a fall. This is the same survival instinct we see in a flower that bends toward sunlight for warmth or a tree whose roots grow around boulders in search of moisture. While it is true that Nature expends tremendous resources to preserve life, instinctual acts of self-preservation taken by themselves don't constitute the "clinging" spoken of in this sutra. Clinging requires attachment—an emotional dependence caused by:

- The fear of annihilation
- The habit of depending on self-effort to sustain our lives
- Relying on sense experiences for happiness
- Past-life recollections of dying

Fear of Annihilation

Although fear of the unknown is terrifying, there exists another, more dreadful prospect: the fear of annihilation. We fear ceasing to exist. However, if we look a little closer at this formidable fear, we see that it is not exactly as it appears. What we actually fear is *being aware* of an eternity of nonexistence. Of course, that means we are not truly annihilated, but this is how the mind tends to conceive of death without an afterlife.

Fear of annihilation persists in part because most of us have never experienced (or, more precisely, do not remember experiencing) other, more subtle modes of existence that exist beyond the body-mind and the physical world.

Self-Effort

While cooperating with the body's instinct for survival by eating a good diet, exercising, reducing stress, and having regular medical care is good and reasonable, we get in the habit of thinking that survival depends on self-effort alone. This self-centered attitude pushes us beyond the body's biological impulse for self-preservation into a craving for the continuation of physical life that is at once sentimental and passionate.

Sense Experience

What is it about this material universe that captivates us so?

We are mesmerized by the distractions and attractions of the world and become reluctant to vacate the premises. We cling to this playhouse of life because we have come to recognize sense experiences as the only apparent gateways to happiness. Indeed, there is an addictive quality to the sensory pleasures of the world. It's difficult to abandon this misdirected search for happiness even though we have been burned many times before. The irony is that although it is our nature to seek joy, we learn to settle for little bits of pleasure instead.

Now let's examine the cyclical nature of this clinging.

Past-Life Recollections of Dying

"Flowing by its own potency," in this sutra is a reference to reincarnation. It means that clinging to life exists and persists due to our past experiences with dying. We fear the process of dying because we have already experienced the pain that separating from life can bring—pain that is the result of being taken away from the things and people to which we cling for happiness. It is the pain of being separated from our attachments.

When we leave this earthly arena, the pain passes, and we experience life in a subtler body and on another plane of existence. When our time there runs out, we cling to *that* life, only to be reborn here. Once again we are separated from an existence to which we have become attached.

In truth, death is not to be feared at all. It's a natural and safe transformation that continues our spiritual journey toward Self-realization. Freed from the limitations of the body, the soul gains wonderful perspectives on life.

Yet clinging to life runs so deeply that it exists even in the wise. Studying scriptures and philosophy is not enough to eliminate it. Only light can remove the darkness. Only the experience that comes from Self-realization can completely erase this fear. When we attain realization of our True Identity as Purusha, we will know that we exist on a level beyond matter and beyond the transitory comings and goings of all things physical.

Now let's look at this sutra from a different viewpoint. Consider that instead of clinging to bodily life, we cling to a familiar lifestyle. In this sense we could understand this sutra as a way of helping us to prepare for the dramatic changes that our lives will undergo, by adhering to the principles of the eight limbs that will be introduced in sutra 2.29. Change, even if it is beneficial, can be stressful. Yogis need to be prepared to let go of any conceptions of who they are and what life is about. They need to be primed for the transformation that results from the yogic life. They are like snakes constantly shedding their skins, being reborn as new and better beings.

2.10. In their subtle form, these obstacles can be destroyed by resolving them back into their original cause (the ego).

The "subtle form" referred to here are the "dormant" and "feeble" stages (*see sutra* 2.4) of the obstacles mentioned in sutra 2.3. Dormant and feeble refer to activities of the obstacles that are too fine to be clearly identified by the intellect or that exist on the subconscious level as samskaras.

Resolving the obstacles to their original cause refers to the experience of Self-realization in which the mind is transcended and ignorance eradicated. Since ignorance gave birth to the obstacles and sustains them, when it is dispelled by the light of the Self, the obstacles can no longer exist.

2.11. In the active state, they can be destroyed by meditation.

Obstacles in the active state are referred to in sutra 2.4 as "intercepted" and "sustained": those obstructions that have noticeable presence and impact on the conscious mind. Meditation (dhyana) averts awareness away from the obstacles, which will gradually wither from lack of attention.

Related Sutra: 1.29: *Examines a parallel idea; referring to mantra repetition, it states: "From this practice, the awareness turns inward, and the distracting obstacles vanish."*

2.12. The womb of karmas has its roots in these obstacles, and the karmas bring experiences in the seen (present) or in the unseen (future) births.

"What goes around comes around." Karma is the universal law of cause and effect; action and reaction. Actions and experiences are linked. This principle is also found in the Bible: "*Do not be deceived. God cannot be ignored. A man reaps what he sows*" (Galatians 6.7). Our thoughts, words, and deeds determine our experience in life.

As a central tenet in Hindu thought, karma was probably as familiar to Sri Patanjali's students as the concept of sin is for those in a Judeo-Christian-influenced society. They most likely learned that karma is the universal law of cause and effect and understood that their karma binds them by embroiling them in the world of relative, material existence. The relentless cycles of action and reaction would also be recognized as the cause of reincarnation. However, the notion that karma is rooted in the obstacles, which are in turn grounded in ignorance—that karma cannot operate without ignorance—might have been unsettling or perhaps a revelation. It meant that they couldn't blame an impersonal, immeasurable, cosmic payback system—or anyone else for that matter—for their bad luck or suffering. They confronted then what we confront now: that all experiences of pleasure and pain are and have always been in our own hands (*see sutra* 2.14, "*The karmas bear fruits of pleasure and pain caused by merit and demerit*"). Though this information may clarify the "what and how" of karma, it does not explain the "why."

Karma is the cosmic law that makes learning possible. Every encounter with a piece of information is a cause that has an effect on our lives. The law of cause and effect allows us to learn from our experiences: Rain falls (cause); seeds sprout (effect), certain herbs lower blood pressure; deep, regulated breathing calms the mind; too much cheesecake causes a stomachache; stress causes a headache. Knowledge is the result of observing relationships—the impact that objects, circumstances, and actions make on each other. Karma is the cosmic mechanism that God instituted to teach us. Its ultimate aim is to guide us to enlightenment.

PADA TWO

Related Sutras: 1.24: "Ishwara is the supreme Purusha, unaffected by any…actions, fruits of actions…" and 3.23, 4.6–4.9, 4.30: For more details regarding the nature of karma. (Also see Karma in the Glossary and in the Sutras-by-Subject Index.)

2.13. With the existence of the root, there will also be fruits: the births of different species of life, their life spans, and experiences.

This sutra expands on the previous one.

The Root

Ignorance gives birth to egoism, the limited "I." The birth of the ego creates a metaphysical "big bang." First "I" comes into being. That "I" has to be somewhere. The only place "I" can be is *here*. When *here* appears, *there* surfaces. A cascade of dualities follows: *you, it, up, down, in, out, good, bad*, and so on. The appearance of the entire universe rests on the existence of "I."

The Fruits: Births of Different Species of Life, Life Spans, and Experiences

Our past thoughts, words, and deeds have produced who we are now. What we do now determines who we will be tomorrow. Karma determines whether we will be male or female, rich or poor, a genius or dull-witted—even whether we will be in a human form. It also determines the lengths of our lives and the experiences that come to us.

This does not mean that we have no control over what happens in our lives. Our choices create new karmas all the time. The future is rooted in our present thoughts, words, and deeds and exists as a universe of infinite possibilities.

2.14. The karmas bear fruits of pleasure and pain caused by merit and demerit.

This sutra expands on the last word of the previous one—experiences. The nature of the experiences we will someday have: our successes and failures, the obstacles and unexpected blessings we will encounter, the friends and foes, and how much we might suffer or rejoice are all contained in that simple word.

Meritorious acts bring pleasurable experiences; negative acts bring painful ones. Therefore what we experience is based on our own past actions—in this life or a past one. Meritorious acts include those based on the moral and ethical principles of yama and niyama and the "four locks and four keys" (*see sutras* 2.29 *and* 1.33).

The next sutra takes us beyond the daily concerns of pleasure and pain.

2.15. To one of discrimination, everything is painful indeed, due to its consequences: the anxiety and fear over losing what is gained; the resulting impressions left in the mind to create renewed cravings; and the conflict among the activities of the gunas, which control the mind.

This sutra explains the inner workings of disappointment, longing, and suffering. It presents essentially the same message as the first two of Lord Buddha's Four Noble Truths: in life, suffering is inevitable; and second, there is a cause for that suffering. (Looking ahead, the next sutra is similar to the third of the Four Noble Truths: there is a way out of that suffering; and in this Pada, sutra 2.26 presents discriminative discernment as the way to remove ignorance.)

Use of the word "discrimination" in this sutra might lead us to misinterpret this sutra to mean that there is an inverse relationship between one's discriminative capacity and happiness. In other words, the more refined our perceptions become, the less happy we will be. This sutra does not reject the joys of life. Instead, the insight that "everything is painful" comes to those whose concerns (ambitions, focus, and objectives) have risen above the search for transitory pleasure and the avoidance of pain. Their interest has made a radical shift in favor of the search for *permanent* fulfillment. It is as if they had been on a long journey and now wish for nothing more—can think of nothing more inviting—than their own home.

Most of us have had the experience of travel. Even in the midst of exotic locales and wonderful diversions, there were times when all we wanted was to go home. We missed the security, familiarity, and even the routine. Home is where our loved ones reside, where symbols of what is important to us fill the rooms. Disney World, Atlantic City, Rome, and the pyramids of Egypt are all wonderful places to visit, but they sink to second place when the longing to return home arises.

At some point in the spiritual journey, long-lost memories begin to stir, inspiring what amounts to almost a restlessness. Desires for worldly pleasures are replaced by a longing to return to our spiritual home, to rest in our own Self. The diversions of the world are fine, but they are not enough to satisfy us anymore; they simply cannot fulfill our yearning to return home. In the presence of that yearning, what we once experienced as pleasures are now perceived as distractions, delays in going home. It is in this context that everything becomes painful to one of discrimination.

And why is it that "everything" is painful?

The Anxiety and Fear over Losing What Is Gained

In life there are no guarantees (other than the disease, old age, and death that Lord Buddha warned are inevitable). Even if our ambition and hard work earn us a coveted material possession or a position of power or status, we know that there are many ways it could be snatched from us. Gain often comes with a high price tag: our peace, our health, our relationships. We mistakenly believe that worldly gains will bring lasting fulfillment. An unbiased assessment of life reveals that although our attainments may have brought temporary satisfaction, they were accompanied by the inevitable fears of the possibility (in fact, the inevitability) of loss.

Many years ago, a friend of mine coveted a particular model of sports car. In his dreams, it was jet black with a pure white interior. He worked long and hard delivering stationery supplies to save enough for this pricey item.

When he had finally saved enough, he was dismayed when the dealer informed him that there was only one black model in the world and it was the property of the owner of the company. In deference to the owner, they didn't produce any others like that. Undeterred from his dream, he bought a white version with a white interior.

The day he picked up his treasure, he drove straight from the dealer's lot to an upscale auto body shop. There, they completely disassembled the body, sanded off the paint to the bare metal and, in a multilayered extravaganza, painted it glossy jet black. It was a makeover that took four weeks.

A few days after receiving his newly painted, only-the-second-one-in-the-world version of the sports car, he came to my house to pick me up. I looked forward to seeing his flashy new car. It was raining heavily as he pulled up in front of my house and honked his horn. I rushed down, clutching an umbrella against the driving rain and strong wind. I opened the door and was about to speak words of congratulations, when he looked up and said, in a deadpan delivery, "Take off your shoes."

"What!"

"Take off you shoes before you get in."

I could see his resolve was Gibraltar-like. Folding my umbrella, I fumbled off my shoes and sank into the tiny leather seat. I made the trip with him, gingerly holding cold, wet shoes in my hands.

Now, this is the question: Was he enjoying his new car? Don't his actions remind you of anxiety and fear over losing what is gained? He feared losing his new car's clean white perfection. Due to his attachment, the car, instead of being a source of joy, made him uneasy. It became a source of stress. What joy he might have felt was diminished by anxiety.

The Resulting Impressions Left in the Mind to Create Renewed Cravings

It is our common experience that cravings often follow pleasurable experiences. There was a potato chip company that made a fortune selling its chips with the slogan, "Bet you can't eat just one." Pleasurable experiences cry out for repeat performances: one chip won't do the trick. Not only that, but memory of the enjoyable snack will return as a craving to duplicate the experience. If I believe that the chips made me happy, a subconscious impression is formed linking the chips to an experience of happiness. That is why simply fulfilling desires can never eliminate them.

The same subtle mechanism exists for painful experiences. The only difference is that the craving expresses as a desire to stay away from the painful situations.

The Conflict among the Activities of the Gunas, Which Control the Mind

Like a lawyer, Sri Patanjali closes the last loophole. There is no way out of this clause. Even if there is no anxiety over losing what we have gained, and no renewed cravings, our mind is still a part of nature and is bound to change. Sometimes, even before the outside circumstance changes, our mind may change. We become bored, restless, or suspicious—the mind simply changes. We may not fret much about keeping our new car perfect, but after a while, it may no longer provide the rush of pleasure it did when we first brought it home. Maybe now our mind turns toward upgrading our TV—a craving for something more lavish: a big-screen, surround-sound, home theater system.

The mind changes because of the constant interplay of the three gunas, with one temporarily dominating for a while and then giving way to another. That is why there can be no security, no lasting comfort gained by merely feeding the senses. The fourteenth chapter of the Bhagavad Gita presents a clear description of the gunas and their impact on the mind. Here are relevant verses:

> Sattwa binds you to happiness; rajas binds you to compulsive behavior; and tamas, by veiling your mind, binds you to confused thinking and bad judgment. Sometimes, Arjuna, sattwa arises above rajas and tamas and predominates. Sometimes, rajas is above sattwa and tamas, and tamas sometimes is above sattwa and rajas. When the light of wisdom shines through all the gates of the body, this is a sign that sattwa is dominant. Whenever you see greedy behavior, restlessness, or continuous thirsting after one thing or another, Arjuna, these are signs that rajas is dominant. And when tamas is dominant, ignorance, sloth, and indiscriminant thinking arise.
>
> Bhagavad Gita, 14.9–14.13

Related Sutras: 2.18 and 2.19: Expands on the nature of the gunas.

2.16. Pain that has not yet come is avoidable.

A note of hope after what might be experienced as a somewhat pessimistic sutra. If pain is avoidable, it means that there is something we can do to create a better fate for ourselves. The choices we make in life determine our experiences of happiness or suffering.

Related Sutra: 2.14: Examines the connection between karma and pain.

2.17. The cause of that avoidable pain is the union of the Seer (Purusha) and seen (Prakriti).

It might seem paradoxical that Sri Patanjali cites "the union of the Seer and seen" as the cause of pain. After all, isn't union—Yoga—what we're seeking? This sutra seems to suggest that Oneness, instead of bringing the end of ignorance and pain, is the cause of suffering.

It might be clearer if we replace the word "union" with "confusion." *Samyoga*, translated as union, also signifies "correlation or connection." In this context, it represents the fundamental inappropriate or false correlation: mistaking the mind-stuff, which is part of Prakriti, for the Seer. If we believe that we are the mind, we tend to make choices that serve its whims, fears, and habits. We look to sense objects—the "seen"—to bring security, happiness, and wisdom, to give us what they cannot. This mistaken approach to life is the cause of pain and is rooted in ignorance (avidya).

Related Sutras: 2.5: "Ignorance is regarding the impermanent as permanent, the impure as pure, the painful as pleasant, and the non-self as the Self"; 2.24: "The cause of this union is ignorance."

2.18. The seen is of the nature of the gunas: illumination, activity, and inertia. It consists of the elements and sense organs, whose purpose is to provide both experiences and liberation to the Purusha.

The "seen" is Nature or Prakriti (from the verb root, *kr*, "to make or do," and *pra*, forth," "to bring forth"). As the stuff of creation, it is the source of everything that becomes an object of perception for the Self.

The phrase that ends this sutra offers an answer to a question that has intrigued humanity from time immemorial: What is the purpose of life? Our lives are played out on the material stage of the universe. Why should it be so? Why have we been put here? Are all the good and bad times, choices, accidents, successes, and failures in our lives leading us to a goal? Or is life a random series of events, with our free will battling to create comfort, security, and joy from chaos?

For the yogi, each and every event, whether marvelous or difficult to bear, is filled with meaning. Everything that happens is for the purpose of giving experiences to the Purusha. Or, more correctly, the experiences are for the mind, since the Purusha is by nature free. All Yoga theories and practices are for the sake of liberating the individual from the limitations of the ego and the obscuring power of ignorance.

The "experiences" mentioned in this sutra are learning experiences. They are the spiritual lessons that help turn our attention to the Self. There are two main ways we learn from Nature:

- Nature teaches us by exposing its limitations. In this sense, Nature is like a playpen which limits the movement of the child while he plays with his toys. Sooner or later the child tires of the toys and the restriction of the playpen. He turns to the only one who can help—the one who put him there in the first place—his mama. He cries out loud, and the mama drops whatever she is doing and rushes to the side of her baby. Likewise, the transitory nature of worldly pleasures becomes tiresome sooner or later.
- Another way we can learn from Nature is that God cannot help but leave "fingerprints" all over creation. Every aspect of Nature reveals a bit of the Creator's presence to a mind with a receptive, contemplative disposition. From observation of Nature we can find examples of qualities such as strength, patience, caring, selflessness, order, and perseverance that eloquently speak to the existence of a Divine Intelligence.

All of Nature is at our service; ready, willing, and able to teach us the way to liberation.

Related Sutra: 2.21: *"The seen exists only for the sake of the Seer."*

2.19. The stages of the gunas are specific, nonspecific, defined, and undifferentiated.

Sutra 2.17 stated that the cause of our pain is the confusion of the Seer and seen, implying that we cannot always discern the difference between the two. To aid in ending our confusion, we will examine Prakriti's evolution from unmanifest to manifest in four stages. These four stages are signposts that help us trace back our everyday experience of the solid, three-dimensional world we live in to the very doorstep of the Seer.

We will examine these stages from the subtle to the gross.

Undifferentiated

Pure latent Prakriti existing universally. This is unadulterated, undifferentiated matter without any names or forms. When creation begins, we come to the next stage...

Defined

The first product of Prakriti's evolution is the cosmic intelligence: buddhi (mahat). The gunas then begin to express their respective qualities. Next follow the first recognizable, though subtle, expressions of creation...

Nonspecific

The evolution into subtle senses and elements, including the individual's buddhi, ahamkara, and manas. Evolution continues toward the grossest stage. Matter becomes more compounded, finally manifesting as...

Specific

Gross objects; the things we see, feel, touch, smell, taste, and hear with our senses.

These four stages of Prakriti can help us understand the categories of samprajnata and dharmamegha samadhi (*see sutra 4.29 and Samadhi in the Sutras-by-Subject Index*). We find here the gross elements (*specific*) of the vitarka samadhis, the subtle elements, mind and ego-sense of the vichara samadhis (*nonspecific*), the gunas beginning to lose their hold on the practitioner in dharmamegha samadhi (*defined* and *undifferentiated*).

2.20. The Seer is nothing but the power of seeing which, although pure, appears to see through the mind.

The Seer is the power of seeing, awareness itself, consciousness, the Purusha, the Self.

The mind has no consciousness of its own. Its awareness is borrowed from the Seer. This can be compared to the sun's reflection in a mirror. The sun represents the Self; the mirror corresponds to the mind. The entire globe of the sun, though immeasurable in relation to a mirror, can be reflected in it. However, we cannot properly say that the sun is contained in the mirror. The sun is not limited nor its nature altered by being reflected. It remains untouched and pure.

Related Sutras: 4.18–4.25: Elaborate on the principle presented in this sutra.

2.21. The seen exists only for the sake of the Seer.

Using devotee's language, we might say that the purpose of creation—why life exists at all—is to serve the purpose of its Creator, which we know is the liberation of the individual (*see sutra* 2.18).

There is no simple, satisfying answer as to why life is this way. The response to this question lies outside the grasp of the mind. It is one of many spiritual puzzles, the solutions to which we will discover not by use of logic but by transcending ignorance.

2.22. Although destroyed for him who has attained liberation, it (the seen) exists for others, being common to them.

Objects enjoy an existence that does not rely on any individual's perception of them. The tree outside my window exists whether or not I perceive it, since any person walking by my home will experience the same tree. So this sutra is not talking about the destruction of the universe. It *is* describing a change in the realized yogi's relationship with the universe. Before liberation, Prakriti created a limitless storehouse of sense objects that the mind craved and that we mistakenly believed could bring happiness. With the attainment of liberation, Prakriti loses its central place in life, no longer holding the same relevance.

In short, before Self-realization; Nature is the center of our universe. We know it as a solid reality whose inviolable laws govern our lives. Meanwhile, the Self—what we intellectually believe to be the true center of existence—is experienced as an elusive dream. With liberation, the tables are turned: Nature is experienced as the dream, while the Self is the rock-solid reality.

2.23. The union of Owner (Purusha) and owned (Prakriti) causes the recognition of the nature and powers of them both.

In this sutra, Sri Patanjali substitutes the words "Owner" and "owned" for Seer and seen. This change of words suggests a purposefulness to the relationship.

The Purusha and Prakriti are allies in the phenomenon we experience as life. This alliance forms the foundation for acquiring knowledge. The fundamental consciousness that is the Purusha allows for the perception of objects to take place. And it is the ability of the mind to discern the changing nature of Prakriti that leads to gaining knowledge about and realization of the Purusha.

(See Purusha and Prakriti in the Sutras-by-Subject Index.)

2.24. The cause of this union is ignorance.

In the previous sutra, the union of Owner and owned sounded like a nice situation, a source of knowledge. And on the relative level, it is. But regardless of how much we learn about the universe and study the nature of the Self, as long as we remain ignorant of our True Identity, we are subject to suffering.

Sri Patanjali doesn't overtly deny that the universe is full of beauty to appreciate and wonders worth exploring. Yet we cannot ignore the fact that Nature remains bound by the limitations of its own laws. Sri Swami Vivekananda very eloquently expressed this in his poem, "Song of the Free":

> The beauteous earth, the glorious sun
> The calm sweet moon, the spangled sky,
> Causation's laws do make them run;
> They live in bonds, in bonds they die.

Until we attain liberation we, as part of Nature, are fettered as well.

2.25. Without this ignorance, no such union occurs. This is the independence of the Seer.

Yoga practices gradually remove ignorance. With the departure of ignorance, the alliance between Purusha and Prakriti ends and, along with it, the mistaken identification of self for Self. The cause of suffering is dismantled and we become liberated beings, *jivanmuktas.* (See sutra 4.34, which discusses this state in more detail).

The previous eleven sutras (2.15–2.25) presented an important, dynamic, and at times a seemingly paradoxical understanding of the

PADA TWO

relationship between the Purusha and Nature. It might prove helpful to review them.

After learning that everything is painful and that the pain can be avoided, we discover that the cause of pain is the union (confusion) of the Seer and seen. But the seen is not stereotyped as a villain. It is Nature expressing in different stages. Though our interaction with it does often result in painful experiences, it also serves to liberate the Purusha, whose nature is pure consciousness. Prakriti's alliance with the Purusha, though founded on ignorance, is the foundation for knowledge of them both.

When ignorance is erased, the purpose of the seen is ended. Now perceived in a radically new light, it ceases to exist (in the sense of not having any personal relevance) for the yogi. With the elimination of ignorance, the Seer is free. There is no more pain for a realized yogi.

2.26. Uninterrupted discriminative discernment is the method for its removal.

Discriminative discernment, viveka, is an innate faculty. In day-to-day life, we know it as the ability to discern the unique characteristics of an object or the distinctions between two or more objects. Ordinarily, our discriminative capacity is occupied with a constant stream of pertinent and nonpertinent thoughts: perceptions of objects, events, wishes, and people that flow into consciousness. But to pierce through ignorance, to perceive the Self as our True Identity, viveka requires a high order of clear, steady focus and the absence of selfish attachment. The more one-pointed our minds become, the more refined, subtle, and complete our ability to "see" becomes. As we continue with meditation, prayer, nonattachment and study, we will be developing not only nirodha but viveka as well.

Viveka is the shifting of awareness from the object of perception to the power of perception itself (Purusha). Ultimately it is pure consciousness knowing itself as distinct from any object or experience.

(See Viveka in the Sutras-by-Subject Index.)

Experience It

The practice of viveka includes recollecting the Truth behind appearances, searching for that which is changeless in that which changes. It is also learning to confront pain in a new way. When disturbed by negative emotions or physical pain, we can ask ourselves who or what it is that feels the pain. "Is it me or my lower back?" "Am I sad, or is it just my mind?" This kind of analysis refines viveka.

2.27. One's wisdom in the final stage is sevenfold.

The practice of viveka changes the way we perceive life. Our perception will reveal a different self and universe from those we knew before.

Sri Patanjali does not list the sevenfold wisdom, though the sage Vyasa (*see Glossary*) does in his commentary. Vyasa's addition, commented on below, is included in many translations.

Through the practice of viveka, what is to be avoided (the causes of suffering) is recognized. Therefore, there is nothing more to be known on this subject.

For students skillful in viveka, there are no lingering questions regarding how and where happiness will be found. The course has been examined, considered, and set. Now all that is left is the journey home.

The causes of suffering having been identified, they are progressively weakened.

This refers to the overcoming of attachments and aversions through the practice of discernment and analysis. When the craving to attain or to avoid anything begins its exit, we can be sure that ignorance is vanishing as well. (*See sutra 2.3, where attachment and aversion are introduced.*)

Through samadhi, the causes of suffering are eliminated. There is nothing more to be gained in this arca.

Samadhi arrests the causes of suffering. They no longer influence the yogi's perceptions.

This and the following stage foreshadow the benefits of dharmamegha samadhi, in which all afflictions and karmas cease (*see sutras 4.29 and 4.30*).

Mastery in viveka having been reached, there is nothing else self-effort can accomplish.

This is the end stage of practice. Self-effort can take the yogi no further. The causes of suffering have been identified, examined, understood, restrained, and then overcome through samadhi.

The following three stages are the natural outcome of the first four and can be regarded as a further explication of sutra 4.34, which describes the final state of independence: Self-realization.

Sattwa dominates the functioning of the mind-stuff.

Sattwa prevails when the ego subsides. It is illumination, clarity, joy, and peace. It is the reflection of the Purusha on the tranquil mind. (*See sutras 1.17, sananda samadhi, absorption on sattwa element; 3.36, the distinction between Purusha and sattwa; and 3.50, how making the distinction between sattwa and Purusha leads to omniscience.*)

The gunas, having fulfilled their purpose, lose their foothold like stones falling from a mountain peak and incline toward reabsorption into Prakriti.

The feeling of "doership" is no longer falsely attached to the Purusha. The activities of the buddhi become quiet, and the subconscious impression fall away. In essence, mental functioning comes to a standstill. Nirodha is perfected. (*See sutras 4.25 and 4.26, which describe the "pull" of the Absolute; also sutra 4.34, which describes the reabsorption of the gunas into Prakriti.*)

The Purusha is realized as independent from the gunas (constituents of nature).

The artificial limitations imposed by ignorance and the ego vanish.

2.28. By the practice of the limbs of Yoga, the impurities dwindle away and there dawns the light of wisdom leading to discriminative discernment.

Notice the sequence of events:

- The practices of the limbs of Yoga remove impurities. Yoga practices do not bring anything new; they remove what is unwanted or unnecessary.
- As the impurities dwindle, wisdom emerges, indicating that wisdom is already within. In this sutra, the light of wisdom (*jnanadipti*) refers to insights into spiritual truths. In terms of Yoga practice, wisdom allows for the ability to recognize the goal, set our course on the right track, and keep it there.
- Wisdom leads to viveka, which we saw in sutra 2.26 is the method for the removal of ignorance.

The next sutra expands and refines our understanding of what is meant by Yoga practice.

2.29. The eight limbs of Yoga are:
1. **yama – abstinence**
2. **niyama – observance**
3. **asana – posture**
4. **pranayama – breath control**
5. **pratyahara – sense withdrawal**
6. **dharana – concentration**
7. **dhyana – meditation**
8. **samadhi – contemplation, absorption, or superconscious state**

The eight limbs seamlessly integrate selfless, active participation in life with introspection and contemplation. This exquisite balance is designed to encourage self-knowledge, expand and transform consciousness and culminate in Self-realization.

Students familiar with the teachings of Buddhism may have detected principles of a Buddhistic nature being developed in the last fourteen sutras. It is interesting to compare the two.

Lord Buddha's Four Noble Truths:
Suffering is inevitable due to disease, old age, and death
Suffering arises from craving
Suffering ceases when attachment to cravings ceases
Freedom from suffering is possible by practicing the Eightfold Path

The Yoga Sutras:
Everything is painful due to fear of losing what is gained, renewed cravings, and the fluctuations of the gunas that control the mind (2.15)
The pain that has not yet come can be avoided (2.16)
The cause of the avoidable pain is the confusion of the Seer with the seen (2.17)
The cause of this union is ignorance (2.24)
Ignorance can be removed by viveka (2.26)
The practice of the eight limbs of Yoga brings viveka (2.28)

Both agree that if you are alive, you will face pain. They also agree that pain can be avoided. Where they differ is that Lord Buddha identifies cravings as the cause of pain, rather than ignorance. In the Buddhist model, when cravings cease, so does suffering. Sri Patanjali's emphasis is different. He identifies ignorance as the cause of suffering and viveka as the means to eliminate it. Of course, it is ignorance—the mistaking of the body-mind for the Self—that leads to cravings, and viveka needs a nonattached mind (a mind free from craving) in order to attain objectivity in discernment.

2.30. Yama consists of nonviolence, truthfulness, nonstealing, continence, and nongreed.

What attitudes precede the actions of the enlightened? Ones that are born of selfless motivations, wisdom, and love, that seek the welfare of everyone involved. These same attitudes—listed here as the yamas—are virtues that strengthen and purify the mind.

The principles of yama might not satisfy someone fond of a dos and don'ts list. They are more properly understood as preparations for actions—attitudes that bring clarity, focus, and objectivity to bear on all situations.

If we allow these principles to guide, cajole, and correct us, we will gradually know them well enough to call them friends. We will be privy to their nature, intent, power, and significance—their spirit. The yamas can be truly understood only when we perceive the spirit behind the "letter of the law."

Nonviolence (Ahimsa)

Nonviolence is supreme among all the yamas, never to be violated. It is to be applied to human beings, animals, and so-called inanimate objects.

Violence is a reaction to fear—a key symptom of the dominance that egoism and ignorance have over the mind. Violence is not defined by any particular destructive act but by the *desire* to see another harmed. That is why nonviolence includes refraining from harm in thought as well as in word and deed. To avoid doing harm while harboring hateful or spiteful thoughts does not satisfy the spirit of ahimsa. Consider the following example.

Imagine there is a rooftop sniper shooting at innocent citizens below. Negotiators are unsuccessful in their attempts to talk him down, but he must be stopped because he is endangering lives. A police sharpshooter is called to the scene. He shoots the sniper in the leg and puts him out of commission. The question is: Did the sharpshooter violate the principle of ahimsa?

Our instinctive response might be "yes"; but from this account, we cannot know for certain. He did shoot the sniper, and ahimsa teaches us to refrain from harming others. But the yogic perspective is more interested in the motivation than the action. If the sharpshooter held hateful thoughts regarding the sniper, it was a violent act. But would our assessment differ if he had neutral thoughts, only thoughts of doing his duty? Or if his only motivation was to protect others? In these cases, the sharpshooter would be following ahimsa even while shooting the sniper. Meanwhile, onlookers not involved in any action but harboring hateful, destructive thoughts would have violated the spirit of ahimsa. This example demonstrates one reason why it is so very difficult to judge the actions of others; we are seldom privy to their intent or motivation.

In considering ahimsa (and the other yamas), does the end justify the means? The results of our acts have an impact on our lives and the lives of others, so they do count. But even when an action brings benefit to others, *we* lose, because any act based on violent intent sinks us deeper into ignorance. And since repetition makes habit, every violent act helps create and maintain a streak of violence in us. Anger-based violence may seem to be an instinctive motivator—it certainly is common enough—but it is unnecessary. To do what is right and good, to act in a way that fosters well-being and harmony, should be motivation enough. Yogis' actions should bring no harm to anybody, including themselves, and benefit to somebody.

Perfecting nonviolence requires patience, courage, strength, faith, and deep understanding. That is why simply practicing this one precept, even if no other spiritual exercises are practiced, is highly valued.

Truthfulness (Satya)

When examining truthfulness, we again need to consider subtle implications.

Truthful in all ways. Truthfulness should be observed in thought, word, and deed.

We normally understand truthfulness to mean that our words should correlate to our actions and thoughts. This is a good foundation for understanding truthfulness, but it is not complete. First we need to test truth against nonviolence.

Truthfulness measured against nonviolence. Ahimsa is the first yama Sri Patanjali lists and so is the touchstone for determining behavior. Even truthful words, if they cause harm to another, should not be spoken. However, before giving up our course of action, we could consider if there is a more auspicious moment for doing what is needed, or a more appropriate approach. In any case, it is always advisable to do some soul-searching to determine if the desire to act is motivated by an interest in the welfare of others or by a need to vent our frustrations or punish someone with whom we have problems. Motives that are tainted by selfishness obstruct the experience of the Self by maintaining or strengthening the influence of ignorance over the mind.

How can we tell if we are doing harm or just causing temporary discomfort? First, we need to discriminate between the two. Discomfort indicates the struggle of the individual to adapt and adjust. To do harm is to destroy or inhibit proper functioning.

We know that there are times (such as when teachers discipline misbehaving students) when words can cause pain but the intent ultimately brings benefit. The opposite is also true. There are times when people use sweet words (as in con games) in order to deceive others. Their behavior may feel good at first but will cause harm later.

We may not experience the consequences of our actions until much later. If we do not know the nature of the tree, we need to wait until it bears fruit. In order to perfect truthfulness, yogis need patience to observe the ultimate outcome of acts, clarity to make the proper assessment of their outcome, and accurate recall not to forget the lessons of experience. Fortunately, patience, clarity, and good memory are also products of the Yoga practices.

A deeper look at truthfulness. Yogis should strictly adhere to all the principles of yama (*see sutra 2.31, in which the yamas are referred to as* "Great Vows"). Yet consider this from the Thirukkural, a scripture of South India: "*Even a falsehood is treated as truth if it brings no harm to anyone and some benefit to someone*" (Kural 292). This quote might make us a little uncomfortable at first. It seems to allow the use of falsehoods for the sake of expediency. In a seeming paradox, the same scripture praises the absence of falsehoods: *"No prestige surpasses the absence of falsehood; all other virtues flow from it effortlessly"* (Kural 296). Can we reconcile the two?

The ultimate intent behind following any virtue is to bring harmony to the individual and to his or her environment. Violence is the ultimate weapon of disharmony. It strengthens ignorance and divides people from each other and their environment. That is the reason why all virtues are tested against ahimsa. Therefore, if our words foster a new or deeper harmony (expressing as peace, joy, love, accord, cooperation) without harming anyone, they are words that not only uphold nonviolence but reflect the intent of all virtues. But as was said before, it is essential to discern if our words and actions are bringing harm or harmony.

Nonstealing (Asteya)

Most of us would never rob a bank or hold up a convenience store. For most people stealing is more subtle. It is often preceded by a sense of unfairness and lack and exists against a background of looking to externals for happiness.

Many people expend a great deal of time and energy focused on what others have. They can become jealous, restless, and unhappy, rationalizing that it is unfair for some to live in luxury while they dwell in modest apartments. They work hard and consider themselves to be decent people but feel that they have been cheated by life. So, taking matters in their own hands, they attempt to make matters more "equitable." They think it is okay to steal a little. Maybe it's on their income tax returns, or taking a modest amount of supplies from the office, padding their time sheet, or extending their break time every day. It is still stealing and it unfailingly sinks them deeper into ignorance.

One day, we will realize that God has attended to every minute detail and given us exactly what we need at each moment to grow. At that point, we will not feel lack but abundance. Lord Jesus taught, *"I have come that you may have life and have it in abundance"* (John 10.10). He was not talking about having more things, but that most sought-after of possessions: complete satisfaction, utter fulfillment, the absence of want.

One of the most subtle forms of stealing comes when we steal ideas from others. Though this could take the form of outright plagiarism, it more often assumes the more benign character of improperly (often subtly) accepting credit for someone else's ideas to advance our career or status among our peers. The difficulty with this is not only that we may deprive others of the recognition they deserve, but that we perpetuate an unconscious expectation that receiving acknowledgments can treat a sagging self-image. We become attached to acknowledgment, thinking it will make us happy.

It's helpful to remember that to some degree, all of our ideas are stimulated by the teachers, authors, musicians, role models, and others who serve as inspirations in our lives. Both inwardly and outwardly, it is appropriate to give credit where credit is due. In the end, the ultimate credit should go to God, the giver not only of our sources of inspiration but of our intelligence, strength, and abilities as well.

Continence (Brahmacharya)

Spiritual pursuits make significant demands on time, attention, and energy. In Yoga, as in almost any other worthwhile endeavor, the only way to ensure success is to dedicate our resources to the goals we have set before us. That is why continence, the avoidance of non-productive expenditures of energy, has always held a central position in Yoga practice.

Each and every act and thought is an outflow of energy. Some thoughts and actions offer beneficial dividends, while others simply drain our resources. In the name of continence, we are asked to be wise investors.

A common rendering of brahmacharya, the word translated as continence, is celibacy, an interpretation that may be a little misleading. While brahmacharya includes sexual continence, it has a broader connotation. Translated literally, brahmacharya is "path to Brahman." Brahman means "greater than the greatest," and is often translated as Absolute Reality or God. For our purposes, it is the same reality as the Purusha. In practice, brahmacharya means to expend our energy on activities that are conducive to the attainment of Self-realization. Therefore it is misleading to limit it to celibacy. Too much (or too little) talking breaks this vow, as do extremes in eating, sleeping, working, and so on. This same principle is expounded in the Bhagavad Gita, 6.16 and 6.17:

It is impossible to practice Yoga effectively if you eat or sleep either too much or too little. But if you are moderate in eating, playing, sleeping, staying awake, and avoiding extremes in everything you do, you will see that these Yoga practices eliminate all your pain and suffering.

How did celibacy come to be almost a synonym for brahmacharya? Ancient yogis studied various categories of activities and realized that of all of them, the sex act uses the most energy. Yogic tradition states that it takes sixty morsels of food to make one drop of blood and sixty drops of blood to make one drop of semen. This underscores how concentrated and powerful sexual energy is and the importance of using it properly. In women, the sex act also involves expenditure of energy, but not as much as in men. For them, childbirth is the great spender of vital energy. This does not imply that women should refrain from having children; we should simply understand the processes at work.

So, *is* celibacy required of Yoga students? This question was asked of Sri Swami Satchidananda at a talk given at Rutgers University in 1974 to an audience of 350, mostly college students.

After he spoke, there was time for questions and answers. A young woman posed the first question. She stood up rather nervously and asked: "Is it really necessary for a person who wants to practice Yoga to be celibate?"

The question immediately caught the attention of the young crowd. They became still.

Sri Swamiji looked very indrawn. He leaned back, his head tilting downward in a gesture that suggested contemplation. After a few moments, he leaned forward, looked up and said....

"Well..." and again leaned back.

The crowd became even more still and attentive. You could feel the anticipation building. Sri Swamiji leaned forward again.

"I would say... " Once again he leaned back into his seat and paused.

You could hear the creaking of seats as a large number of those in attendance leaned forward in anticipation.

"In matters of sex..."

It was almost too much. He looked downward and rested against the back of his seat. After a few moments he looked up, leaned forward, and said…

"Be efficient."

A standing ovation spontaneously erupted. His dramatic pauses had allowed their attention to focus and their doubts and anxieties over this subject to surface. His answer was at once intriguing and liberating. After the crowd quieted he explained what "efficient" meant. He made an analogy to enjoying a meal.

If you really want to enjoy a meal, how would you do it? One thing is that you don't want to spoil your appetite by snacking; it will inhibit healthy hunger, and good digestion will be compromised as well.

Another point: no one goes to much trouble when eating alone. You enjoy food better with someone you really love and care for, someone you have a committed partnership with. And what would you prepare? Not just anything, but something special. You shop for the best ingredients to prepare their favorite dishes. With all care you prepare the meal. And when it comes time to eat, you put out your best tablecloth and dinnerware. Maybe have some flowers and candles on the table, too. Then when you sit to eat, you eat until you are satisfied. Enjoying a meal like this gives the maximum enjoyment, and you also don't get hungry soon afterward because you are satisfied.

God has put the sexual hunger in us just like the hunger for food. Sex is not forbidden to yogis unless they have taken monastic vows, as swamis (monks) have done. For the rest, the householders, it is fine. But it should be done with a yogic approach. There should be meaning to the relationship, a committed partner with whom love, caring, and a common life vision is shared. There is no energy lost or spiritual gain wasted in such a loving union. In this context, the sex act is not just for satisfying the flesh, but is an expression of the love that is within.

We should also take care not to overindulge. Moderation not only prevents us from wasting our energy but is necessary for the healthy enjoyment of sex. If we examine this point, we will recognize from our own life experiences that anything we have overdone loses most of its appeal and leaves us feeling drained and unsatisfied. It is no different with the sex act.

Sexual activity should be treated with the respect and care that it deserves. We are dealing with very powerful and refined energies, the wasting of which can impede our growth, the overuse of which can harm us, but whose conservation brings immense spiritual benefit.

When sexual energy is intelligently conserved (not repressed), it is naturally transmuted to a more refined energy called *ojas*. Ojas is a potent healing energy that helps overcome physical disorders and strengthens the subtle and gross nervous systems. It bestows physical stamina and lucidity to the entire thought process and is therefore a great aid to concentration, making sustained, deep meditation possible.

When conserved, ojas becomes even more refined and is referred to as *tejas* (splendor; brilliance), a subtle form of prana. It is ojas and especially tejas that distinguish the teaching of great spiritual masters from ordinary teachers. Spiritual teaching is different from any other form of instruction in that it is not the mere imparting of ideas or even methods of analysis but the transmission of this most subtle and precious vital energy from teacher to student. It is this process that awakens the forgotten truth of the Self in the student. Tejas is the serene radiance and compelling glint in the eye of those that are spiritually realized.

However, abstinence does not a master make. Many great masters of the past and present lived a married life. Brahmacharya in the context of married life is not about abstinence but about not being bound by craving, observing moderation in sexual activity, and finding other, richer avenues to express and receive love.

Nongreed (Aparigraha)

Greed bespeaks a basic craving, an unsatisfied state of mind. Unfulfilled craving gives birth to greed, and it is this inner gnawing to find fulfillment that leads to the other vices.

This yama can also be understood as not accepting gifts. Though we might consider it impolite to refuse gifts, something other than manners is at work here: Does the acceptance of the gift bring about a feeling of obligation in the mind of the receiver? If so, and neutrality is lost, then it is better to decline the gift. If not, you can accept it with loving gratitude. We see the problem of the obligatory gifts in politics. In these cases the recipient's judgment and even freedom to act from conscience can be compromised.

2.31. These Great Vows are universal, not limited by class, place, time, or circumstance.

This sutra emphasizes the importance of the yamas. They are even accentuated over the niyamas, since they apply to everyone, whether or not they are spiritual seekers. These are the guiding principles for anyone regardless of occupation, status, locale, the time of day, year, or life, or what the context is. Since they transcend all circumstances and challenges, they are as valid today as they were thousands of years ago.

2.32. Niyama consists of purity, contentment, accepting but not causing pain, study, and worship of God (self-surrender).

The word *niyama* indicates the essential principles that govern spiritual growth. While the yamas are universal—for everyone in all circumstances and stages of life—the niyamas are particularly important practices for spiritual seekers who wish to prepare the mind for Self-realization.

Purity (Saucha)

This refers to purity on the physical and mental levels. To achieve it, we need to regulate what is allowed into our bodies and minds as well as to clean any toxic material already present.

Most of us have occasionally hampered our digestion by eating food in unhealthy quantities or of poor nutritional quality. This leads to incomplete digestion, with the partially digested food becoming toxic when it stays in the body too long. In order to cleanse the body of the toxins that are already present, yogis use the postures, cleansing practices, and breathing techniques of Hatha Yoga. Then, to help maintain the toxin-free body, a vegetarian diet consisting of light, easily digested foods is suggested.

We can understand mental toxins in a similar way. Mental toxins rob the mind of its energy and focus and incline it toward unhappiness and anger. Sources of mental toxins include:

- Thoughts or experiences that have not been completely digested, i.e., unresolved, misperceived, or not assessed properly
- Anything we cling to because of selfish attachments
- Vices, such as the opposites of the yamas

All of the above can exist as samskaras (latent impressions). Activated by external or internal cues, they influence activity on the conscious level. Often they are unseen motivators seemingly beyond our control

To cleanse mental toxins, yogis carefully monitor what is allowed to go in the mind, while practices such as meditation, self-analysis, and prayer clean the toxins from past activities.

Contentment (Santosha)

There can be no contentment where there is craving. The mind that focuses on acquisition or achievement withdraws from the present by shifting attention from what it has and what is available to it to hopes of a future fulfillment of a desire. The mind also has a tendency to relive the past, to dwell in a land of regrets and missed opportunities, or to worry about future needs and wants.

Contentment is the ability to live in the present moment, outside the continuous passage of time. The moment is precious because it reflects the infinite possibilities that exist outside the confines of time. Every moment holds the information, guidance, and support we need to succeed and grow spiritually. It has been said that God is either "now, here," or "nowhere." When our thoughts and actions are rooted in the moment, we come closer to the experience of the Absolute.

Over time, contentment develops the faith that the Divine Consciousness animating all life will provide what we need (though not necessarily what satisfies our greed). *"Consider the lilies of the field, they toil not, they spin not, but are arrayed in a splendor even greater than King Solomon's"* (Luke 12.27). Contentment, because it develops faith and steadies the mind, is enough to take us to Self-realization.

The final three principles of niyama were already discussed at the beginning of this chapter, so our discussion here will be brief (*see sutra* 2.1).

Accepting But Not Causing Pain (Tapas)

Tapas suggests a state of spiritual maturity. It asks us to recognize and accept life's inevitable occurrences of pain. We are challenged to refrain from striking out in fear, anger, or retaliation when pain does arrive. There is no blame attributed to anyone or anything, no shaking of angry fists at the heavens. Instead there is the acceptance of pain as the teacher of vital lessons. Yet tapas should not be misunderstood as a passive, do-nothing-and-trust-in-God resignation in the face of injustice. Mahatma Gandhi is a good example of this. He and his followers were well aware that they would have to face many painful situations, yet they accepted the harsh treatment without returning harm or even expressing hateful thoughts to the British. By adhering to nonviolence and truthfulness, they were able to liberate India.

Study (Svadhyaya)

Raja Yoga seeks to have a complete and harmonious development of the individual. It is a system in which the teachings act as checks on an exaggerated growth of any aspect of the personality.

By including study as one of the fundamental teachings, it is clear that Sri Patanjali does not expect his students to travel the path to enlightenment fueled by vague feelings, blind faith, or superstition but by understanding.

In addition to scriptural study, traditionally this niyama includes the study of the lives of sages and saints, the repetition of mantras, and the study of the nature—the ways of life—of human, animal, and plant.

The fact that mantra repetition is included as a form of learning implies that study means something more than the accumulation of facts and the ability to reason. It recognizes that a mind focused on any object will penetrate it to find deeper levels of understanding. Therefore our education attains depth as well as breadth. Repetitive study also strengthens the ability of the mind to meditate.

Worship of God or Self-Surrender (Ishwara Pranidhana)

We tend to think of worship as prayer and ritual. But in focusing on the externals, we may miss the attitude behind the actions. Self-surrender is the inner environment in which worship flourishes.

Self-surrender is the willing dedication of time, energy, and abilities to a person, cause, or achievement in hopes of receiving a valued reward. It's no different for those who "worship" fame, fortune, and so on. They, too, must sacrifice their time, energy, and skills in order to achieve what they desire. Worship of God requires that we give ourselves completely—that we willingly sacrifice our selfishness. In this surrender, nothing can be held back. But the rewards are incredible. The great saint, Maanikkavaachakar wrote this after his experience of enlightenment:

> God, I thought You are all wise, that You are omniscient. Now I see that you are a little foolish. You are not a good businessman. I worked and prayed and finally was able to surrender to You completely. And what did You give me in return? You. It's not good business. What are You going to do with me? I am nothing special. But, I have You and with You, I have everything.

The practice of self-surrender includes dedicated service—performing actions for the welfare of others without selfish expectations. In yogic terms, this is known as the path of Karma Yoga. The ego gives up a little ignorance with every dedicated act.

Related Sutras: 1.23–1.27: *List characteristics of Ishwara.*

We will consider the next two sutras together.

2.33. When disturbed by negative thoughts, opposite (positive) ones should be thought of. This is pratipaksha bhavana.

2.34. When negative thoughts or acts such as violence and so on are caused to be done, or even approved of, whether incited by greed, anger, or infatuation, whether indulged in with mild, medium, or extreme intensity, they are based on ignorance and bring certain pain. Reflecting thus is also pratipaksha bhavana.

This is the second time that Sri Patanjali presents the causes of certain pain (*see sutra* 2.15: *"To one of discrimination, everything is painful indeed, due to . . ."*). In both sutras, ignorance is the source.

Negative thoughts or acts refer to those that are in opposition to the yamas and niyamas. For eliminating negativity, Yoga offers two invaluable techniques: a remedy to take when in the midst of negative episodes, and a preventative that immunizes the mind from their recurrence.

Suppression is not used to eliminate negative thoughts or acts, since suppressed thoughts eventually return with doubled force. And when we are in the middle of a moment of struggle, it does little good to try to analyze the situation. The mind, neither clear nor calm, is unfit for self-analysis. If we cannot regain our composure by suppression or analysis, what can we do?

Immediately take the mind to an elevated place; focus attention on thoughts that can counter the negativity. We could reflect on peace when anger emerges, love when thoughts of intolerance appear, or contentment when greed arises. Or we could simply cultivate one potent thought to counter all negativity. If we have a great reverence for Lord Jesus, we could invoke his name, image, or example for every disturbing situation. Or call forth images of the patience of Mahatma Gandhi or the compassion of Lord Buddha. Perhaps we might think of an experience that elevated us—a pilgrimage we took, for example. Those who have a personal mantra could use that as the counterforce for all negative impulses. Any thought or image will work if it has a powerful uplifting association with it.

Pratipaksha bhavana is a practice that requires skill. The more we use it, the better we become at it. As the opposing thought gains in strength, the ability to counter negative thoughts and actions becomes easier.

When the mind is too disturbed even to shift its attention elsewhere, we can move our bodies to a more positive space or temporarily leave until we calm down. For example, if we are tempted to indulge in a cigarette when someone at a party lights up, we can leave until the feeling passes.

The second facet of pratipaksha bhavana (sutra 2.34) is utilized when the episode of negativity has passed. This is the appropriate time for self-analysis. Over time we will discover the motivation behind the negative impulses and gain inspiration for avoiding them by contemplating their undesirable consequences.

On this level of pratipaksha bhavana, Sri Patanjali gives us no wiggle room. Negative, selfish behavior has no place for a yogi because it brings pain. Let's look at his argument in detail. When negative thoughts or acts are. . .

Caused to Be Done, or even Approved Of

It is a violation of the principles of Yoga to engage in negative acts or passively allow others to do so. This sutra leaves no doubt that yogis are called upon to be responsible citizens; they are not passive bystanders on the sidelines of life.

Incited by Greed, Anger, or Infatuation

Greed. It doesn't matter what motivates the negative act. It isn't difficult to find people who believe that wanting is equivalent to an entitlement, a right. They don't like the discomfort of craving and regard their distress as proof of entitlement. That "proof" can become the basis for rationalizing greedy or selfish behavior. The craving to possess or achieve cannot be used as an excuse for negative thoughts or acts, no matter how strong the desire or how long the yearning.

Anger. We sometimes hear about righteous anger. If we are wronged and lose our temper, emotions of retaliation or revenge are often regarded as acceptable. Anger in this sense is even considered beneficial to society. There are numerous historical examples in which anger directed toward injustices inspired wrongs to be corrected. Still, Sri Patanjali does not approve righteous anger for his students. There are two reasons why anger is not a good source of motivation: it harms the individual, and it ignores better motives.

Individual harm. Anger disturbs the equanimity of the individual. After outbursts of anger, the body shakes as if it has experienced a trauma (it has). Toxins are released into the system, bile pours out, and the entire nervous system is thrown into imbalance. Furthermore, judgment and rational thought are compromised. How many times have we apologized to someone after an outburst of anger by saying, "I'm sorry, I was angry and didn't know what I was doing." Not knowing what we are doing is like a type of insanity. Is loss of rationality really how we wish to direct our moral and ethical choices?

Better motives. Righteous anger is elevated to a virtue because by habit or nature our responses have become limited: we either become angry at an injustice or are unmoved or uncaring. Anger is rajasic; not caring is tamasic. To be untouched by another's suffering is the lowest state. At least the angry individual has a heart that can be moved. Yet even this is not the highest response. The option usually missed is sattwa. The sattwic response is to acknowledge the injustice, keep the mind clear and focused, and correct the injustice in the most effective manner. To correct an injustice does not require the sacrifice of equanimity, ethics, or morals.

Infatuation. The word translated as infatuation, *moha*, suggests a state of delusion, an almost total loss of perspective based on prolonged, deep, or complex selfish emotions. Delusion causes us to forget the lessons of experience.

Under the influence of moha, we slip from the path, at least temporarily losing what progress we have made. The Bhagavad Gita presents a clear description of this process, beginning with the simple and seemingly innocent act of thinking about objects and culminating with the loss of the spiritual gains that have been made:

> From brooding on sense objects, attachments to them arises. Out of that attachment, personal desire is born. And from desire, anger appears. Anger confuses the thinking process, which in turn, disturbs memory. When memory fails, reasoning is ruined. And when reason is gone, one is lost.
>
> Bhagavad Gita 2.62 and 2.63

Indulged in with Mild, Medium, or Extreme Intensity

A wrong act is a wrong act. All acts that are born of ignorance strengthen ignorance. Just as that tiny, delicate patch of skin, the eyelid, can block the sun, so too can a little greed, anger, or lust keep us from Self-realization.

Sri Patanjali next tells us what perfection in the yamas and niyamas and the rest of the eight limbs looks like.

2.35. In the presence of one firmly established in nonviolence, all hostilities cease.

The mindful struggle to overcome gross and subtle aggressive tendencies is an advanced study in the psychology of violence. Through these personal struggles, yogis experience for themselves that fear breeds anger and that anger ruins our peace and clarity. Therefore, yogis understand the pain that violence brings and know that this pain is something we all share. Their empathy for the suffering of others naturally brings compassion. Over time, compassion gives birth to a love and understanding so pure that it lifts the mind to a place of peace beyond any tranquility we had imagined. Then, in a process similar to osmosis, the powerful healing energy of love and understanding flows from an area of greater to lesser concentration. The calming influence of selfless love is a powerful and palpable natural emanation flowing from the hearts of those perfected in nonviolence to the hearts of others. Fear and discord vanish in their presence.

It is then that we will see fulfilled in us the beatitude from the Sermon on the Mount: *"Blessed are the peacemakers, for they shall be called the children of God"* (Mark 5.9).

2.36. To one established in truthfulness, actions and their results become subservient.

The yogi achieves unity with truth. There can be no question of uttering anything not meant to be. Whatever she says *is* the truth. Her thoughts, like feathers blown by the breeze, are easily moved by every whisper of the Divine Will.

2.37. To one established in nonstealing, all wealth comes.

In addition to keeping our hands out of unauthorized cookie jars, perfection in nonstealing includes not improperly benefiting from another's thoughts or ideas. Nonstealing brings about a shift from incessant craving for more to contentment with what we are given and finally to generosity. Generosity is what leads to the wealth mentioned in this sutra. The more we selflessly give, the more we receive. It's the law of karma and good business, too.

On a higher level, real wealth is not defined by having piles of money or possessions. The accumulation of material wealth, though offering a feeling of security, is never deeply satisfying. Without peace, love, and happiness, even if we are wealthy, we won't be fulfilled. At the same time, there are others who have little in the way of material goods but, because they possess peace of mind, feel their life is full and rich.

Sri Swami Satchidananda tells the story a rickshaw man whom he tried to hire. He describes seeing this simple man lounging on the ground, leaning against his rickshaw, smoking a *bidi*, an herbal cigarette. He was obviously poor, yet he seemed utterly without a care in the world, completely unconcerned with attracting customers. His appearance of absolute contentment was so striking that it enticed Sri Swamiji to try to hire him to take him home. The driver declined, saying that he had pulled enough for the day's food. He even refused the offer of higher payment for his services, simply repeating that he had pulled enough for the day's food. He sat like a king, emanating a great peace. With what little he had, he was truly wealthy.

Our wealth is defined not only by material possessions but more importantly by our relationship to them.

2.38. To one established in continence, vigor is gained.

When we don't waste energy, we gain vigor. It is not simply that we will have more energy, but the quality of it will be more subtle, stable, and healing. It is the kind of energy that others will feel in our presence, naturally radiating like light or heat.

2.39. To one established in nongreed, a thorough illumination of the how and why of one's birth comes.

When free of greed, we gain the ability to see how our desires affect what we experience in life. We will discover not only how cravings brought certain experiences in this birth but how powerful past desires propelled us from our past life into this one.

2.40. By purification, the body's protective impulses are awakened, as well as a disinclination for detrimental contact with others.

This is the first of two sutras that discuss the benefits of purity. Here, Sri Patanjali is addressing purity from a physical viewpoint.

There is some confusion surrounding this sutra, primarily regarding the translation of the term, *jugupsa*, usually translated as "disgust." Let's look at a word-for-word translation:

Sauchat, "purification"

Svanga, "one's own body"

Jugupsa, "that which inspires protection," derived from, *ju*, "to urge, inspire, further," *gup*, "to guard, protect, preserve," and *sa* = "procuring, bestowing"

When jugupsa is defined as disgust, it should be understood as similar to our senses' instinctive rejection of anything that is toxic to the body. We would instinctively spit out a mouthful of crude oil, for example. Disgust should not be confused with personal preference. A dislike for red cabbage is not disgust. No matter how objectionable it is to our taste buds, the rejection of red cabbage for dinner is a matter of personal preference.

It is not likely that jugupsa in this sutra was meant to suggest what we mean today when we use the word "disgust." After all, even the wicked people, toward whom Sri Patanjali recommends we maintain equanimity, seem to get off easier than our bodies (*see sutra* 1.33, "*By cultivating attitudes of . . . equanimity toward the nonvirtuous . . .*"). Are we being asked to believe that as a result of perfection in physical purity, we will come to finally regard our body as repugnant, something to be shunned?

Jugupsa is an expression of the protective intelligence inherent in every individual. There is a principle central to Ayurveda, the healing science of India, which states that until our bodies are well purified, we will tend to crave the foods and activities that entrench and even aggravate our imbalances. We will be attracted to things that are bad for us. It is only when purification has restored the natural balance that we begin to be drawn to that which is beneficial while turning away from that which is harmful. For example, if a lit cigarette were held near a baby's nose, it would squint and withdraw from the smoke. This natural impulse arises from the inborn capacity of clean lungs to discriminate what is acceptable to breathe from that which is harmful. However, to smokers whose lungs have long ago lost their natural capacity to discriminate between what is harmful and what is healthy, that same whiff of smoke awakens in them a craving to breathe even more deeply.

As a result of physical purification, the body's protective instincts become fully awakened and alert. Unhindered by the influences of entrenched toxins, they become engaged in the business of warning us away from foods, drinks, and activities that are detrimental to our health. And, just as important, our immune systems can now work at their optimum level, improving the body's defense against disease.

Paraih, "with others, alien, adverse"

Asamsargah, "noncontact, noncontamination"

With these definitions in mind, we are ready to explore this sutra.

We can understand how a pure, healthy body can better protect itself from diseases. But what does "disinclination for detrimental contact with others" mean?

A shift in perception takes place due to purification. We become acutely aware of the body's continuous production of toxins, the aches and pains and diseases. Of course, we may have been aware of all these facts before but ordinarily not in this way or to this extent. The "untidy" and "cumbersome" aspects of living in a physical body now stand in stark contrast to the Self, which, partially due to the process of purification, becomes clearer in our minds and dearer to our hearts.

Under these circumstances, the body, though understood as an important vehicle for work and play, is also no longer where our heart abides. Just as the prospect of living in our car wouldn't be desirable, we would never exchange the realization that the Self is our home for the state of identifying ourselves as the body. In other words, the body is not an appealing place to call home.

Sri Patanjali doesn't explain exactly what he means by "contact." It certainly could be referring to sexual relations, but it could as easily refer to any unhealthy relationship—or both. It could also refer to a vain primping and preening of one's own body, a preoccupation with physical beauty.

In regard to physical attractions, as a result of purity our vision evolves to "see" the inner being, the spirit of the individual, rather than focusing on the appearance of the flesh. Or, as Sri Swami Satchidananda often would say, "We learn to see and appreciate the Cosmic beauty, rather than the cosmetic beauty." For much of the world, the fleshly garment of an individual is the standard by which they are often judged. The sage Ashtavakra heard only laughter at his deformities when he entered the court of a great king. Ignoring those who scorned him for his physical disabilities, he looked into the king's eyes and said, "Sire, your court is filled with individuals whose vision cannot see beyond the flesh. Like butchers, they only see meat."

Purification frees us from obsessing over things sexual. For those who are in committed, loving relationships, sexual activities can still be a vital aspect of their relationship. But as a result of purification, sexual intercourse solely for its own sake becomes unappealing, since sex without commitment, caring, and love is ultimately an empty and lonely act. In this case, sex offers no real meaning and is too superficial to bring any lasting fulfillment. There is no love expressed, no support and caring, in fact, no real intimacy or joy— only tension and release (*see commentary on continence in sutra* 2.30).

The gift of purification is that without being attached to or obsessed with the physical beauty or even the health of our own body or the bodies of others, we are free to perceive our body as the vehicle for Self-realization.

The same inborn intelligence, if allowed to operate without the restrictions imposed by an impure mind, would protect us from "psychological toxins" such as backbiting, gossip, and other hurtful behaviors. As a result of purification, our innate intelligence is awakened and actively protects us from harmful relationships.

2.41. Moreover, one gains purity of sattwa, cheerfulness of mind, one-pointedness, mastery over the senses, and fitness for Self-realization.

Having examined the benefits of physical purity, Sri Patanjali now discusses the benefits of mental purity.

The list of benefits of mental purity given in this sutra includes two items that are reminiscent of the two-pronged approach for achieving nirodha presented in sutra 1.12: practice and nonattachment. In this sutra we learn that purity fosters one-pointedness of mind (*see sutra* 1.13) and mastery over the senses (*see sutras* 1.15 *and* 1.16).

As we examine the benefits of purity listed in this sutra, we can better understand why Lord Jesus taught that by purity alone God can be known: "*Blessed are the pure in heart, for they shall see God*" (Matthew 5.8). Purity is like a fishnet that pulls together all the major facets of Yoga practice.

Purity of Sattwa

Recall that sattwa is also referred to as buddhi (*see commentary on sutra 1.2*). Sattwa's nature is tranquility, balance, and illumination. When the sattwic aspect of the mind is purified, the discriminative faculty can function at its highest level. The mind regains its natural ability to penetrate the object of its attention to its depths

Cheerfulness of Mind

Cheerfulness is a characteristic of sattwa. Cheerfulness is included not simply because it is an anticipated outcome of practice but because a cheerful mind has the energy and perseverance necessary to proceed to the highest states of spiritual experience.

(*See sutra 1.17, regarding sa-ananda, the blissful samadhi.*)

One-pointedness

This is another quality inherent in sattwa. One-pointedness precedes samadhi (*see sutras 3.11 and 3.12, which describe the role one-pointedness plays in developing samadhi*).

Mastery over the Senses

In sutra 1.15, nonattachment was introduced as "the manifestation of self-mastery in one who is free from craving for objects seen or heard about." In sutra 2.41, mental purity is identified as a way to attain nonattachment.

Recall that in the commentary on sutra 2.32, mental impurities were listed as thoughts or experiences that are unresolved, misperceived, or not assessed properly, or as selfish attachments or vices. To cleanse these mental impurities, yogis monitor what is allowed to go in the mind, while practices such as meditation, self-analysis, and prayer clean out current impurities. One result of this mental cleansing is that our love-hate relationship with sense objects is recognized for what it is: a short-term emotional event, the endlessly played drama of infatuation—of desire, striving, and acquisition (or failure to acquire).

What naturally follows from sense-mastery is a shift in priorities. Our values change from the acquisition of objects, power, or status to seeking the experience of spiritual values such as clarity, serenity, selfless love, faith, joy not dependent on externals, and Self-realization.

Fitness for Self-realization

To sum up the benefits of mental purity, the mind will be:

- Lucid, tranquil, and balanced
- Cheerful and energetic
- Focused
- Free from attachments

If you review sutra 2.28, you will find that Sri Patanjali correlates the dwindling of impurities to the attainment of viveka, and in sutra 2.26 he tells us that viveka is the method for the removal of ignorance. In other words, if the mind is purified, it is ready for Self-realization. This illustrates the interconnectedness of spiritual principles. They enhance, amplify, and balance each other. Grasp onto any link in the chain; keep pulling and you will attain the goal.

2.42. By contentment, supreme joy is gained.

Contentment is perfected in the absence of cravings. It is the experience that nothing is lacking, that everything that happens is an integral part of a Divine Plan. The result is a joy that transcends transitory pleasures and almost perfectly reflects the supreme bliss of the Self.

Joy is not an accident or a blessing that is arbitrarily bestowed by a capricious Deity. It is the outcome of cultivating a vision of life that "sees" the unity of the Self behind the diversity of names and forms.

Related Sutra: 1.16: "When there is nonthirst for even the gunas (constituents of Nature) due to realization of the Purusha, that is supreme nonattachment."

2.43. By austerity, impurities of body and senses are destroyed and occult powers gained.

Austerity is the struggle to live according to the principles we have set before ourselves and to accept whatever life brings our way. It is a process that strengthens and purifies us.

In addition to physical toxins, impurities include the obstacles of sutra 1.30, anything that opposes the spirit of the yamas and niyamas (*sutras 2.30 and 2.32*), and the source of all impurities, ignorance of the Self (*sutras 2.3 and 2.4, the klesas*).

Related Sutras: 2.1 and 2.32: Discuss austerity (tapas); 4.1: Details the various ways the occult powers may come about.

2.44. Through study comes communion with one's chosen deity.

There are three important ideas to consider in this sutra: *deity*, *chosen*, and *communion*.

Deity

The *Yoga Sutras* don't advocate any particular form of God to worship because the yogi understands every deity as being a manifestation of Ishwara and worthy of veneration. Therefore every name and form of God can be a gateway to higher spiritual experiences.

Chosen

The chosen deity, *ishta devata*, is a common characteristic of Hinduism. Seekers are free to choose whatever name and form appeals to them as objects of their devotion (*this is reminiscent of sutra 1.39, in which Sri Patanjali states we can choose any object of meditation we like*).

It is understood that there are certain qualities prominently associated with a particular deity that may deeply resonate in the devotee. The freedom to worship God in any form we choose offers the advantage of being able more easily to cultivate a loving relationship with the Divine. Where the heart is, there also will be our energy, our thought, and our actions. Love is never idle. In this case, it begets sadhana and communion with the Absolute.

Communion

The receptivity and one-pointedness developed through study absorb the mind in whatever aspect of the Absolute the seeker has formed a devoted relationship with. This experience can also result from repetition of a mantra that is linked to the seeker's object of devotion.

Communion with one's chosen deity also suggests imbibing the qualities associated with that deity.

Related Sutras: 2.1 and 2.32: Which mention study.

2.45. By total surrender to Ishwara, samadhi is attained.

Every spiritual path one day brings us face-to-face with the unadulterated ego. We perceive it in all its stubborn glory. But if we wish to realize the infinite Self as our True Identity, we need to transcend the limitation that is the ego. The problem is that efforts to transcend the ego often cause it to reassert itself emphatically as the fear that we will cease to exist if we proceed.

Surrender to Ishwara is the easiest way to overcome this obstacle because it is not based on having the will power to overcome the threat of annihilation in order to transcend the ego. Instead, the ego becomes absorbed in loving reverence and willingly moves toward union with the beloved Divine.

Related Sutra: 1.23: The first time surrender to Ishwara as a means to attaining samadhi is mentioned.
(Also see *Mind and Self* and *Purusha* in the *Sutras-by-Subject* Index.)

2.46. Asana is a steady, comfortable posture.

This refers to formal seated meditation postures and suggests that we should find or cultivate a posture that leaves us free to focus the mind and breath without the interference of aches, pains, or restlessness.

The bending and stretching postures of Hatha Yoga are important means to achieving "asana."

2.47. By lessening the natural tendency for restlessness and by meditating on the infinite, posture is mastered.

When we sit in a comfortable, steady asana and focus on the Infinite, we experience a natural lessening of restlessness. It happens when we focus on something immovable and whose boundaries are immeasurable to us.

There is also a symbolic meaning to this sutra. Ananta (the word translated as "infinite") is also the name of the cosmic snake, the symbol for the power of Lord Vishnu. Lord Vishnu is often depicted as seated on Ananta, whose many hooded heads spread open to form a canopy over the Lord's head. All around Lord Vishnu are the waters of life—a churning, rolling, restless ocean. Lord Vishnu is the Self, and Ananta represents the power of the universe under His feet and at His service. These symbols demonstrate that we attain Divine mastery (symbolized by Lord Vishnu) when we bring the natural tendency for restlessness (the churning ocean of energy or prana) under our control by meditating and tapping into the infinite source of inner power (represented by Ananta).

2.48. Thereafter, one is undisturbed by dualities.

To penetrate the deeper reality of the Self, the mind needs to be unfettered from dualities—heat and cold, up and down, in and out, and so on. This is an important prerequisite for the subtler experiences of pranayama, sense withdrawal, and meditation.

This sutra suggests that the purpose of the practice of asana is not simply a physical one but a mental one as well.

2.49. That (firm posture) being acquired, the movements of inhalation and exhalation should be controlled. This is pranayama.

Pranayama is mastery of prana, the universal life force, *through* the breath. The movements of the breath reflect the state of prana in the body-mind. Irregular breathing is indicative of imbalances or blockages in the flow of prana. Through regulation of the breath, the prana flows in the appropriate measure and locations. Blockages are removed, increasing energy and improving health.

In sutra 2.15, we learned that it is impossible to be permanently happy unless the gunas are controlled: "To one of discrimination, everything is painful indeed, due to its consequences...the constant conflict among the activities of the gunas, which control the mind." Pranayama is of vital importance for this endeavor because it helps brings the gunas to a balanced state.

In Pada One, we were introduced to a connection between the breath and mind. Disturbed breathing was given as a symptom of the "shaking of the chitta" (*see sutras* 1.30 *and* 1.31). Because of the mind-breath connection, it follows that if the obstacles cause the breathing to become irregular, regulation of the breath can diminish the activity of the obstacles.

(*See Pranayama in the Sutras-by-Subject Index.*)

2.50. The modifications of the life-breath are external, internal, or stationary. They are to be regulated by space, time, and number and are either long or short.

Generally, our breath rotates between three different movements in relation to the body: toward it, away from it, and fixed (the breathing mechanisms become still).

Space refers to the point of mental focus during the practice. Where the attention goes, the prana flows. The attention is directed either to areas such as the base of the spine or between the eyebrows, or perhaps, when healing is intended, to where the practitioner feels there is a lack of prana.

Time means the length of time for the inhalation, exhalation, and retention of the breath.

Number refers to the number of repetitions and rounds of the specific practice.

The three modifications that the breath takes—inhalation, exhalation, and retention—can be manipulated and regulated to foster progress in pranayama practice.

Note: the advanced practice of pranayama, especially breath retention, should be learned and practiced under the guidance of a qualified teacher.

2.51. There is a fourth kind of pranayama that occurs during concentration on an internal or external object.

Sri Patanjali doesn't provide details on what this fourth type of pranayama might be, though it most likely refers to a natural, effortless state of breath suspension that occurs during deep meditation, called *kevala kumbhaka*. Since the breath reflects the state of the body and mind, if the body is completely still and relaxed and the mind becomes quiet and clear, the breath naturally stops for a while.

2.52. As its result, the veil over the inner light is destroyed.

Prakasa, translated as inner light, refers to a quality of the sattwa guna. It shines forth when tamas, or darkness, disperses.

All our thoughts can be categorized according to the qualities of the gunas—tamas, rajas, and sattwa (*see Gunas in the Glossary*). Thoughts that are characterized by dullness, carelessness, or lack of attentiveness are tamasic and are characterized as being heavy and restraining movement. Rajasic thoughts are restless and conceal the Self by uneven attention and powerful emotions. The practice of pranayama helps counteract the inertia of tamas and the restlessness of rajas. When rajas and tamas decline, sattwa predominates. Though the veils covering the Self are now more transparent, the fullness of the Self is still concealed by the engaging but transitory happiness of sattwa.

The mind finds the inner light captivating . . .

2.53. And the mind becomes fit for concentration.

More sattwa means more peace, clarity, and steadiness in meditation. The mind finds joy in the practice since it experiences something nice. Focusing the mind becomes easier.

2.54. When the senses withdraw themselves from the objects and imitate, as it were, the nature of the mind-stuff, this is pratyahara.

The senses do not function independently of the mind; therefore, when the attention is pulled inward, they disconnect from their objects and also go within.

The senses are portals through which input reaches the mind-stuff. But perception occurs only when the mind is "joined" to the senses. Without the union of mind and senses, no perception can take place. For example, we do not notice sounds outside our living room when the mind is absorbed in a thrilling novel. The sound vibrations still reach the ears, but since the mind is engaged elsewhere, they make no conscious impression on the individual awareness.

The mind has learned to ignore most sense input when performing tasks; it is how we are able to be productive and get work done with relative efficiency. Yet the mind resists blocking out all sense input—an ability needed to achieve deeper states of meditation. This is why pratyahara is practiced. Pratyahara brings the senses back to their source: the essential nature of the mind. This pure sattwic aspect of mind is characterized by tranquility, clarity, illumination, intelligence, and the ability to discriminate.

Pratyahara neutralizes the mind's predominant occupation with sensory input. What remains after success in pratyahara are subconscious impressions (samskaras) arising as memories that don't require input from the outside world. Pratyahara eliminates an entire category of mental impressions—sensory awareness—allowing the mind to examine more subtle aspects of mental content and activity.

This leaves one more aspect of pratyahara to consider: How do we achieve it?

Since we already know that the senses follow the lead of the mind, the question becomes: When disconnecting the mind from sense objects, where should the attention be re-directed? Consider the following quotations from the Bhagavad Gita:

> But the yogi learns to control the senses by meditating on me [Lord Krishna symbolizing the Self] as the highest goal. As the senses come under control, the yogi's wisdom becomes steady. (2.61)

> Then sit and calm the mind and senses by concentrating on one thing; thus you practice Yoga [meditation] for self-purification. (6.12)

In both instances, control of the senses is attained not by pulling the mind away from the sense object but by redirecting attention toward something elevating (*see sutras* 1.34–1.39, *which suggest various objects for meditation*). One of the benefits of redirection is that it cultivates nonattachment by replacing transitory sense satisfactions with the deeper, more satisfying contentment of the sattwic mind.

The practice of pratyahara is an education in the proper use of the senses. It requires and cultivates discipline, discrimination, memory, and courage: discipline to shift attention from sense objects; discrimination to assess the appropriate use of the senses and to understand the motives behind the compulsion to remain engaged in objects that catch the senses' attention; memory to examine the benefits and liabilities resulting from the use, abuse, and overuse of the senses; and courage to temporarily give up indulging a particular sense in order serve the purpose of Self-realization.

Finally, let's put pratyahara in the context of the eight limbs, as part of a process of progressive interiorization:

- Yama and niyama help maintain equanimity of mind in interactions.

- Asana helps the mind become impervious to the effects of dualities.
- Pranayama removes the veil that covers the light of consciousness, preparing it for concentration (dharana). It makes the mind energetic and alert while further stilling the activities of the vrittis.
- Pratyahara brings attention within by withdrawing attention from ambient sounds, odors, or other sensory stimuli.

Pratyahara not only prepares the mind for meditation but also enhances the enjoyment of life through the senses. Gone are regrets of overindulgence or misuse. Pratyahara brings the freedom of mastery.

2.55. Then follows supreme mastery over the senses.

The practitioner can withdraw the senses at will as a tortoise pulls in its limbs. Temptations and cravings are dealt with not by suppression but by redirecting the attention to a more beneficial place and holding it steady.

It's important to understand that sense-mastery is not a practice of deprivation. Instead it is the gateway to greater joy:

> The happiness we can receive by mastery lasts longer than temporary joys. We should all become masters. That is true freedom and real victory. If you are free from your own mind and senses, nothing can bind you: then you are really free.
>
> Sri Swami Satchidananda

Pada Two Review

1. Kriya Yoga, the essential preparatory practices of Yoga, is given:
   - Accepting pain as help for purification
   - Study of spiritual works
   - Surrender to God

2. The practices of Kriya Yoga help to minimize obstacles (the klesas) and pave the way for the experience of samadhi.

3. The klesas are presented:
   - Ignorance: regarding the impermanent as permanent, the impure as pure, the painful as pleasant, and the non-Self as the Self
   - Egoism: identification of the power of seeing with the instrument of seeing
   - Attachment: that which follows identification with pleasurable experiences
   - Aversion: that which follows identification with painful experiences
   - Clinging to bodily life

4. The klesas are rooted in ignorance.

5. Ignorance and the other klesas can be eliminated through meditation, uninterrupted discriminative discernment (viveka), and samadhi.

6. The law of karma is introduced as the cause for our experiences in the present and future births. Specifically, karma is responsible for experiences of:
   - Pleasure and pain
   - Birth into different species
   - Life span
   - General life occurrences

Karma cannot exist without ignorance.

7. In sutra 2.15, Sri Patanjali demonstrates that any experience grounded in ignorance brings pain. He cites three factors: fear and anxiety over potential loss; the inability completely or permanently to satisfy cravings (which are induced by pleasurable experiences); and the inevitability for the mind (except for the highest samadhi) to find rest due to the influence of the activities of the gunas.

8. Sri Patanjali again addresses the topic of ignorance, defining it as the confusion of the nature of the Seer and seen. To help put an end to this confusion, he lists the essential qualities of both, ending with the assertion that the seen exists solely for the purposes of the Seer.

9. Since we should be ready to understand and engage in Yoga practice more fully, the eight limbs of Raja Yoga are presented, a complete and balanced program for Self-realization that cultivates the uninterrupted discriminative discernment necessary to remove ignorance:
  • Yama (abstinence)
  • Niyama (observance)
  • Asana (posture)
  • Pranayama (breath control)
  • Pratyahara (sense withdrawal)
  • Dharana (concentration)
  • Dhyana (meditation)
  • Samadhi (absorption, superconscious state)

10. The yamas and niyamas are defined:
  • Yama, referred to as the "Great Vows," constitutes the moral and ethical code vital for everyone to follow
  • Niyama is composed of principles especially important for seekers

11. Pratipaksha bhavana, the practice of replacing negative thoughts with positive ones, is introduced as an aid to the practice of yama and niyama, though it is also effective as an aid for meditation practice and in any disturbing life situation.

12. The rest of this pada details the benefits that result from perfecting each of the first five limbs of ashtanga (the eight-limbed) Yoga.

What to Do

Examine the nature of painful experiences. See how many instances you can recall when a situation you initially considered painful turned out to be a blessing in disguise.

Formulate a plan of study of sacred works, not only continuing with the sutras but perhaps incorporating writings from other traditions as well.

Practice surrender to God through selfless service, worship, and prayer. For those students who have rejected a particular faith tradition, it might be beneficial to review at least some of its fundamental teachings, prayers, customs, and practices. All faiths contain the same essential, universal teachings. Can you find any similarities with the *Yoga Sutras*? Many students of Yoga have experienced a newfound appreciation for the faith tradition in which they were raised. Developing a deep interfaith-based vision of spirituality is certainly in keeping with the sprit of the *Yoga Sutras*.

Contemplate sutra 2.15, "everything is painful indeed," as a reminder of the consequences of believing that anything other than Self-realization offers permanent happiness. But don't forget sutra 2.16, "the pain that has not yet come can be avoided," and that the ultimate cause of pain is ignorance.

Memorize the yamas and niyamas and the eight limbs. Take one yama and one niyama per week to practice. You could log your experiences in a diary.

Begin or continue with your practice of asana, pranayama, and meditation.

Pada Three
Vibhuti Pada: Portion on Accomplishments

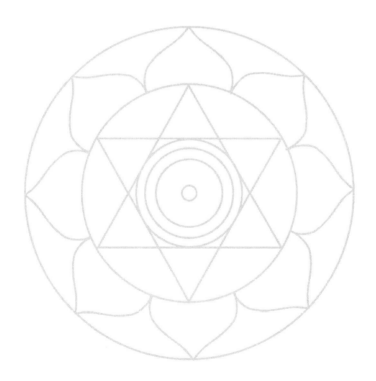

Inside Pada Three

A passing glance at Pada Three might lead one to believe that it is basically a list of the extraordinary accomplishments that can result from the practice of Yoga. But scratch the surface a bit, and we will discover that this chapter presents Sri Patanjali as research scientist, dissecting the nature of the material world and explaining its relationship to the mind and the Purusha. Sri Patanjali urges us to understand Nature well, to master it, and then to realize the Spirit that lies beyond it.

The remarkable powers listed in this section are the outcome of a mind that has attained laser-like focus and that has begun penetrating the layers of Nature. They only *seem* amazing because we do not see the true nature of our world.

The first three sutras of this Pada complete the concepts presented in Pada Two. Having reached this point in the studies of the sutras, you possess all the practical day-to-day theories and practices you need to experience Self-realization. However, there is an incredible wealth of valuable information and inspiration in the last two books of the *Yoga Sutras*. In Padas Three and Four we discover—among many other teachings—the nature of consciousness, both individual and cosmic; the latent powers of the mind; and the inner workings of karma.

Key Principles:
- *Parinama*: the stages of development in nirodha and samadhi
- *Samyama*: a practice that yields mastery over aspects of Nature. (*See definition of samyama in Key Practices below.*)
- Nonattachment to siddhis as a necessary precursor to Self-realization

Key Practices:
- Concentration (*dharana*): the focusing of attention
- Meditation (*dhyana*): a mind with steady attention; the word is also commonly used to refer to the entire process of concentration, meditation proper, and samadhi

- Samadhi: the state of unity or absorption with the object of contemplation
- Samyama: the combined practice of concentration, meditation, and samadhi upon any object

Other Key Terms:
- *Ekagrata*: one-pointedness
- *Siddhis*: accomplishments, yogic powers

PADA THREE

Pada Three
Vibhuti Pada: Portion on Accomplishments

The first twelve sutras of Pada Three describe the stages leading to perfection in nirodha:
- Sutras 1—8 present the major stages of mental mastery that practitioners will experience
- Sutras 9—12 provide a detailed description of the progression from dharana to dhyana and finally to samadhi

It is a process that leads to Self-realization.

3.1. Dharana is the binding of the mind to one place, object, or idea.

In dharana (concentration), the mind directs its attention to a fixed point: any place, object, or idea the practitioner chooses. Of course, the mind is not in the habit of attentively focusing on one point. It wants to run here and there, and does. Many times during a meditation session, the mind will quietly slither away, initially undetected. Each time the mind's wandering ways are discovered, the practitioner lets go of the wayward thoughts and refocuses on the object of meditation. Over time, the mind wanders less frequently and becomes increasingly still, clear, and powerful.

Letting go of distracting thoughts is a hallmark of many Yoga practices. For example, this technique is similar to the method of redirection used in pratipaksha bhavana, pratyahara, and the practice of the four locks and four keys. Therefore, regularity in these practices will serve as a support for advancement in dharana.

Related Sutras: 1.33, 2.33, and 2.54: Discuss the four locks and four keys, pratipaksha bhavana, and pratyahara, all of which are important aids to attaining dharana.

3.2. Dhyana is the continuous flow of cognition toward that object.

When dharana becomes continuous, it automatically becomes dhyana, the state of meditation proper. During the time the mind is in the meditative state, no other thoughts intrude. At this stage, the web-weaving vritti activity of the mind winds down to a halt, and the natural penetrating quality of the mind becomes more apparent. With dhyana, the process of communion with the object of meditation begins in earnest.

It is noteworthy that while it takes effort to *achieve* dhyana, when *in* that state, no further struggle is involved. Meditation is the natural, easy, and unbroken flow of attention toward the chosen object. The mind in meditation is peaceful, clear, and one-pointed.

In fact, only when the mind has attained all three criteria at the same time can we say that there is a state of meditation.

Peaceful

Peaceful means that there is a reduction in mental activity or that whatever activity remains is tranquil and orderly. The meditator experiences a serene mental landscape. However nice this may be, a peaceful feeling alone is insufficient to describe the state of meditation. The mind can be peaceful while in a semi-focused, lazy reverie on a summer's eve.

Clear

This indicates that the meditator is acutely aware of whatever thoughts are in the mind. But clarity does not ensure peace. The mind can also be quite clear while harboring negative thoughts such as envy. It can also be clear and hyperactive at the same time.

One-pointed

This is a state of mind, begun in meditation, in which only one thought is sustained in the individual's awareness. However, the mind can attain a type of one-pointed focus (more like a temporary obsession with a particular vritti or stream of thoughts) on disturbing images or thoughts that can upset our peace.

Only when the mind has attained all three criteria at the same time can we say that there is a state of meditation.

Another sign of a mind in meditation is losing track of time, thinking that only a very short time has passed when in fact the time elapsed has been longer. Of course, a snooze could achieve the same effect, but a sleeping mind does not fulfill the threefold criteria of peace, clarity, and one-pointedness.

However, the most infallible sign of progress in meditation is that we become more peaceful, more content, more loving and giving.

A mind that withstands the assaults of life while maintaining its inner peace has gained in spiritual maturity.

3.3. Samadhi is the same meditation when the mind-stuff, as if devoid of its own form, reflects the object alone.

If the goal of the practice of meditation is to gain knowledge of the object of meditation that is immediate, unbiased, and whole, then the mind has to reach a state where it completely, even if temporarily, gives up whatever form it is holding in favor of that of the chosen object. The mind, having surrendered any resistance to union with the object of meditation, completely and accurately reflects the form of that object in the same way that an undistorted and perfectly clean mirror holds the full and exact reflection of our face.

The samadhi presented in this sutra does not describe the highest samadhi, nirbija samadhi, in which all latent subconscious impressions are also wiped out.

Related Sutra: 1.41: *Offers a good, less technical definition of samadhi based on this same idea.*

3.4. The practice of these three (dharana, dhyana, and samadhi) upon one object is called samyama.

Samyama means to be perfectly controlled.

Union with the object of meditation occurs when the mind penetrates it through successive progression from dharana to dhyana and finally to samadhi. In samyama, the mind dives deeply into any object or idea. In the process, it gains complete knowledge of the object of attention, down to its most subtle aspects.

3.5. By mastery of samyama, knowledge born of intuitive insight shines forth.

The word for "shines forth" is *prajnalokah*. It is composed of *prajna*, "intuitive insight or wisdom," and *alokah*, "brilliance, light."

The knowledge gained by samyama is direct and intuitive. It is a bursting-forth of the light—the reality or essential nature—of the object of meditation. The inception, evolution, and dissolution of any object are fully revealed.

Samyama is a skill that helps make a practitioner fit for the transcendent knowledge of the Self.

3.6. Its practice is accomplished in stages.

Knowing that there are several stages of accomplishment, we can surmise that there are various signposts to help guide and reassure us on the path. These will be discussed in sutras 3.9—3.12.

This sutra may also be a gentle admonishment directed to students who, upon hearing of the amazing benefits of the practice of samyama, think they could start their practice at this level. Everyone must begin at the beginning. At the same time, it encourages those who feel that the practice of samyama is too difficult to achieve by reminding them that the longest journey begins with a single step.

This sutra could be understood in another light. Let's look at the Sanskrit:

Tasya, "its" (samyama)

Bhumisu, "stages," rooted in bhumi, "ground, earth, field, site, territory."

Viniyogah, "practice, application, progression." It can mean "to direct."

This sutra can be translated: "It (intuitive knowledge gained from samyama) can be applied to any field (of examination)."

Related Sutras: 1.17: *The four stages of samprajnata samadhi*; 1.42–44: *Savitarka, nirvitarka savichara, nirvichara samadhis*; 3.9–12: *Development of one-pointedness and samadhi*.

3.7. These three (dharana, dhyana and samadhi) are more internal than the preceding five limbs.

To practice the yamas and niyamas, you need the outside world. To practice asana and pranayama, you need the body, which is composed of the gross elements. Pratyahara only makes sense in relation to a world external to the senses. But to practice these last three limbs, the practitioner must go within and begin to work with and explore consciousness itself. That is why these limbs are considered more internal.

3.8. Even these three are external to the seedless samadhi.

Until nirbija samadhi, subconscious impressions remain as seeds that can activate the influence of ignorance on mental functioning. In nirbija samadhi, the entirety of individual consciousness, including the subconscious, becomes still and pure.

All other samadhis are external when compared to nirbija samadhi.

Related Sutra: 1.51: *Describes nirbija, the seedless samadhi.*

Development in Nirodha: Notes on Sutras 3.9 to 3.12

The next four sutras deserve a preface because they summarize and expand on the core principle of Yoga practice introduced in sutra 1.2: nirodha. Nirodha, which can be understood as the process of shifting from object-oriented consciousness to awareness of the inner organ (the mind), is a shift that culminates in the realization of the source of consciousness, the Purusha. Yet the degree of nirodha necessary to achieve Self-realization can seem like a mountain that looks more massive and imposing as we near it.

The primary obstruction to the development of nirodha is the inclination of the mind to be restless and outwardly directed. This mode of functioning, the predominant characteristic of ordinary awareness, has its roots in subconscious impressions that were created by—and remain under—the influence of ignorance. That is why development of nirodha involves restructuring the subconscious mind to allow for a profound change in the way the mind perceives and understands itself and its experiences in the world.

We generally function under the sway of a web of subconscious impressions and a mode of mental behavior that generates and sustains a false sense of self-identity based on:

- The desire to have contact with objects that are regarded as separate from one's self in order to understand and either pursue or avoid them

- The expectation that these experiences will bring permanent happiness
- A sense of selfhood built upon identification with pleasurable and painful experiences in the world

Sri Patanjali uses the word *vyutthana*, "externalization," to characterize this mode of mental behavior and the impressions that support it.

First, let's examine the foundation of the subconscious: samskaras (*see Samskaras in the Sutras-by-Subject Index*). Samskaras are mental modifications that sink to the bottom of the mental lake, where they become potential activators to further thought activity. Samskaras form the deep inner structure of the mind that influences all thought processes. They determine much of what constitutes our personality, habits, and behavior and have a strong sway over the choices we make. They constantly trigger conscious mental activity, which in turn creates new impressions or strengthens ones already lying in the subconscious.

Samskaras become dominant factors in determining our character when similar ones bind together to form subconscious tendencies and traits (*see Vasanas in the Glossary*). For example, impressions of fear gather together to predispose us to further occasions of fear that in turn create and strengthen impressions of fear. It is a vicious cycle that is broken by nirodha (*see sutra 4.11, which details the factors that keep samskaras active*).

Every moment of stillness, focus, and clarity creates impressions of nirodha. Each instance of nirodha—of redirecting attention inwards—predisposes the practitioner to another. Once firmly grounded in the subconscious, impressions of nirodha completely transform how we perceive the world and our self-identity.

Samskaras of nirodha take root more quickly and decisively when moments of nirodha are vivid, marked by enthusiastic and energetic efforts. When impressions of nirodha grow sufficiently in number and strength, they permeate the subconscious, replacing impressions of externalization. Over time, samskaras of nirodha become the dominant influence on the mind's functioning (*see sutras 1.14 and 1.21*). When this occurs, the mind naturally attains a clear, steady focus and objectivity in its

PADA THREE

perceptions. It turns within effortlessly and with great zeal as it searches for the source of consciousness—the Purusha. If vyutthana is the obstacle, nirodha is the solution.

Nirodha gains its ascendancy over subconscious activity not primarily through occasional dramatic breakthroughs but in small, steady steps. This idea of progressive transformation is central to understanding how advancement is made in Yoga and it appears several times in the sutras.

In the introductory sutras of this pada, Sri Patanjali stated that samadhi isn't achieved all at once. Rather, it is a continuum of ever-increasing mental focus that progresses from concentration to meditation to samadhi. Then, after presenting samyama (concentration, meditation, and samadhi taken together) as the way to gain intuitive insight, he again emphasizes that progress is made in stages (*see sutra* 3.6). Now, in sutras 3.9 to 3.12, development in nirodha is presented as a product of transforming the subconscious through regularity and repetition. (To complete the topic of transformation, in sutra 3.13 we discover how time and environment affect evolution.)

There is a mysterious or subtle aspect to our advancement toward Self-realization. Most of our efforts produce results that are not apparent because they work on a subconscious level. There are times when we may become discouraged, feeling that little or no progress is being made. This group of sutras helps practitioners realize that most progress is made out of the reach of their conscious awareness.

Persistence and faith pay off: each instance of practice, every moment of nirodha, surely adds to the restructuring of the subconscious mind, leading to the transformation of the individual into a liberated yogi.

3.9. Impressions of externalization are subdued by the appearance of impressions of nirodha. As the mind begins to be permeated by moments of nirodha, there is development in nirodha.

Like the sunrise which always overpowers the darkness of night, nirodha unfailingly counteracts vyutthana, externalization.

Our efforts are like powerful seeds that do most of their work out of sight. No effort in Yoga is ever wasted. Our practices plant and nourish seeds of nirodha, of stillness and clarity. In time they will sprout, grow, and blossom.

It is apparent that practices such as meditation, prayer, study, and self-analysis develop nirodha. But nirodha really gains momentum when we create the inner environment in which nirodha thrives. In practical terms, this means looking to principles of sacred wisdom as the standard by which we make choices and by which we adjust our perception of life and the world. By adopting sacred standards as our guidelines for living, we create an inner universe where fears, anxieties, and restlessness are diminished by faith, compassion, and clear, steady focus (*see sutra 1.7, which lists "authoritative testimony" as a source of valid knowledge*).

Development in nirodha is greatly accelerated when we live our lives guided by the principles found in the yamas and niyamas. Once we include guidelines such as these in our lives, Yoga practice ceases to be limited to a couple of hours a day. The advantage of this is that more and more of our thoughts and acts add to our momentum towards liberation.

3.10. When impressions of nirodha become strong and pervasive, the mind-stuff attains a calm flow of nirodha.

This describes a mind that through regular, devoted effort has achieved effortlessness in nirodha. There is no more strain, no coercing the mind. A powerful subconscious momentum towards Self-realization has been created. Such a mind finds it natural to look within for fulfillment, to be more peaceful, focused, and selfless. The doors to wisdom begin to open, and faith increases.

Related Sutra: 1.14: *Describes how habits are created.*

3.11. The mind-stuff transforms toward samadhi when distracted-ness dwindles and one-pointedness arises.

As the time in nirodha is repeated and prolonged, the mind-stuff begins to lose the habit of shifting attention from object to object. It is said to be attaining ekagrata, one-pointedness. One-pointedness marks the beginning of development in samadhi, samadhi parinama.

Samadhi brings significant changes in the mental environment. It's almost like renovating a house, adding a new floor, more rooms, windows, and closets. We see fresh vistas through new openings and suddenly find storage places for everything. Our newly refurbished house impacts our lives on many practical and emotional levels. Similarly, the mind undergoing the transforming process of samadhi begins to operate in a state of heightened receptivity that opens it to subtle influences, knowledge, and experiences.

3.12. Then again, when the subsiding and arising images are identical, there is one-pointedness (ekagrata parinama).

Even when the mind has attained one-pointedness, thought waves still arise, though in a unique manner. There is a continuous flow of attention toward the object of attention in which subsiding and arising thought waves are identical. It's like filming a bowl of fruit when neither the bowl nor the camera is moved. Each frame is indistinguishable from the last. The effect would be essentially the same as a still photograph.

When the mind achieves one-pointedness, it takes the form of the object of meditation. Seer and seen become one (*see sutras 1.41 and 1.43, which describe this experience*). Even the thought "I am meditating" disappears. This idea was echoed by Saint Anthony of Egypt (251–356 C.E.), known as the founder of monasticism in Christianity, when he wrote, "*The prayer of the mind is not perfect until one no longer realizes himself or the fact that he is praying.*"

The practitioner then also receives knowledge of the forces (the subtle elements, for example) that brought the object into being.

Time loses its meaning in this state. We mark time essentially by noting changes. If no change is noticed, we cannot perceive the passage of time. Loosening the bonds of time brings us one step closer to awareness of the eternal present.

3.13. By what has been said (in sutras 3.9–3.12) the transformations of the form, characteristics, and condition of the elements and sense organs are explained.

This sutra focuses on the effects of time and environment on evolution. It gives us a glimpse into the three major tracks along which objects in Nature—including the mind—change.

Form

This refers to the gross form of an object.

From the undifferentiated ocean of Prakriti an object manifests. The first stage is the interaction of the gunas, which produces the gross elements, *bhutas*, (ether, air, fire, water, earth). The gross elements come together into material objects, making Prakriti visible to our senses.

Characteristics

Having come into being, the form of the newly created object is altered due to the ever-shifting mix of the gunas.

Over the course of time, characteristics that have only been implied (latent potentialities) in an object or entity are revealed. The oak tree is implied in the acorn. It manifests as a tree only within the context of the succession of the individual changes we call time. From seed to seedling, to mature tree, to firewood and ash, each stage reveals something about the nature of the oak tree.

Each object has its own unique internal clock determined by the mix and interplay of the gunas.

Condition

This refers to the state the object is in: coming into being, strengthening, whole, deteriorating, or dissolving out of being. Every object passes through all five stages unless acted upon by an outside force. The orderly succession of evolutionary changes can be altered by its environment, which can enhance, hamper, interrupt, or halt it. The natural evolution of the oak tree can be altered by factors such as lightning, weather, fire, or human or other outside interventions.

The three factors mentioned in this sutra—form, character, and condition—can also explain how nirodha, environment, and effort interact to bring about the transformation of the mind.

The evolutionary parallels between sense objects and the mind may not be immediately apparent, because we usually regard the transformation of the mind as an act of individual will, while evolution in Nature is considered to be governed by laws such as Darwin's natural selection and survival of the fittest or by Divine Will (*see commentary on sutra 4.3 for a yogic view of evolution*).

PADA THREE

We've just learned that the form and the characteristics of an object are determined by the unique combination of elements that created it. Once it has come into being, its life span and condition are subject to the influence of time and environment. The degree of the object's susceptibility to factors of environment and time is also determined by the combination of elements that make up that object. In all cases, time, environment and other external forces help reveal something of the latent potentials or hidden qualities of the object.

For example, a cup can be made of clay, paper, or quartz. The rate of change we can perceive in the cups is determined by the material they are made of and by the influence of external forces. For example, a clay cup lasts longer than a paper one, unless the clay cup is in a harsh environment and the paper cup is in a sealed, climate-controlled vault.

Now let's apply this understanding to development of nirodha one-pointedness. A mind swayed by externalization is not stable. It is like a paper cup in a harsh environment. Changes happen quickly because the mind is easily distracted and influenced by externals.

As the mind develops nirodha, it becomes more sattwic, more stable, more able to withstand distractions and restless roaming. It is like the clay cup. Due to nirodha, the mind is populated and influenced by samskaras and modifications that have ceased identifying with and yearning for fulfillment from external experiences. The influence of outside forces is reduced. When the mind focuses within, it is less frequently disturbed by restless promptings from the subconscious and becomes more focused on understanding the nature of consciousness and self-identity, intent on following them both back to their source. However, though it has been transformed by nirodha, the mind is still under the sway of the three gunas.

As the mind continues its progression, it finally reaches a state of steady one-pointedness, the most stable state it can know. It is like a quartz cup sealed in a climate-controlled vault. The utter stability, clarity, and objective discernment of nirodha are the natural manifestations of the mind's potentials waiting to unfold in time.

How do we get to this stable condition from where we are now? The mind is transformed by a synergism of self-effort (the increasing influence of nirodha through practice and nonattachment) and environmental factors (life experiences and lifestyle choices) which remove obstacles to evolution (*see sutra* 4.3). Therefore, knowing the power of regularity, students of Yoga are resolute in engaging in daily practices. Through regular practice alone, habits that are not conducive to spiritual growth naturally begin to fall away. At the same time, progress can be accelerated when practice is performed in a favorable environment. It is beneficial to turn our attention to various aspects of life such as living quarters, livelihood, diet, recreation, and physical activities. Our examination of these factors may lead us to make adjustments in our environment and lifestyle to maximize the effects of effort and minimize any distracting influences.

3.14. The substratum (Prakriti) continues to exist, although by nature it goes through latent, uprising, and unmanifested phases.

Prakriti remains a constant. It is the substratum of all the changes and phases that objects pass through. Latent (*santa* or quieted) refers to the form(s) of the object now in the past, uprising indicates the present phase, and unmanifested refers to an object's potential, the transformations yet to come.

3.15. The succession of these different phases is the cause of the differences in stages of evolution.

The effects of time and environment on an object, which happen in an orderly and predictable manner, are the reasons we see changes (what we call evolution) in objects in Nature.

The reason we see changes in objects is because the interplay of the gunas brings changes in the perceivable form of objects; characteristics that have existed in the past (latent) appear in the present (uprising) and wait to express in the future (unmanifested).

The use of the term "evolution" implies direction. Does Sri Patanjali give any clues as to the nature of this direction?

> The seen is of the nature of the gunas: illumination, activity, and inertia. It consists of the elements and sense organs, whose purpose is to provide both experiences and liberation to the Purusha (*sutra* 2.18).

PADA THREE

The seen exists only for the sake of the Seer (*sutra* 2.21).

It is for the Seer's purpose that Prakriti exists, and that purpose is the liberation of the individual.

Next begins a series of sutras that detail various *siddhis* (attainments) from the practice of samyama; the technique of applying dharana, dhyana, and samadhi toward any object.

3.16. By practicing samyama on the three stages of evolution comes knowledge of past and future.

By focusing on the inner workings of evolution (the birth, development, and subsiding of objects in Nature), the yogi can directly perceive the origin and evolutionary direction of any object or event.

Before continuing with the list of attainments, let's pause to examine why so many sutras revolve around this the practice of samyama.

Directly or indirectly, all questions proceed from one: Who am I? This one question gives birth to countless others, such as: What is the nature of life and the cosmos? When did it start? What is time? What is the purpose of life? Everything we study, observe, and investigate can reveal a little bit about our nature and purpose.

Today, we look to scientific methodologies, high-tech instruments, computer analyses, and double-blind studies to reveal the mysteries of the universe. Scientific investigation in Sri Patanjali's day may have lacked the advantages of sophisticated instrumentation, but exquisitely subtle observations were made in a different way. The source of matter and the boundaries of the universe were plumbed by harnessing the power of the mind to a remarkable degree.

The primary source for this knowledge can be found in the tenets, stories, parables, and myths of spiritual traditions. The great insights attained by the ancients are often not appreciated as scientific because the language and imagery of scripture is often poetic in nature. The *Yoga Sutras* present teachings on the nature of the universe that range from the most subtle aspects of mind and matter to factors that affect evolution. These teachings are observable phenomena. Since we are not expected to be blind followers, we are provided with a methodology for the scientific investigation of the teachings: a way for the teachings to be verified. The technical term for the method is samyama.

Samyama is a way of obtaining knowledge through experience: direct perception of the highest order. There are no intermediary words, biases, blind spots, faults of logic, no history, no agendas— just the mind confronting an object head-on, penetrating it to its core. The knowledge brought by samyama is therefore different from that obtained by the study of books or everyday experience, which is usually clouded to some degree by the factors mentioned above. Samyama is scientific investigation with no instrument other than the mind, which can then fully focus on, penetrate, and master perceivable objects. The mind can continue probing deeper still, exploring all manner of subtle phenonomena, searching for the cause behind each effect until the source of all matter is known.

Knowledge always brings at least some measure of control. Familiarity with the inner workings of the atom has brought control over it and has unlocked the key to incredible power. Samyama can unlock the secrets of any object and is the way that yogis attain seemingly miraculous powers.

The attainments listed offer a radically different understanding of the nature of reality from that offered up by our ordinary senses. The solidity of matter, the predictability of its nature and character, the powers and limitations of the mind, and ultimately our place in the universe are not what they seem to be. These attainments not only provide insight, they also tear down the false walls of a universe that seemingly binds us, false limitations that prevents us from knowing creation as it truly is and from realizing that we are in fact, the Purusha.

For example, what does it do to your conception of reality when you come across a sutra that states—as fact—that through samyama you can gain the strength of an elephant? (*See sutra* 3.25.) It's likely similar to when you learn that according to modern science, the solidity of matter is an illusion. In truth, objects are composed of relatively vast expanses of space interspersed with a bit of substance. In the former instance, the understanding of the limitations of human physiology is torn down; in the latter case, the solidity of the world of matter. In both cases, the message is the same: there is more to life than meets the eye.

3.17. A word, its meaning, and the idea behind it are normally confused because of superimposition upon one another. By samyama on the word (or sound) produced by any being, knowledge of its meaning is obtained.

We can ascertain the meaning behind any sound or word by samyama. What a great boon to communication! We become privy to the true motivation of any speaker. We could also understand the intent behind the sounds that our pets make.

3.18. By direct perception, through samyama, of one's mental impressions, knowledge of past births is obtained.

Reincarnation is not simply a comforting philosophy or a theory that is believed because it makes rational sense. It is a reality that can be directly perceived (*see sutra 1.7, where direct perception is given as a source of right knowledge*).

By turning our attention inward, directly observing subconscious impressions, and noting when, how, and why they manifest, we will see themes, keynote thoughts—the essential plotline around which our current life was formed. When we directly perceive these themes through samyama, we will find that they originated from past actions and latent impressions of previous births. By following this path even further, we will discover that those past impressions were the product of former incarnations.

Reincarnation completes the law of karma. We need to face the consequences—good or bad—of every act. If circumstances do not permit it this time around, we must be reborn to finish the cycle.

Related Sutras: 3.23 and 4.7: Discuss the different types of karma.

3.19. By samyama on the distinguishing signs of others' bodies, knowledge of their mental images is obtained.

There is the story about Abraham Lincoln that took place when he was interviewing potential personal assistants. After meeting with one man who seemed to be ideal for the position, Mr. Lincoln's advisor asked if he should go ahead and hire the man.

"No, I think we should interview a few more."

"Why? He has impeccable qualifications and experience."

"I didn't like his face," replied the chief executive.

"You didn't like his face! I don't understand. Is that any reason not to hire him? After all, why should he be faulted for how he looks?"

The president replied with a question: "How old is he?"

"Forty years old."

"That's right. Forty years old. Any man forty years old is responsible for his own face."

President Lincoln was utilizing basic human skills. We do it ourselves when we form initial impressions of individuals largely based on two visible factors:

- Their physical structural features, which have manifested due to past karmas (past thoughts and actions help shape our physical features)
- Facial expressions: the way their minds hold those features in place

We have an instinctive reaction (in part due to biological impulses) to the physical appearance of others and form conscious or subconscious impressions concerning at least some aspects of their character. For example, we may be wary of people whose eyes are too close together or instinctively know that the person whose shoulders are habitually hunched up around their ears is a fearful type.

The fact that people's appearance can be so different when they sleep (when the conscious mind releases its hold to the subconscious) demonstrates that the content of the mind helps arrange the physical structures of their face. In other words, the character of the individual determines facial expressions and body language.

By samyama, the yogi can more deeply and accurately tune into all these signs and even more subtle ones to gain knowledge of the nature of the mind of an individual.

3.20. But this does not include the support in the person's mind (such as motive behind the thought, and so on), as that is not the object of the samyama.

By observation of the body, we can know the nature of the mind but not the underlying motives.

3.21. By samyama on the form of one's body (and by) checking the power of perception by intercepting light from the eyes of the observer, the body becomes invisible.

The ancient yogis understood that in order for perception to take place, waves of light need to be taken in by the senses and passed on to the appropriate brain center. The eyes need to catch the light reflected off an object to perceive it. Yogis can intercept the light that reflects off their bodies, making it seem that they have disappeared.

3.22. In the same way, the disappearance of sound (and touch, taste, smell, and so on) is explained.

That the yogi's mastery extends to such subtle areas has already been suggested.

Related Sutra: 1.40: *"Gradually one's mastery in concentration extends from the smallest particle to the greatest magnitude."*

3.23. Karmas are of two kinds: quickly manifesting and slowly manifesting. By samyama on them or on the portents of death, the knowledge of the time of death is obtained.

The yogi can perform samyama on the subconscious karmic seeds waiting to sprout. Some are appropriate to this current life circumstance and come to fruition quickly; others find the current life inconducive to their growth.

Through samyama, yogis directly perceive the karmas that have brought the present life into being and that have been the basis for vital lessons. When the lessons have been completed, the yogis know it is time to graduate from the present birth. After graduation from this birth, they may take another birth in the future, or if they have attained Self-realization, they might simply enjoy their unity with the Absolute.

Knowledge of the time of death can be advantageous, since our last thoughts are especially influential in determining the nature of future births. Spiritual thoughts will help bring a birth favorable to furthering spiritual growth, hankering after material success may bring a materially comfortable birth, and negative thoughts, an undesirable incarnation.

Since our character (based on that which has been most important to us) is revealed in our last moments, we cannot count on being able to forcefully shift our attention to uplifting images and thoughts. However, if our minds have become accustomed to dwelling on high spiritual ideals that are firmly grounded (*see sutra* 1.14), we can be assured that the next incarnation will be especially favorable for continuing our journey to Self-realization.

Related Sutra: 4.8: *"From that (threefold karma), follows the manifestation of only those vasanas (subliminal traits) for which there are favorable conditions for producing their fruits."*

3.24. By samyama on friendliness and other such qualities, the power to transmit them is obtained.

This sutra offers a wonderful way to better our own life and the lives of others. By performing samyama on a desirable quality, such as friendliness, we can attain its benefits.

Spiritual history is filled with stories of sages and saints whose mere presence mysteriously changed the lives of others. Often, without intent or effort, they transmitted these virtuous qualities, just as the sun, without intent, automatically radiates warmth and light.

The four locks and four keys of sutra 1.33 are alluded to here. By extension, we can understand this sutra to imply that we can gain such power with any virtue.

Related Sutras: 2.35–2.38: *Describe the benefits that result from perfection in the first four principles of yama: nonviolence, truthfulness, nonstealing, and continence.*

3.25. By samyama on the strength of elephants and other such animals, their strength is obtained.

The use of an image such as an elephant is only an aid. Any image that relays the idea of great strength could be substituted. The underlying principle is that the infinite power of the universe is available for the focused mind to tap into.

PADA THREE

3.26. By samyama on the light within, the knowledge of the subtle, hidden, and remote is obtained. [Note: subtle as atoms, hidden as treasure, remote as far-distant lands.]

The object of this samyama is not the Self but the light of the Self reflecting on the mind. By virtue of this samyama, the inner senses are illumined, resulting in the capacity to gain knowledge of things that are present but normally not perceivable.

Related Sutra: 1.36: "Or by concentrating on the supreme, ever-blissful Light within."

3.27. By samyama on the sun, knowledge of the entire solar system is obtained.

The sun is the center of the solar system, and all life depends on it. Know the source and you will know the manifestations. By knowing a part, you can know the whole; the whole is reflected in the part. This concept is central to Eastern healing modalities, where, for example, by taking the pulse, observing the tongue, or palpating the abdomen, the practitioner can evaluate all organs and systems. Acupuncturists use points on the ear and the scalp to treat every part of the body, iridologists can evaluate all bodily systems by examining the eyes, and reflexologists treat imbalances in any body part by massaging reflexes on the hands or feet.

3.28. By samyama on the moon comes knowledge of the stars' alignment.

The stars' alignment refers to the constellations.

3.29. By samyama on the pole star comes knowledge of the stars' movements.

The pole star is fixed in the sky; the movements of the stars are known in relation to it. Since we are considering the products of samyama and not simply ordinary observation or study, the knowledge that Sri Patanjali speaks of offers a description not only of what is, but of why. In this case, the yogi may catch a glimpse into the reasons that the stars exist.

3.30. By samyama on the navel plexus, knowledge of the body's constitution is obtained.

The navel is the source point from which we develop in the womb. Oriental medicine teaches that on the energetic level, we continue to be recreated from the navel after birth. From this knowledge there evolved a detailed system for the assessment of the health of the organs and systems of the body by visual and palpatory examination of the abdomen.

3.31. By samyama on the pit of the throat, cessation of hunger and thirst is achieved.

This would be a very practical technique for yogis living in caves, forests, or other remote areas and who often relied on alms for their sustenance.

Some powers, such as this one, are considered not too difficult to achieve. They could also serve as tests for practitioners who wonder how far their mental mastery has progressed.

3.32. By samyama on the kurma nadi, motionlessness in the meditative posture is achieved.

The *nadis* are flows of prana, or vital energy, similar to the meridians of acupuncture. Nadis are a communication and regulation system for the body-mind. *Kurma nadi*, literally, "tortoise-shaped tube," is located below the throat and refers to the function of prana that closes the eyes. This perhaps symbolizes the ability to withdraw the attention from the outside world.

The image of a tortoise suggests that symbolism can be at play in this sutra.

A tortoise is able to withdraw its head and limbs into a protective shell, just as a yogi is able to withdraw the senses from day-to-day concerns, allowing the mind to become still and quiet and preparing it for meditative practices.

In the mythology of India, the world was said to be supported on the back of a cosmic tortoise as it swam through the universe. The tortoise would be understood to represent a powerful, steady foundation.

There is a story of Lord Vishnu, who incarnated as a tortoise to support Mount Mandara, which was needed by the celestial beings to stir up the ocean of life in order to recover the nectar of immortality.

The ocean represents the chitta that is churned by the practice of meditation. The Lord's incarnation as a tortoise represents the Divine as unyielding support. The nectar stands for Self-realization.

Looking at these symbols, we can consider the kurma nadi as a regulatory center for subtle energies that, when activated by the mental focus of samyama, harmonizes the pranic currents in the body, bringing balance and stillness and making the mind fit for Self-realization.

3.33. By samyama on the light at the crown of the head (sahasrara chakra), visions of masters and adepts are obtained.

When the consciousness is lifted to the crown chakra, visions of the great saints and sages will be experienced. Another interpretation is that when consciousness functions from the crown chakra, we obtain the same spiritual vision as the masters have. Sri Patanjali did not leave us with detailed descriptions of these experiences. They are subtle and are best left to experience rather than discussion and analysis.

There are seven major *chakras* (literally, "wheels"), which are subtle centers of consciousness that although not part of the gross anatomy, are located along the spine from the tailbone to the top of the head. They represent levels of evolution:

- The chakra at the base of the spine pertains to self-preservation, our primary impulse as living beings.
- The next chakra, located behind the genitals, is principally concerned with reproduction. Once we feel safe, the desire to procreate arises.
- At the navel is the chakra that governs the assertion of the will and our interactions with others.
- The heart is the fourth chakra, the center of compassion. It is the middle chakra and the center of harmonization of body and mind. It is the core of selfless impulses, the willingness to sacrifice for the welfare of others.
- The throat is the location of the fifth chakra, which pertains to the ability to discern and communicate. It is the center for intellectual pursuits and more complex communication.
- The space between the eyebrows, the third eye, is the seat of the mind and the sense of individuality. Since it is also the center

though which subtle communication takes place, it is also called the "guru chakra."

- Finally, the crown of the head pertains to the superconscious state in which body consciousness is transcended. It is the center of pure universal awareness.

3.34. Or, in the knowledge that dawns by spontaneous intuition (through a life of purity), all the powers come by themselves.

The powers can manifest even if they are not sought after. They may spontaneously appear as the natural result of purity and a selfless, carefree mind. Since the ego is kept out of the mix, this is the best and safest way to attain these powers.

3.35. By samyama on the heart, the knowledge of the mind-stuff is obtained.

The fifth and sixth chakras (intellect and seat of the mind) might seem more likely objects for gaining knowledge of the mind-stuff; instead Sri Patanjali cites the heart, *hridaya*, as the way to attain knowledge of the mind-stuff. The mind is dependent for its existence on the ego, which is better approached through the heart. In this case "heart" refers to the core or "feeling" center of the individual, the place where motives and intent reside.

3.36. The intellect (sattwa) and the Purusha are totally different, the intellect existing for the sake of the Purusha, while the Purusha exists for its own sake. Not distinguishing this is the cause of all experiences. By samyama on this distinction, knowledge of the Purusha is gained.

Although all of creation is one, unified whole, as individuals we come to know only bits and pieces of the totality of life because we have not experienced the distinction between the Purusha and the intellect. The intellect is finite in nature and can learn of the world only through the limited and colored filter of the ego.

Recall that sattwa, translated here as "intellect," is the same as the buddhi (*see Glossary and commentary on sutra* 1.2). The qualities associated with sattwa—tranquility, balance, and illumination—are really reflections of the Purusha on the buddhi. Therefore, to experience the buddhi is to experience a facsimile of the Purusha. Logic is not up to the task of delivering this distinction to the realm of direct perception. The subtlety and power of samyama is needed to be able to discriminate between the self (reflected light) and the Self (light-giver).

Related Sutras: 2.6: "Egoism is the identification of the power of the Seer with that of the instrument of seeing (body-mind)"; 2.12: "The womb of karmas has its root in these obstacles and the karmas bring experiences in the seen (present) or in the unseen (future) births"; 2.20: "The Seer is nothing but the power of seeing"; 2.21: "The seen exists only for the sake of the Seer"; 2.23: "The union of Purusha and Prakriti causes the recognition of the nature and powers of them both"; 2.24: "The cause of this union is ignorance"; 4.25: "To one who sees the distinction between the mind and Atman, thoughts of the mind as Atman cease forever"; 4.26: "Then the mind is inclined toward discrimination and gravitates toward Absoluteness."

3.37. From this knowledge arises superphysical hearing, touching, seeing, tasting, and smelling through spontaneous intuition.

The extrasensory perceptions listed here are a by-product of the samyama on the distinction between the intellect and Purusha.

3.38. These (superphysical senses) are obstacles to (nirbija) samadhi but are siddhis in the externalized state.

These extrasensory powers are expressions of great mental power, but they still exist in the realm of relativity and are obstacles to the interiorization of mind needed for Self-realization. Actually, it's not the powers themselves that are obstacles; it's the attachment to them that obstructs progress. Under the influence of attachment, these powers can tempt egos that are not yet cleansed of selfishness and become a major obstruction to the experience of the highest samadhi.

Why, then, would Sri Patanjali bother to enumerate these extraordinary attainments? One reason is that they are a natural by-product of the search for Self-realization, and it is his responsibility to present the entirety of the spiritual experience. Another reason is that perhaps in his day, seekers might have been dazzled or frightened by charismatic individuals who exhibited these capabilities. Some of these miracle workers, abusing these powers for self-aggrandizement, would have attracted followers who wished to develop those abilities for themselves. Sri Patanjali would not have wanted to see seekers distracted from the path of Self-realization by a search for supernormal powers. So he demonstrates that the basis for these powers is a natural outcome of a clear and deeply focused mind intent on peeling back layers of nature, continually looking for the cause (the more subtle) behind the effect (the more gross). The essential principle is that mind is subtler than other objects, and the subtle is the cause and controller of the more gross.

Since every individual's path to Self-realization is unique in many ways, not all Self-realized individuals attain these powers. However, when they do manifest in the enlightened, it is a case of the Divine Will working through these great souls to accomplish some good.

Related Sutra: 3.51: "By nonattachment even to that (all these siddhis), the seed of bondage is destroyed and thus follows Kaivalya (Independence)."

3.39. By the loosening of the cause of bondage (to the body) and by knowledge of the channels of activity of the mind-stuff, entry into another body is possible.

It might be helpful to break down this sutra phrase by phrase.

By Loosening the Cause of Bondage (to the Body)

This refers to the mind's bondage to the body. It is caused by the ego, which is born of ignorance (*see sutra 2.6, which defines egoism as the identification of the power of the Seer with the instrument of seeing, the body-mind*).

By Knowledge of the Channels of Activity of the Mind-Stuff

Prachara, translated as "channels," suggests a going forth or manifestation. It is the knowledge of how the chitta manifests and works within and through a body: the subtle nerve pathways it uses, the relationship of mind-stuff to the gross physical body, and an understanding of how the chitta moves from body to body at each birth.

Entering into Another (Parasarira) Body

Many translators have rendered parasarira as "another's." This follows the tradition of the commentary by the sage Vyasa. But parasarira could be translated as "another." Therefore this sutra could be referring either to entering another individual's body or to the attainment of an intimate knowledge of the evolutionary journey of the individual's chitta from birth to birth. The latter interpretation is consistent with the discussion of the process of evolution discussed in sutras 3.13 to 3.16.

Yet another interpretation is possible. The "body" referred to could be the astral body. By withdrawing consciousness from the physical body, the yogi would be able to function through the astral body free from the limitations that the physical sheath imposes.

Whatever interpretation is preferred, the important point is that the yogi gains knowledge of the way the mind-stuff moves into, interacts with, and functions through a body. This samyama, therefore, helps to break the false identification with the body.

3.40. By mastery over the udana nerve current (the upward-moving prana), one accomplishes levitation over water, swamps, thorns, and so on and can leave the body at will.

We all have had the experience of our bodies feeling lighter—when we are so happy we feel like dancing or jumping for joy, for example. We even use the term uplifted when describing how we feel upon hearing good news.

In deeper states of meditation, the mind goes within and the prana moves upward, making the body feel light. In fact, it is not an uncommon experience for meditators whose feet have fallen asleep to have them reawaken without changing position just by the ascension of consciousness and a stronger upward movement of the udana prana.

In Christianity there are several examples of saints who spontaneously levitated. This experience came from their deep joy in prayer or worship. One such example was the Franciscan friar, Joseph of Cupertino, who would go into deep ecstatic states during masses, disrupting the service by involuntarily floating around the ceiling of the church. While this example doesn't present an example of *mastery* of the udana current, it does show that when it is strongly activated, as in ecstatic states, similar experiences as those mentioned here can result. However, in the cases of advanced yogis, the udana current can be brought under their conscious control, making the manifestations listed above possible at will.

(*See Prana in the Glossary.*)

3.41. By mastery over the samana nerve current (the equalizing prana) comes radiance that surrounds the body.

The function of *samana* prana is to maintain equilibrium in the body by transforming food into a form usable by the cells and then distinguishing between that and the waste that is to be eliminated.

The samana prana is rooted in the abdomen, the seat of our digestive "fire." By samyama on the samana nerve current, the digestive fire increases in strength and efficiency. The body gains in health and attains a healthy glow.

The fire element is also associated with intelligence, specifically as the capacity to discern what is harmful and what is beneficial. Fire—in the form of light—is associated with discrimination. The processes of transformation and discrimination are also performed on the mental level. The mind needs to digest experiences and discriminate between what is useful (appropriate for assimilation) and what is useless or harmful (to be eliminated).

By this samyama, the fire element becomes focused and refined, greatly augmenting the discriminative capacity of the mind. By this and what has been said above, a special radiance is produced. This radiance could be what we see depicted as halos or auras in spiritual artwork.

(See *Prana* in the Glossary.)

3.42. By samyama on the relationship between ear and ether, supernormal hearing becomes possible.

Ether, *akasha*, is the element associated with sound; therefore it has a special relationship with the ear.

Ether can be thought of as space. It is the first-created of all the subtle elements. We are all probably familiar with the biblical quote, *"In the beginning was the word"* (John 1.1) Before the word could be uttered, there needed to be a place in which to utter it. That place is ether.

3.43. By samyama on the relationship between the body and ether, lightness of cotton fiber is attained, and thus traveling through the ether becomes possible.

Ether (akasha), the subtlest of the elements, is the fundamental building block of the body. When our consciousness can rest on the level of ether, our bodies vibrate at its frequency and can travel by way of etheric currents, the waves of ether that permeate creation.

3.44. (By virtue of samyama on ether) vritti activity that is external to the body is (experienced and) no longer inferred. This is the great bodilessness which destroys the veil over the light of the Self.

The veil, *avarana*, is the same word used by Sri Patanjali in sutra 2.52, "As *its result (of the practice of pranayama) the veil over the inner light is destroyed.*"

This siddhi is a further attainment derived from samyama on the relationship between the body and space (akasha) when the individual experiences the physical borders of the body beginning to blend or expand into the infinite ether around it. The ego-sense begins to experience itself as unfettered to a particular place.

Our identification with the body and mind is so ingrained that breaking it is no easy task. As long as this identification exists, we feel that our thoughts are generated from our body-mind, and therefore the location of our awareness is limited to wherever our body resides. But by samyama on ether, we come to experience the mind as omnipresent and understand that it exists and functions outside the body as well as within it. This is the "great bodilessness" referred to in this sutra.

Redefining Our Self: A Review of Sutras 3.36 to 3.44

If we examine sutras 3.36 to 3.44, we will see that Sri Patanjali has systematically expanded the boundaries (the ways we define and limit) of self-identity;

- In 3.36, we are reminded that the mind and the Self are different and that failure to make that distinction enmeshes us in the cycles of worldly experience. If we can loosen our identification with the body-mind, we will experience a gradual expansion of consciousness.
- Our senses can become superphysical (3.37 *and* 3.42).
- We can function free of the limitations of the physical body (3.39).

- Because our bodies are not the rigid enclosures we imagined, we can develop the capacity to levitate, leave, and enter the body at will and travel by way of etheric currents (3.39 *and* 3.40).
- The increased equilibrium resulting from enhanced transformative and discriminative powers brings a special radiance (3.41).
- Along the way, Sri Patanjali pauses to remind us that these powers are obstacles to the highest samadhi (3.38).
- Finally, we come to sutra 3.44, in which we experience that consciousness was never bound to a particular place. A great veil over the inner Light is lifted.

3.45. Mastery over the gross and subtle elements is gained by samyama on their essential nature, correlations, and purpose.

Let's examine this sutra point-by-point.

Gross and Subtle Elements

The gross elements are all that we can see, touch, smell, hear, and taste. Beneath the level of gross elements is the level of subtle elements. The subtle is the cause of the gross.

Essential Nature

Subtler than the subtle elements, there is the characteristic essence of a thing: the *solidity* of a rock, the *liquidity* of water, the *mobility* of air, for example.

Correlations

Going deeper, we come to the level of the gunas, which are common to all objects. The gunas have an active relationship— a correlation—to the above factors.

Purpose

Finally, behind all matter, from gross to the most subtle, is the purpose—the *why*—of matter. Why do elements exist at all, and why is there an almost infinite number of objects? Sri Patanjali has told us that matter exists for the sake of the Self (*see sutra* 2.21, *"The seen exists only for the sake of the Seer"*).

By samyama on the above points, the yogi achieves mastery over matter.

3.46. From that (mastery over the elements) comes attainment of anima and other siddhis, bodily perfection, and the non-obstruction of bodily functions by the influence of the elements.

The eight major siddhis alluded to are *anima*, "to become very small'; *mahima*, "to become very big"; *laghima*, "to become very light"; *garima*, "to become very heavy"; *prapati*, to reach anywhere"; *prakamya*, "to achieve all one's desires"; *isatva*, "the ability to create anything"; and *vasitva*, "the ability to command and control everything."

The mastery over matter achieved in the previous sutra is what brings these attainments.

In its original form, this sutra only lists three siddhis: becoming minute, bodily perfection, and freedom from afflictions caused by the constituents of Nature (gunas). The rest of the list, handed down through tradition, adds references to mental attainments as well.

3.47. Beauty, grace, strength, and adamantine hardness constitute bodily perfection.

The bodily perfection mentioned in this and the previous sutra is the result of the samyama (*see sutra* 3.45) that brings mastery over the gross and subtle elements.

The practices of Yoga increase, refine, and harmonize the functioning of prana in the body. Each cell becomes charged with powerful spiritual vibrations and operates at optimal efficiency.

In light of this, we might wonder why some great yogis have suffered from physical ailments. What we see as physical ailments are residual karmas that are being allowed to manifest from a time prior to Self-realization.

Great yogis experience that they are not their body. They may fulfill their duty to the body by trying various treatments while remembering that the body is composed of the elements of Prakriti and that whatever is composed of elements will one day dissolve back into those elements. They understand that Nature will take its inevitable course and they accept their physical trials as God's will. Their minds remain at peace.

3.48. Mastery over the sense organs is gained by samyama on the senses as they correlate to the process of perception, the essential nature of the senses, the ego-sense, and to their purpose.

This parallels sutra 3.45. Instead of turning the attention to matter, here the yogi examines the act of perception and how it relates to the ego and the sense organs.

Knowledge leads to mastery. By knowing the essential nature and purpose of the senses, the role they play in the act of perception, and how they work with and help maintain the ego-sense, the yogi gains control over the senses.

This samyama can also provide at least some insight into the fact that the Purusha—not the ego-sense operating through the senses—has consciousness of its own.

3.49. From that, the body gains the power to move as fast as the mind, the ability to function without the aid of the sense organs, and complete mastery over the primary cause (Prakriti).

Complete mastery of matter comes only after mastering the sense organs and ego.

The Power to Move as Fast as the Mind

This is not a reference to the rapid transit of the body through space. That has already been discussed. It refers to the ability of the mind to function without the hindrance that the normal process of perception imposes.

Ability to Function without the Aid of Sense Organs

The senses are gateways for a great deal of knowledge, and the mind uses them in the normal course of perception. But the sense organs are also a limitation, since they can function only within the relativities of gross matter. The mind of the adept, having transcended the physical nature, of which the senses are a part, can function without them. This results in the ability to gain knowledge that is instantaneous, intuitive, and immediate. It is a high order of direct perception.

Complete Mastery over the Primary Cause

The "primary cause" refers to Prakriti.

3.50. By recognition of the distinction between sattwa (the pure reflective aspect of the mind) and the Self, supremacy over all states and forms of existence (omnipotence) is gained, as is omniscience.

The subject of this sutra is the veil that separates the self (ego) from the Self. The distinction between the Self and its reflection in a perfectly clean and undistorted mirror (pure sattwa or buddhi) is very difficult to make. But the benefits are great: it results in mastery over all levels of mind and matter, bringing omnipotence and omniscience. The loosening of the bondage (which we began discussing in 3.36) to the body-mind is almost complete. But we still have those pesky samskaras dwelling in the subconscious, capable of sprouting and causing mischief at any moment.

3.51. By nonattachment even to that (all these siddhis), the seed of bondage is destroyed and thus follows Kaivalya (Independence).

All siddhis are mental phenomena, products of a one-pointed mind. They exist within creation and are limited; therefore the yogi—even when experiencing omnipotence and omniscience—is still in bondage. To attain liberation, the yogi needs to let go of even the desire to know everything and be all-powerful!

How can we achieve nonattachment to such alluring experiences? One way is by practicing Ishwara Pranidhana (surrender to Ishwara) (*see sutras 2.1, 2.32, and 2.45*). By worship of Ishwara, we can transcend the ego along with any and every limitation that could prevent us from experiencing Self-realization.

3.52. The yogi should neither accept nor smile with pride at the admiration of even the celestial beings, as there is the possibility of his getting caught again in the undesirable.

Practitioners who have achieved a high degree of spiritual maturity often attract the admiration of others, whether they are celestial beings or our fellow earth-bound humans. The ego loves to be stroked and praised. We are warned not to let these overtures distract us from attaining Self-realization.

The celestial beings were unenlightened Yoga adepts in a former life. Their overtures may be motivated by envy of the progress the yogi has made.

Enlightenment cannot be achieved until viveka takes us beyond time and matter. The next four sutras offer a detailed description of this profound degree of discriminative discernment.

3.53. By samyama on single moments in sequence comes discriminative knowledge.

Our minds tend to misperceive the distinct individuality of moments as the blur of time. It's like watching a movie. The illusion we fall into (and willingly accept) is that the images are moving, but in reality, what we are viewing is a series of still photos traveling past the light and lens of the projector.

Time is how we perceive change. This samyama unveils time in its most elemental form, as distinct waveforms of Prakriti that gradually unfold their inner nature. Self-realization requires the ability to distinguish between that which undergoes change and that which is changeless (*see sutra* 2.5, *"Ignorance is regarding the impermanent as permanent ..."*).

3.54. Thus the indistinguishable differences between objects that are alike in species, characteristic marks, and positions become distinguishable.

Normally we distinguish the differences between objects utilizing one or more of the above factors.

Species

We can readily distinguish an apple from an orange.

Characteristic Marks

If we have two oranges before us, we look for distinguishing marks: Does one have a greenish tinge or a brand label affixed to it?

Position

Lastly, if the two objects before us are identical in species and characteristics, we can distinguish them by their position in space. One orange is in the refrigerator, the other in your hand.

But what if we lost these three factors? The yogi, whose discriminative discernment has evolved to a remarkable degree, could still discern the difference.

Related Sutra: 4.14: See the commentary, which gives a possible explanation of how this distinction can be made.

3.55. The transcendent discriminative knowledge that simultaneously comprehends all objects in all conditions is the intuitive knowledge (which brings liberation).

This is the zenith of viveka. It is "transcendent" because it goes beyond the omniscience mentioned in sutra 3.50. It is a complete and flawless experience of the entirety of the created universe in all phases, changes, and conditions—past, present, and future—all at once.

3.56. When the tranquil mind attains purity equal to that of the Self, there is Absoluteness.

This is the natural evolution of the discrimination described in 3.55. The mind returns to the state of pure sattwa. When the mirror becomes completely clean and undistorted, it is transparent to the Self. It is then that we can understand how we can, in the words of Lord Jesus, *"Be perfect even as your heavenly father is perfect"* (Matthew 5.48).

Review of Sutras 3.45 to 3.56

This group of sutras can make you dizzy. They are technically worded and a little tricky to understand. As is often the case, the underlying principles are not so thorny. They are detailed accounts of how the practice of samyama leads to the final stages of two Yoga practices that were introduced earlier: discriminative discernment (viveka) (*see sutra* 2.26), and non-attachment (vairagya) (*see sutras* 1.15 *and* 1.16). Then, in sutra 3.56, we arrive at the state of spiritual independence, Kaivalya.

Discriminative Discernment. Discriminative discernment is applied in two contexts:
- In the process of perception—matter, ego-sense, and the Self. This path leads to omnipotence and omniscience. (*See sutras* 3.45, 3.48, *and* 3.50.)
- In the role that time plays in revealing not only the nature

of objects but their impermanence as well. The mind comes to be able to comprehend all objects in all conditions simultaneously. This is another way of speaking of omniscience. (*See sutras 3.53 and 3.55.*)

Discriminative discernment in either context gives the yogi the ability to distinguish between that which changes and that which is changeless—which is what is needed to make the final distinction between the individual self and the Purusha and attain Self-realization.

In sutra 3.45, mastery over the gross and subtle elements is gained by samyama on their essential nature, correlations, and purpose. Sutra 3.48 shifts from the *objects* of perception to the *process* of perception and its principle components, the sense organs and ego. Again, samyama brings mastery. Sutra 3.50 moves from the process of perception to contemplation of the *perceiver*. This involves making the distinction between the pure element of sattwa and the Self (Seer). Making this distinction brings omnipotence and omniscience.

Sutra 3.53 teaches that by making samyama on single moments (which are part of Prakriti), discriminative discernment is strengthened. The yogi comes to understand that we call "time" is central to how we measure perceived changes in sense objects. Sutra 3.55 describes discriminative discernment that is so refined, steady, and subtle that the yogi simultaneously apprehends all matter in all its states. It's something like perceiving an entire movie in a micro-moment, except that the experience of this level of discriminative discernment is infinitely more vast, complex, and amazing. It is what opens to door to Self-realization.

Nonattachment. To be forever free from the delusion that anything outside the realization of the Self can bring lasting fulfillment is the second factor necessary to attain enlightenment. This is reflected in sutra 3.51 where we are taught that we need to be nonattached not only to the siddhis but to the lofty gains described in the five sutras listed above. Only then can we experience Independence, Self-realization.

Independence. We are finally free. Sutra 3.56 states that the distinction between that which changes and that which is changeless was made possible by the mind attaining purity equal to that of the Self. The mind has become perfectly still, clear, and tranquil. It has become a faultless mirror capable of reflecting the fullness of the Self.

For individuals who stand firm in their resolve to realize the highest, the reward is almost unthinkably great: the end of suffering, doubt, and craving, which evaporate like a nightmare upon awakening. Those who persevere experience the complete and utter fulfillment of realizing their true identity as the eternal Self. They experience peace, joy, and love everywhere and at all times.

Pada Three Review

1. Sri Patanjali finishes the discussion of the eight limbs with dharana (concentration), dhyana (meditation), and samadhi (absorption), the more internal of the eight limbs. The three limbs are presented as a continuum, a process of gradual development in mental mastery.

2. As a preparation for the presentation of the extraordinary powers that may result from the practice of Yoga, Sri Patanjali explains that everything we experience as life is nothing other than the interaction and relationship of waves of Prakriti.

3. The remainder of Pada Three consists primarily of a listing of the various siddhis (accomplishments or powers). Sri Patanjali does not hesitate to provide this list but states that although most people would consider them alluring wonders, attachment to them is an obstacle to nirbija samadhi.

The list of siddhis is a list of attainments that cover a wide range of categories, including:
- The immediately practical (relieving hunger and thirst)
- The inner workings of the natural world (the arrangement and movement of stars and planets)
- Apparently superhuman abilities (becoming invisible, flying)
- Almost unimaginable mental feats (the ability to comprehend all objects in all conditions)

4. This section ends with a description of the final stages that lead to the ultimate goal: the direct experience of the Absolute.

PADA THREE

What to Do

Continue with your practices.

Try to deepen your meditation. You could extend the time a little or add another sitting.

If your practices seem stalled or stale, find ways to reinspire yourself. Reading uplifting spiritual books or chanting are good options. One of the best is to associate with other seekers. Environment is stronger than will.

Become more aware of how your mind behaves during the course of the day. Find opportunities to practice keeping the mind focused and nonattached in every situation.

Constantly remind yourself of the goals you have set. Write them down, post them on your refrigerator, hang them near your phone or computer—do anything you can think of to keep yourself on track.

Don't let any setbacks stop you. Every great yogi has suffered through difficult times before achieving success. Let your challenges inspire you to unfold your best—your untapped strength and creativity.

Pada Four
Kaivalya Pada: Portion on Absoluteness

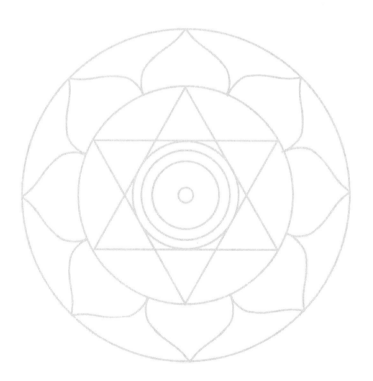

Inside Pada Four

The final pada covers a fascinating array of subjects, all leading to the experience of the highest enlightenment. Like a great lawyer, Sri Patanjali's summation is masterful, emphasizing the important aspects of his philosophy while uncovering the drama that characterizes and enlivens spiritual life.

The subject of evolution is addressed, as is the reality of the outside world. This leads to a magnificent set of sutras that draw the distinction between the mind, which has no consciousness of its own, and the Purusha, consciousness itself.

Then, beginning with sutra 4.29, he sprints to the very brink of Self-realization by introducing *dharmamegha samadhi*, a state experienced by the yogi who has achieved perfect discrimination. At this stage the seeker experiences an almost irresistible pull toward union with the Absolute.

Key Principles:
- Cause of evolution
- The inner workings of subconscious impressions
- Contrasting the mind with the Purusha

Key Practices:
- Making the distinction between the mind and the Atman

Other Key Terms:
- *Vasanas*: subconscious traits; desires
- *Dharmamegha samadhi*: cloud of dharma samadhi
- *Siddhi*: accomplishment, occult power, any unusual faculty or capability

Pada Four
Kaivalya Pada: Portion on Absoluteness

The first eleven sutras address evolution, paying particular attention to the role that our actions play in the process of change.

4.1. Siddhis are born of practices performed in previous births, or by herbs, mantra repetition, asceticism, or samadhi.

Before moving on to new topics, Sri Patanjali briefly summarizes the various means given in the last pada for attaining the siddhis.

Previous Births

God has not arbitrarily given gifts to people who are born with siddhis. They put forth efforts in previous births and are now experiencing the fruits of their labors.

Herbs

There are and have always been those who seek a chemical short-cut to spiritual achievements.

Mantra Repetition

Although the concentrated repetition of any mantra can bring siddhis as a side effect, this sutra is probably referring to the use of mantras that are meant to produce specific results. There are mantras that can heal, manifest certain events or objects, or bring many other siddhis.

Asceticism

Those who willingly accept suffering and engage in a rigorous course of spiritual practices develop great mental strength and may experience siddhis as an outcome of their disciplines.

Samadhi

Through the stillness, depth, and purity of samadhi, the siddhis may also come.

The main teaching is that siddhis should not be the goal. In an impure mind, siddhis can feed the ego. However, if they come as a natural by-product of a selfless, dedicated practice,

PADA FOUR

they will have manifested when it is natural and beneficial for them to do so.

The next two sutras deal with evolution through reincarnation.

4.2. The transformation of one species into another is brought about by the inflow of nature.

The force of evolution is innate to all beings and objects. It is the nature of Prakriti to reveal latent potentialities from birth to rebirth: from embryo to fetus, to birth, maturation, old age, death, and then rebirth.

Since *jati*, translated as "species," also means "birth," this sutra also refers to the gradual process of evolution that takes place from birth to birth for an individual.

4.3. Incidental events do not directly cause natural evolution; they just remove the obstacles as a farmer (removes the obstacles in a watercourse running to his field).

Within the sinner, the saint waits to manifest. The heart of the Buddha lies within everyone. Our nature is Divine; nothing needs to be added to reach enlightenment. Instead, all our effort is focused on removing the obstacles that have been barring the expression of our divinity. The latent qualities—the potentialities—of every object in Prakriti naturally express when obstacles are removed. Evolution, then, is a manifestation of the inherent nature of every object and being.

Natural selection and survival of the fittest—the theory that competition is the prime mover of evolution—provide an incomplete understanding of the cause of evolution. If competition for food, shelter, and reproduction ceased, evolution would still continue due to other influences. The sun, rain, and soil help the seed unfold its hidden nature as a flower. Likewise, our interactions with others—good or bad—help bring out our strengths and weaknesses. Every climatic, political, spiritual, astronomical, biological, artistic, and commercial event is an "incidental event," an occurrence that can remove obstacles to evolution.

The topic of evolution continues over the next three sutras with a discussion of the development of individual consciousness.

4.4. Individualized consciousness proceeds from the primary ego-sense.

Understanding this sutra is easier if we review the Sanskrit first:

Nirmana chittani asmita matrat. Nirmana from *ma*, "to measure, to allocate, apportion, make, create"; *chittani*, "multiple individual consciousnesses, mind-stuffs"; *asmita*, "ego-sense"; *matrat*, "alone, primary, from only."

There are two schools of thought regarding the meaning of this and the two sutras that follow. The first school examines these sutras in the context of evolution; the second school regards these sutras as an extension of the discussion of the siddhis.

From an evolutionary point of view, these three sutras are understood as describing the origin of individual consciousness and its relation to the unconditioned consciousness that is the Purusha. So in this context, nirmana chittani is regarded as the "individualized mind-stuffs" that evolve from asmita matrat, the "primordial ego" (*mahat* in Sankhya philosophy). Asmita matrat is unparticularized "I-am-ness" which makes the phenomenon of all individuality possible.

The second school of thought is influenced by the sage Vyasa's commentary. His interpretation, based on the understanding that these sutras are an extension of the discussion of the siddhis, relies on different shades of meaning for the same words. Nirmana chittani is interpreted as "artificially created mind-stuffs," and asmita matrat refers to the yogi's own ego as the source of those "manufactured" minds. These sutras are therefore seen to be discussing the ability of yogis to consciously create other minds for the purpose of accelerating the purging of their past karmas or for increasing their ability to serve others.

4.5. Although the activities of the individualized minds may differ, one consciousness is the initiator of them all.

Chitta ekam, translated as "original mind-stuff," is another way of referring to the principle of asmita matrat.

Asmita matrat creates the appearance of many individual consciousnesses with separate "lives" and activities. In truth, there is only one all-pervading awareness behind all egos. The pure, undivided consciousness of the Purusha pervades all of Prakriti's manifestations.

4.6. Of these (the different activities in the individual minds), what is born from meditation is without residue.

The residue referred to in this sutra is subconscious impressions, samskaras, which spur the mind to relentless activity.

Vritti activity leaves an accumulation of impressions—memories—that dwell in the subconscious mind. Since selfish desires lurk behind most vritti activity, the resulting subconscious accumulations are a source of future pain; they nudge the mind toward a never-ending search for new diversions. The samskaras left by most mental activity are like a sack of karmic seeds waiting to sprout.

Thoughts that arise out of meditation are different. The impressions left by meditation encourage deeper excursions into equanimity and stillness. The whirling of the vrittis cease as the mind settles on one object. The samskaras left by meditation are unified in purpose; they lead to the transcendence of ignorance. In meditation, the landscape of the mind is not marred by longings but marked by an organic movement toward Self-realization. These samskaras leave no accumulation; they are without residue.

We now come to the last in this series of sutras on evolution. This time, the emphasis is on karma (cause and effect) and its relationship with desires, subconscious impressions, and the evolution of individual character traits.

4.7. The karma of the yogi is neither white (good) nor black (bad); for others there are three kinds (good, bad, and mixed).

Yogis who have eliminated ignorance do not create any karma—good or bad. They are liberated beings. Their actions no longer serve to further their evolution, since their efforts have already led them to the highest spiritual state.

Those in whom ignorance continues to perform its illusory dance must face the consequences of the karma that ego-centered actions have created: pleasurable, painful, or mixed.

Related Sutra: 2.12: "The womb of karmas has its root in these obstacles, and the karmas bring experiences in the seen (present) or in the unseen (future) births."

4.8. From that (threefold karma) follows the manifestation of only those vasanas (subliminal traits) for which there are favorable conditions for producing their fruits.

To understand this sutra, it will be useful to briefly discuss three principles:

Samskaras: subconscious impressions

Karmasaya: depository of karmic residue

Vasanas: subliminal personality traits, tendencies, and potentialities that form and help maintain patterns of habit

Samskaras

Every thought, word, and deed (whether done consciously or unconsciously) becomes a samskara. Samskaras function as subliminal activators, constantly propelling the conscious mind into further thought and action.

Karmasaya

No action is without its reaction. All reactions are stored as subtle impressions in the subconscious mind. The receptacle for karma is called the karmasaya. There are three kinds of karma found in the karmasaya: those being expressed and exhausted in this birth (*prarabdha karma*); new karma created during this birth (*agami karma*); and latent karma waiting to be fulfilled in future births (*sancita karma*).

Vasanas

Vasanas are a subcategory of samskaras. They are subconscious impressions that come together, irrespective of their order of creation, to create a subset of impressions: a "family" of related impressions. Since vasanas induce a person to repeat actions, they are sometimes referred to as subtle desires.

Vasanas form individual personality traits and patterns of habit. They represent self-identity formed under the influence of ignorance (avidya). In other words, personality traits can exist only in an environment which supports the ego-sense and the mistaken belief that we are not the Purusha.

The coming-together of related vasanas is the process that brings forth the karma of this birth (prarabdha karma) from the karmasaya. The vasanas are, in effect, channels through which the evolutionary force of Prakriti manifests, expressing as the birth of the individual and the experiences that will be encountered in that life.

PADA FOUR

This explains why we don't always face the results of our current actions in this birth. Karmas need the proper environment to come to fruition. Therefore some of the karmas we must face are kept in abeyance by the time (the point in history) of our birth and by our current environment, social status, and place. The time necessary for the fulfillment of these karmas could extend from minutes or hours to days, years, or lifetimes. Only when the circumstances are appropriate will a karma surface.

The practical teaching of this sutra is that environment is an extremely important factor in spiritual growth. Vasanas of gambling will find the surroundings of a monastery inhospitable. On the other hand, spiritual vasanas will have a difficult time germinating in Las Vegas casinos.

(*See Glossary to compare Vasanas to Samskaras. Also see Samskaras in the Sutra-by-Subject Index and sutra 4.24.*)

Experience It

As the saying goes, "As you think, so you become." It is very beneficial to create a home environment that supports Yoga practice.

With this in mind, stroll through the rooms of your home. Note the kind of pictures and decorations that adorn your living space. Take an inventory of your music and book collection, noting which types you have on hand. Is your environment uplifting? Does it inspire you to be a better—more loving, compassionate, clear-thinking—person?

Yogis can benefit by taking a hint from those who aspire to Olympic gold. The walls of their rooms are crowded with pictures of past champions. The first thing they see upon awakening and the last thing they see before retiring will be their heroes and heroines. Similarly, our living space should contain at least some pictures, paintings, or statues of great sages and saints, deities, serene landscapes, or uplifting sayings.

We should also take care concerning the people with whom we socialize. Do our associates partake in negative activities: gossiping, backbiting, and so on? Do they influence our thinking and behavior in ways that do not support Yoga's objective of having an easeful body, a peaceful mind, and a useful life?

We do not have to abandon our associations in order to practice Yoga, but we should heighten our awareness of the influence they have on our happiness. A nonconducive environment, if sufficiently detrimental, can undermine our spiritual life. On the other hand, practice and nonattachment performed in the proper environment produce fruits most quickly.

4.9. Vasanas, though separated (from their manifestation) by birth, place, or time, have an uninterrupted relationship (to each other and the individual) due to the seamlessness of subconscious memory and samskaras.

This sutra sounds more complicated than it is.

Vasanas—which make up the characteristics of our personality—do not necessarily manifest in the order that they were created but move to the front of the line according to their intensity. Their intensity, in turn, is the result of experiences that have a deep and powerful impact on the mind.

Even though the manifestation of vasanas is not a chronologically ordered process, there is a continuous thread of individuality that links lifetimes of personalities. This has implications in regard to the cause and effect of karma. Because of the continuity of individuality, every person will face the karmas he or she has created. Although manifestations of karmas can be shared by groups (as in all the baseball fans at a particular game experiencing a rain-out), they never transfer from person to person.

Let's break down this important sutra further.

Vasanas

These are personality traits—tendencies—and were discussed in detail in the previous sutra.

Separated (from Their Manifestation) by Birth, Place or Time

As mentioned above, vasanas do not manifest in the order in which they are created. Some of the characteristics, habits, and tendencies that appear in this life may have originated many incarnations ago. Vasanas manifest when certain samskaras attain a "critical mass," when they are strengthened through repeated acts, or when a particular samskara is strong enough to gain momentum. It becomes like a whirlpool that sucks in similar samskaras, thereby becoming an influential player in building the subconscious structure of the personality.

Have an Uninterrupted Relationship

Even though the vasanas do not appear in the order of their origin, they maintain an unbroken connection to the individual that created them through the samskaras that follow the individual from birth to rebirth.

Samskaras are the thread that links together the experiences of all our past lives. Even when all conscious thought vanishes, there remains the subtle subliminal structure of the mind and the strands of samskaras that have woven themselves around it. This subconscious aspect of the mind follows us from birth to rebirth until Self-realization.

Due to the Seamlessness of Subconscious Memory and Samskaras

The word "memory" can be a little misleading in this phrase. It might be easier to think of memory not as the recollection of people, places, or things but as the remnants of action. Memories are the subset of samskaras that form the tendencies and personality traits carried into a given lifetime. In other words, there is a unity between subconscious memory and vasanas—a seamlessness in their relationship.

An analogy may help make this process even clearer. We've all seen movies that do not tell their story in chronological order. Not only that, but the story line shifts locales and character focus. But even though we temporarily leave behind an aspect of the story, we know that in the end the plot will tie together loose ends and then take us to a climax and logical conclusion. Vasanas are like the scene we are currently watching. And just as the script is the storehouse for all the scenes, samskaras are the pool from which vasanas are taken. The screen is Prakriti, the film is our lifetimes, and the light that illumines it all is the Purusha. It is just so with our own lives. All of who we are (and have been and will be) and what we experience works together to bring us to Self-realization.

4.10. Since the desire to live is eternal, vasanas are also beginningless.

The urge to live is a reflection of our eternal nature, which is existence itself. The impulse to manifest the infinite, everlasting nature of the Self is also the force behind the desire to procreate. Having children to a large extent fosters a sense that somehow we will continue beyond the years of our physical body. It is one of our everyday links to eternity.

Asishah, translated as "desire to live," can also mean "primordial will." We could then understand this sutra to refer to the will of God, which continually creates out of the store of Prakriti, then reabsorbs those manifestations into the unmanifest form. The subconscious impressions, being a part of Prakriti, are therefore also eternal.

4.11. The vasanas, being held together by cause, effect, basis, and support, disappear with the disappearance of these four.

This sutra examines the factors that bind vasanas to the individual. If we know what keeps vasanas operative, impelling us to take birth after birth, we can find a way to break the chain reaction of cause and effect which binds us.

Cause

Ignorance is the root of all subconscious impressions.

Related Sutras: 2.3 and 2.4: Discuss ignorance.

Effect

The fruits of our actions.

Related Sutra: 2.14: "The karmas bear fruits of pleasure and pain caused by merit and demerit."

Basis

The mind, which is the storehouse for all impressions.

Support

The existence of external objects that stimulate the mind to form vrittis.

Now that we know what holds vasanas together, how do we make them disappear?

Ignorance is the cause for the continuing existence of vasanas and the root of all obstacles; by overcoming ignorance through meditation and samadhi, we overcome the limitations of vasanas (*see sutras 2.10 and 2.11, "In their subtle form, these obstacles can be destroyed by resolving them back into their original cause (the ego)"; "In the active state, they can be destroyed by meditation"*).

The next six sutras offer a fascinating glimpse into the nature of sense objects, their relationship to time, and the fact that they exist independently of an individual's perception of them.

4.12. The past and future exist as the essential nature (of Prakriti) to manifest (perceptible) changes in an object's characteristics.

All potential forms of an object are within it from its inception. They exist within it as latent seeds. The previous forms of an object dissolve into the past and become dormant potentialities. The future form of an object will be the manifestation of an object's intrinsic characteristics that express according to the conditions in its environment and the external forces that act upon it. The full-grown oak rests in the acorn, as does the old diseased tree that will be cut down for making mulch. Yet within the mature oak the seed hides, waiting to appear. The seed carries within it the essence of the past, its familial predecessors, and the potentialities for all future manifestations.

Contemplating this sutra can help foster nonattachment. Our beautiful, reliable new car has hidden within it the old, dented jalopy in need of constant repair. It will manifest under the influence of time, environment, and circumstance. Anything new will someday be old and will express different qualities due to its age. And just as only a mature tree can pass on its genes to a new generation, what is aged today helps bring forth what is new tomorrow. The message is: It is wise to not hold on tightly to anything. Allow Nature to do her work and experience the beauty inherent in the flow of life.

Related Sutra: 3.55: Describes the direct perception of this phenomenon.

4.13. Whether manifested or subtle, these characteristics belong to the nature of the gunas.

The three gunas are constantly interacting with each other, with the balance among the three always shifting. Therefore the visible characteristics of the object vary over time.

The interplay of the gunas governs the manifestation, evolution, and dissolution of all objects.

Related Sutras: 2.18: "The seen is of the nature of the gunas: illumination, activity, and inertia. It consists of the elements and sense organs, whose purpose is to provide both experiences and liberation to the Purusha"; 2.19: "The stages of the gunas are specific, nonspecific, defined, and indefinable."

4.14. The reality of things is due to the uniformity of the gunas' transformation.

The "uniformity of the gunas' transformation" refers to the unique characteristics that follow an object from creation to dissolution. This distinctiveness remains consistent through all transformations until it naturally disintegrates into its component parts or is suddenly and drastically altered by an external agent. All change remains coordinated and uniform with those unique characteristics. A rock doesn't suddenly change into wood. Its rock-ness is a uniform quality that follows it from mountain to boulder to tiny pebble.

Over the decades of a human body's life, countless millions of cells are born, function, and then die. Your liver today is composed of a set of cells entirely different from seven years ago. Yet it remains a liver; *your* liver. The liver maintains its liver-ness. Its purpose and function remain the same.

Going a step further, consider that your renovated liver is composed of elements you took in from the food and water you ingested. Cellular bits of potato, apple, and lettuce are now your liver. Your food, in fact, has become your body. Of course, this happens with every organ in the body. The sense of your individual uniqueness did not fade as cells died away and were replaced.

What force gives continuity to your body, keeping its essential character distinct and intact? After eating ten-years'-worth of salad, why don't you transform into a head of iceberg lettuce, becoming cool, green, and leaflike? From a spiritual perspective, we can say that what gives and maintains individuality is purpose. Sri Patanjali teaches that all of Nature (Prakriti) exists for the purposes of the Seer (Purusha) (*see sutra 2.21, "The seen exists only for the sake of the Seer"*). This suggests that there is a specific intent for everything in creation. And that intent, the purpose for everything in creation, is to "provide both experiences and liberation to the Purusha" (*see sutra* 2.18). Intent is the infrastructure that remains intact, maintaining the uniqueness of a being or object through all its physical changes.

In sutra 3.54, we examined the ability to distinguish between indistinguishable objects. This power is possible because every object retains its own unique essence, or individuality—its reason for being (*see sutra* 3.54, "*Thus the indistinguishable differences between objects that are alike in species, characteristic marks, and positions become distinguishable*").

4.15. Due to differences in various minds, perception of even the same object may vary.

Though in the next sutra Sri Patanjali asserts that objects have a reality outside of individual perception, he leaves room for diverse experiences or interpretations of that reality. The differences in perception are due to the particularities (the limitations and biases based on past experiences) of the content of the various minds.

4.16. Nor does an object's existence depend upon a single mind, for if it did, what would become of that object when that mind did not perceive it?

Some schools of philosophy assert that there is no reality external to the individual's mind. If this were true, then when that mind turned its attention to another object, the original object would cease to exist and would not be perceivable to anyone else. Sri Patanjali offers an alternate perspective to that philosophical point.

Laying the Foundation for the Next Ten Sutras

The next ten sutras lead to the very doorstep of Self-realization, a state called dharmamegha samadhi. In order to achieve it, we need to be able to perceive the distinction between the limited awareness of the individual mind and the unlimited consciousness of the Purusha.

Before going on, it will be helpful to review the groundwork that has prepared us for these final steps.

- Pada Three discussed the siddhis: ways of understanding the relationship of matter to mind and the supremacy of mind over matter.
- The beginning of Pada Four continued the examination of matter by presenting the yogic view on evolution, including reincarnation.
- Matter was described as having a reality (an evolutionary life) independent of the mind.
- Evolution was also discussed as it related to the inherent urge and power of Prakriti to express latent potentials.
- On the more subtle level, the individual mind, the organ of perception, was seen to have the primordial ego, asmita matrat (*see sutra* 4.4) as its basis. The principle of ego as the foundation for individual minds (along with the other two facets of the mind, manas and buddhi) was introduced in the commentary on sutra 1.2.
- Meanwhile, if we examine our past karma as the immediate cause of the circumstances of our life and our experiences in it, we will come to understand our life in a more meaningful way.

In short, at this point we should have a good working understanding of matter, cause and effect, and the nature of the mind.

4.17. An object is known or unknown depending on whether or not the mind gets colored by it.

The universe is a series of waves of Prakriti which express as names and forms. The names and forms change appearance during their evolution and then dissolve back into the undifferentiated stuff of matter. These movements within Prakriti attract the mind through the senses like a snake charmer mesmerizing a cobra.

Perception takes place when an object attracts the attention of the mind through the senses. The senses pass on those impressions to the manas (recording faculty of the mind) which then conveys their presence to the buddhi (discriminative faculty) and ahamkara (the ego, which claims the impressions as its own). In other words, perception occurs when the mind gets colored by stimuli from the outside world. Subjectively, this experience makes it seem as if the mind has a consciousness of its own. In truth, our individual consciousness is the "borrowed" reflection of the Purusha on the mind. This is analogous to a mirror which can borrow the light of the sun and reflect it into a room. This basic misperception—that our mind's "own" consciousness (which is tantamount to avidya)—is what has been preventing us from realizing our True Identity as the Purusha.

Related sutras: 2.5 and 2.6: In which ignorance and egoism are defined.

4.18. The modifications of the mind-stuff are always known to the changeless Purusha, who is its lord.

In the previous sutra, we learned that individual perception is dependent on stimulation from outside sources. Therefore it is neither steady nor comprehensive. This is in stark contrast to the consciousness of the Purusha, which is unchanging and unlimited. The principle here is that changes in the mind-stuff are played against a background of pure, still, omnipresent consciousness.

The Sanskrit word translated as "Lord" is *prabhu*, which indicates something that comes first in a lineage—a progenitor. It reminds us that all thought processes came after or are born from the Purusha. The Purusha, which is unchanging awareness itself, is aware of all the changes that the mind-stuff undergoes.

Mental modifications (vrittis) occupy almost all of the mind's time, whether awake, asleep, or dreaming. For perception to occur, contrast is required. For example, most of us have been seated on a train, waiting while it picks up and discharges passengers. Next to us is another train, which is also not moving. We look out our window and suddenly notice motion. For a few moments, we are not sure whether it is our train or the other that is moving.

There are two ways to tell if our train is moving. We experience the contrast between sitting still or moving if we feel our bodies being pressed into our seat back or if we peek through the windows and notice the walls of the train station "moving" away from us. Either way, we would perceive that it is our train that is pulling away from the station. In both cases, perception occurs against a contrasting factor.

To take another example, we may decide it is time to repaint our kitchen the same shade of white we used last time it was painted. As we roll on the new paint, we might have a hard time telling where we left off, since the colors are the same. We lean this way and that and twist our heads to the side to catch the reflection of light off the wall. When we distinguish the wet from the dry, we can easily resume painting. Again, we need contrast to have perception.

Now, let's apply the principle of contrast to the topic of awareness and the ability to perceive. We are aware that we are thinking—that our mind is entertaining thoughts. How do we know? If every aspect of who we are were engaged in the thought process, there would be no one to witness it. There has to be some aspect or element that is *not* thinking, that is *not* involved in the thought process, but simply witnessing it all. That aspect is the Purusha, which is unchanging, unlimited awareness.

Sri Patanjali knows that students need to be convinced of truths before accepting them, so in the next five sutras he offers philosophical proofs of the principle presented in this sutra.

4.19. The mind-stuff is not self-luminous because it is an object of perception by the Purusha.

The mind is an object of perception (*drisyatvat*, literally, "has a seeable nature.") by the Purusha.

|The capacity of awareness that the mind has is a reflected power. It is analogous to moonlight, which is a reflection of the light of the sun. The light reflected off the moon can still help illumine our planet, but the light it gives is not its own.

The next sutra expands this proof.

4.20. The mind-stuff cannot perceive both subject and object simultaneously (which proves it is not self-luminous).

The mind-stuff can act as subject when it perceives objects or it can be an object of perception itself, but it cannot do both at once, which proves that it is not self-luminous.

I can direct the light of a flashlight on an object or on myself but not on both at the same time. At any given moment, either the object or my body will be in darkness. This is in contrast to the Purusha, which is light itself. It never knows the darkness of ignorance.

In daily life it may seem as if the mind (chitta) can be self-aware and aware of an object simultaneously. For example, I might be aware of my displeasure at the cold wind nipping my cheeks and the colorful Christmas displays I spot as I walk downtown, but not at the same moment. The subjective feeling of dual awareness is due the incredible speed at which the mind can travel back and forth between two thoughts.

4.21. If perception of one mind by another is postulated, we would have to assume an endless number of them, and the result would be confusion of memory.

This sutra provides another proof of the nonsentient nature of the mind. It is kind of a "buck stops here" argument for those who would propose that there is one aspect of the mind that specializes in watching while another goes through the various thought processes.

Let's suppose that one part of our mind witnesses another part of our mind. That means that when I smell a honeysuckle, there is a part of my mind that registers the flower, the scent, and the sniffing and still another aspect of my mind that watches all of this. But we *know* that we know. If this is true, if we are conscious of one part of the mind watching another, there must be an additional facet of the mind to watch the watcher. Perhaps this too, is true. The mind is a subtle and mysterious creature. Maybe there is still another aspect of the mind that serves as the witness. But, again, we know that we know. Is there yet another aspect of the mind?

Could this be how perception takes place? It's not really possible. We would be overwhelmed by an infinite number of parts of mind— each behaving like a tiny ego—watching one another. Which "mini-ego" would store memories? And how could we access those memories? Without access to memory, it is impossible to learn or think coherently.

Logic compels us to stop somewhere. That somewhere needs to be outside the processes of thought. We end our search with the Purusha, not as analyzer, creative thinker, or questioner, but simply as the unchanging, unwavering, nonjudgmental witness. Again we are reminded that the consciousness that seems to be an inherent property of the mind is but a reflection of the unbounded, unconditioned consciousness that is the Purusha.

4.22. When the unchanging consciousness of the Purusha reflects on the mind-stuff, the function of cognition (buddhi) becomes possible.

This sutra explains the foundation of individual consciousness.

Buddhi (also called mahat) is the first of the evolutionary manifestations of Prakriti. Being the most pure and subtle aspect of matter, it has a special "nearness" to the Purusha, which allows it to reflect the consciousness of the Purusha clearly. This is what gives buddhi the appearance of self-consciousness.

The countless minds in the universe are born of the reflection of the one Self. The following analogy may help demonstrate how this is so.

You have just washed and waxed your car. Soon afterward, a brief thunderstorm rumbles through. It is a brief storm, and a few minutes later the sunlight reemerges. On the hood of your car you notice many droplets of water. Each and every drop reflects the entire globe of the sun. Though we can view the sun in each drop, we cannot state that the totality of the sun is contained in that droplet of water. Nor can we say that the sun is affected (limited) by being reflected in the droplets. Yet the light we see and the light we use to perceive the reflected sun is the light of the sun itself. Each mind is like a droplet of water capable of reflecting light. The mind is held together by the ego, just as each drop of water is held together by surface tension.

4.23. The mind-stuff, when colored by both Seer and seen, understands everything.

The mind, in effect sits on the border between the Seer and seen. The mind-stuff, though technically part of the seen, "borrows" the power of perception from the Self. It is then in a position to get colored by or become aware of external objects. Thus we have the potential to understand all objects.

4.24. Though colored by countless subliminal traits (vasanas), the mind-stuff exists for the sake of another (the Purusha) because it can act only in association with It.

Our daily experiences might lead us to conclude that the mind exists to satisfy desires, that our bodies and minds were given to us for our own sakes—to achieve our personal goals. Daily we develop cravings and put out effort to fulfill them. When we're successful, we feel better or, more accurately, relieved. The entire process feels so natural that other purposes for the mind's existence may seem remote.

Although it may seem foreign to our daily experience of life, the mind does not exist solely to satisfy personal desires. The mind, as with everything created within Prakriti, exists to fulfill a higher purpose than personal gratification. The mind exists to serve as the immediate link to the realization of our immortal nature. Like the apple tree which fulfills its ultimate purpose when it reproduces its source, the seed from which it came, everything within Prakriti finds completion by "returning" to its source: the Purusha That's why the Purusha is referred to as prabhu—the originator—in sutra 4.18.

It is only at the level of the mind that the ultimate purpose for the existence of the mind—Self-realization—can be experienced. But the direct experience of the Self cannot be attained by logic, by amassing information, or by satisfying sense desires. In addition to these mental functions, the mind has another ability. Like a flawless mirror that perfectly reveals the sun, a still, clear mind reflects the fullness of the Self.

Related Sutras: 2.18: States that Prakriti exists to provide both experiences and liberation to the Purusha. Remember, the mind is a part of Prakriti; 4.8–4.11: More on vasanas.

4.25. To one who sees the distinction between the mind and the Atman, thoughts of the mind as Atman cease forever.

This distinction requires the ability to discern the difference between the original and a perfect copy, that is, the undistorted image of the Purusha reflected on the sattwic mind versus the Purusha itself. They look almost exactly the same. To make matters more challenging, we need to transcend the attachments we have to the reflection. We have believed for lifetimes that the reflection is who we are. It is hard to let go of that identification.

"To one who sees" refers to a deepening or shift in perception. The misidentification of Self with the mind can be said to be the product of sustained one-pointed illusion. In fact, the word translated as "thoughts," bhavana, suggests something that is the product of imagination or meditation.

Related Sutras: 2.28: States that discriminative discernment is born from the practice of the eight limbs; 3.53 and 3.54: To see other ways we can attain such discriminative discernment: "By samyama on single moments in sequence comes discriminative knowledge"; "Thus the indistinguishable differences between objects that are alike in species, characteristic marks, and positions become distinguishable."

4.26. Then the mind-stuff is inclined toward discrimination and gravitates toward Absoluteness.

There is great beauty and power in this sutra. The words in Sanskrit translated as "gravitates" are *"prak"* and *"bharam"* mean to move a weight forward, implying something like a river flowing to its home, to the ocean. If we can make the profound discriminative step that the previous sutra describes, if we can discern/experience the distinction between the mind and Self, we will experience the alluring whirlpool-like force of the Absolute guiding us toward spiritual freedom. The mind is being "moved toward the front," away from the "weight" of ignorance and forward to its source. We will feel the strength of the Self lightening our burden. We will be drawn by that power toward the state of perfect union. You would not be wrong to regard this force as love or grace.

It's not that God waits for this moment to bestow grace on us. That grace is always present and available, guiding us in countless ways. But we can't always recognize or feel it. Our mind needs to be still, clear, and free of attachment to recognize its presence.

Is there a practical benefit that we attain when we feel the pull of the Absolute? Our conscience—our inner guidance system— becomes unfailingly reliable, with virtually every prompting being an intuitive nudge that accelerates our approach to Self-realization. We will be able to distinguish a prompting from the Absolute as opposed to the call of the ego. Finally, that perplexing question, How can I know God's will? will come to a resolution. After years of feeling our way through a dark tunnel, we are now led by a clear vision of light— a light that we imagined, pursued, and theorized about but now recognize. There is no doubt; we are returning home.

4.27. In between, distracting thoughts may arise due to past impressions.

When we forget that we are the Self and fall back into misidentifi-

cation with the mind, distracting thoughts—born of ignorance—
again arise.

Related Sutra: 1.4: "At other times (the Self appears to) assume the forms of the
mental modifications."

4.28. They can be removed, as in the case of the obstacles explained before.

Sri Patanjali refers to earlier sutras in order to tie together a few
philosophical points before his final description of the highest
samadhi and finishing his treatise.

Related Sutras:

The obstacles: 1.30: "Disease, dullness, doubt, carelessness, laziness, sensuality, false perception, failure to reach firm ground, and slipping from the ground
gained—these distractions of the mind-stuff are the obstacles"; 2.3: "Ignorance,
egoism, attachment, aversion, and clinging to bodily life are the five obstacles."

The methods for their removal: 1.27–29: "The expression of Ishwara is the mystic
sound OM." "To repeat it in a meditative way reveals its meaning"; "From this practice, the awareness turns inward and the distracting obstacles vanish."; 1.32: "The
concentration on a single subject (or the use of one technique) is the best way to prevent the obstacles and their accompaniments"; 2.1 and 2.2: "Accepting pain as help
for purification, study, and surrender to the Supreme Being constitute Yoga in practice"; "They help us minimize the obstacles and attain samadhi"; 2.10 and 2.11: "In
their subtle form, these obstacles [from sutra 2.3] can be destroyed by resolving them
back into their original cause (the ego)"; In their active state, they can be destroyed by
meditation"; 2.26: "Uninterrupted discriminative discernment is the method for its
[ignorance] removal." Recall that Sri Patanjali presents the eight limbs of Yoga as the
way to attain uninterrupted discriminative discernment (sutra 2.28). Let's also
remember that back in sutra 1.12, we were given the broad-spectrum yogic "pills" of
practice and nonattachment to overcome the pitfalls of vritti activity. Yoga practice
includes any act that brings steadiness, clarity, and objectivity to the mind.

The last six sutras begin a countdown to the highest spiritual
experience.

4.29. The yogi, who has no self-interest in even the most exalted states, remains in a state of constant discriminative discernment called dharmamegha (cloud of dharma) samadhi.

We have already covered a number of different categories of samadhi. Dharmamegha samadhi is not necessarily a separate type. It is more or less a synonym for asamprajnata samadhi. But it is also a slow-motion, freeze-frame view of the maturation of asamprajnata samadhi into full Self-realization.

Before examining dharmamegha samadhi further, let's review the conditions that precede it:

- Nirodha has been developed to the point where lower levels of samadhi have been experienced, leading the yogi to the source of individual perception (*see sutra* 1.17, *samprajnata or cognitive samadhi*).

- The yogi loses interest in a search for or attachment to any and all rewards—spiritual as well as worldly. This represents *param vairagya*, the supreme state of nonattachment discussed in sutra 1.16.

- Viveka, the discriminative faculty, has reached its highest expression: the unwavering awareness of the distinction between that which changes (Prakriti) and that which is change-less (Purusha) (*see sutra* 2.26, *which introduces viveka as the means to overcome ignorance*).

- The functioning of the gunas has reached its most refined level: purified sattwa has lead to omniscience (*see sutra* 3.50); purified rajas has lead to unattached activity (*see sutra* 4.29); and tamas, cleansed of excessive heaviness, leads to a stable body capable of perfectly relaxed stillness that does not unduly impose its presence on the contemplative mind (*see sutras* 2.47 *and* 2.48 *regarding perfection in asana*).

- The pull of the Absolute that began with discerning the distinction between the mind and Self is now practically irresistible. The mind, purified of ignorance, virtually flies toward union with the Absolute as an iron bar, free of thick, encrusted rust and mud, is inextricably drawn by the force of a powerful magnet.

This brings us to defining dharmamegha samadhi. The first challenge we face in examining this state is in translating the word "dharma." It is a term brimming with important meanings, most of which fall into one of two categories:

- Virtue, law, duty, goal of life, and righteousness

- Form, characteristic, or function (the word is used this way in sutras 3.13 and 4.12)

Regardless of which definition of dharma is used, dharmamegha samadhi is the stage before nirbija samadhi, the highest enlightenment: Self-realization.

Dharmamegha Samadhi with Dharma as Virtue

Viewing dharma as virtue suggests that dharmamegha samadhi eradicates any last vestiges of ignorance, the confusion between Seer (Purusha) and seen (Prakriti). The elimination of ignorance is the highest virtue, since it brings negative behavior to an end. In addition, those individuals who experience the pull of the Absolute (the ever-present assistance of the Divine) would experience all virtues being rained down on them from "above" (*see sutra* 4.26).

Dharmamegha Samadhi with Dharma as Form

Considering dharma as "form" and then combining it with the word megha, gives a different slant on this samadhi. *Megha*, cloud, is traditionally used to refer to a state of consciousness free from any forms, characteristics, or functions. Therefore dharmamegha samadhi is the samadhi in which mind-stuff is being freed from the limitations of form. It is the condition in which the actions of the gunas are experienced as immaterial to pure consciousness, leaving the mind completely free from the bonds of Prakriti. This understanding of dharmamegha samadhi is supported by sutra 4.34, which describes the gunas as terminating their sequences of transformation for the practitioner and reabsorbing themselves into Prakriti. This state is referred to as the "supreme state of Independence."

When we examine both renderings of "dharma," we will find that they offer equally valid glimpses into the moments before complete liberation. Here's why: prior to dharmamegha samadhi, our experience and understanding of life and the universe could be expressed as an equation:

$$me + all\ beings\ and\ objects = life\ and\ the\ universe$$

"Me," represents the false notion of self held in place by ignorance (which also obstructs the inflow of virtue). "All other beings and objects" represents Prakriti, with all its names, forms, and functions. What happens in dharmamegha samadhi is that our experience of "life and the universe" changes because we experience the other two parts of the equation (me and all other beings and objects) dissolving into Oneness.

Furthermore, the outcome is the same regardless of which interpretation is preferred. There is a permanent shift in identity from one based on the activities and structures of the mind-stuff to the pure, unchanging awareness that is the Purusha.

The miracle of Raja Yoga is that the preparation for this state consisted not of heroic efforts at self-denial or torturing of the body and mind but of simple, powerful practices.

4.30. From that samadhi all afflictions and karmas cease.

Dharmamegha samadhi ends all afflictions and removes the practitioner from the wheel of cause and effect. The yogi becomes a *jivanmukta*, a being liberated while still in the body; an experience that lies ahead for all of us, though we know not when.

In describing the benefits of dharmamegha samadhi, Sri Patanjali uses the same words he used to describe attributes of Ishwara. Compare this sutra to sutra 1.24, in which qualities of Ishwara include being un-affected by afflictions, actions, or the fruits of actions. Is Sri Patanjali hinting that at the level of dharmamegha samadhi, we realize that we are, or are in some significant way, identical to Ishwara, the Supreme Purusha? Are we really beyond all afflictions: ignorance, egoism, attach-ment, aversion, and clinging to bodily life? (*see sutra* 2.3). Could it be that we are in reality free of all karmic entanglements? Are we truly that free?

Yes, and more. With dharmamegha samadhi we realize this degree of freedom because ignorance loses its influence on our minds.

Related Sutras: 2.3–2.9: The klesas (obstacles); 2.10, 2.11, and 2.26: The methods for the removal of the klesas; 2.27: "One's wisdom in the final stage is sevenfold." The last three stages listed in this sutra describe an experience similar to that discussed here.

4.31. Then all the coverings and impurities of knowledge are totally removed. Because of the infinity of this knowledge, what remains to be known is almost nothing.

Dharmamegha samadhi removes all the impurities that obscure knowledge. In this sutra, "knowledge" should not be misunderstood to be information gained through the senses or conceptualization.

Here "knowledge" stands for the direct intuitive experience that is dharmamegha samadhi. Therefore the "infinity of this knowledge" does not refer to an endless expansion of facts but the reflection of the Purusha—pure unbounded consciousness, the witness of all phenomena—on a pure sattwic mind.

This sutra says that *"what remains to be known is almost nothing."* What's left to be known is the answer to these questions: What is the experience of awareness when it is devoid of content and location (ego) and outside of time? Who am I when the only "I" that I now know vanishes?

Related Sutra: 3.55: "The transcendent discriminative knowledge that simultaneously comprehends all objects in all conditions is the intuitive knowledge (which brings liberation)."

4.32. Then the gunas terminate their sequence of transformation because they have fulfilled their purpose.

The gunas are like teachers who give us the lessons we need to go beyond ignorance. Once the lessons are learned and the exams passed, we no longer have to study that same subject again. Our minds become free from the limitations of Nature. The measure of Prakriti that composed the individual body and mind—that was until now experienced as our self-identity, a solid three-dimensional reality—begins to dissolve into the experience of consciousness as the one freestanding, unchanging reality. The relativities of time and space melt into a cosmic oneness, the perfect pure awareness of the Self.

Related Sutra: 2.18: "The seen is of the nature of the gunas... whose purpose is to provide both experiences and liberation to the Purusha."

4.33. The sequence (of transformation) and its counterpart, moments in time, can be recognized at the end of their transformations.

All the efforts the yogi has put forth have been directed at eradicating ignorance: the misperception, the illusion, that self-identity is limited to the body-mind. This illusion has been aided by the ego's fascination with the dance of Prakriti, the never-ending play of objects and events that enchant the mind's attention. It's not so much that the ego is gullible (although it may well be and often is); rather it is that Prakriti's show is so convincing. It is a show whose very nature is perfectly designed to fool our senses, causing errors in perception. (But remember that this show is not a malicious practical joke; it is a drama meant to entertain and educate us—to give us the experiences we need to attain Self-realization.) For example, when we look at a twig, our senses perceive it as a continuous piece of matter. Our perception of the twig's solidity doesn't change even if we know that science has proven that the twig in our hand is mostly vast expanses of empty space interspersed with the minutest of particles which in fact have no material existence.

This sutra teaches that change, which is how we perceive time, is in reality a number of distinct successive states correlated to moments, the shortest measure of time. It's something like those old cartoon flipbooks in which a series of sequential drawings are bound together in a small book. The difference from one picture to the next is so slight that we might not notice any variation. But when we quickly flip the series in front of our eyes, we perceive change. The cartoon figures *seem* to move. Each individual drawing is a distinct state that flits past our eyes riding on moments of time. We experience the powerful illusion that this process can create every time we go to the movies.

Just as with the cartoon flipbooks, motion pictures are in reality a succession of still pictures, each slightly different, projected in quick succession on a screen. It is because we perceive motion in the pictures that we can become involved in the story being portrayed. And we may remain happily seduced by the illusion of motion until something happens to interrupt the flow of individual pictures moving past the projector's light or that shifts our attention from the screen. Whether it's a technical malfunction, a loud sneeze nearby, the inviting aroma of warm popcorn, or a friend's insistent tap on the shoulder, the result is the same. Our attention leaves the "movie world" and is thrown back to us and our environment. In other words, we return to the "real world." The Yoga practices are meant to bring us to a similar experience with regard to Prakriti.

Reflect for a moment that through such practices as meditation (*sutras* 3.1–3.3), nonattachment (*sutras* 1.15 *and* 1.16), self-surrender or devotion and total dedication to Ishwara (*sutra* 1.23),

PADA FOUR

229

uninterrupted discriminative discernment (*sutra* 2.26), study and accepting pain as a help for purification (*sutra* 2.1), we have come to this amazing moment; the moment when Prakriti—Nature—dissolves. It loses its seeming solidity, its seeming unyielding influence on our senses. Yogis directly perceive that their false selfhood was constructed from the play of Prakriti and the influence of ignorance. They are now prepared to relinquish the misperceived self-identity, which has brought great suffering, in favor of Self-realization, which brings permanent joy.

4.34. Thus the supreme state of Independence manifests, while the gunas reabsorb themselves into Prakriti, having no more purpose to serve the Purusha. Or, to look at it from another angle, the power of consciousness settles in its own nature.

For the fully realized yogi, the Self as True Identity is directly experienced as an unshakable reality. Ignorance has vanished. The misidentification of the Purusha with the Prakriti is forever gone; the yogi "sees" the true nature of existence and is completely free of all limitation and pain.

We will end our exploration of the *Yoga Sutras of Patanjali* with the inspiring words of two great Raja Yogis, Sri Swami Vivekananda and Sri Swami Satchidananda.

From Sri Swami Vivekananda's *Raja Yoga* and his commentary on this sutra:

> Nature's task is done, this unselfish task which our sweet nurse, nature, has imposed upon herself. She gently takes the self-forgetting soul by the hand, as it were, and shows it all the experiences in the universe, all manifestations, bringing it higher and higher through the various bodies, till its lost glory comes back, and it remembers its own nature. Then the kind mother goes back the same way she came, for others who also have lost their way in the trackless desert of life. Thus is she working without beginning and without end; and thus, through pleasure and pain, through good and evil, the infinite river of souls is flowing into the ocean of perfection, of self-realization.

From *The Yoga Sutras of Patanjali*, Sri Swami Satchidananda's commentary on this sutra:

> Scriptures talking of the Self are just for the sake of our intellectual understanding. But the practical truth for the ego is very simple. Just learn to be selfless. Learn to lead a dedicated life. Whatever you do, do it for others. The dedicated ever enjoy peace.... The entire life is an open book, a scripture. Read it. Learn while digging a pit or chopping some wood or cooking some food. If you can't learn from your daily activities, how are you going to understand the scriptures?

Related Sutra: 1.3: *"Then [after achieving nirodha] the Seer (Self) abides in Its own nature."*

May you be blessed to grow and prosper in the path of Raja Yoga. May you remain steadfast and joyful in all your endeavors. May you soon experience Self-realization and forever enjoy the unbounded peace and joy that is your True Identity. And may you share that peace and joy with one and all.

Pada Four Review

1. Sri Patanjali addresses the topic of evolution. It is a power intrinsic to all beings and objects that rushes forth whenever obstacles are removed.

2. Karma is discussed again, this time in more depth. We learn that most people have mixed karmas: some bring pleasant experiences and some bring pain. A karma will come to fruition only under favorable circumstances.

3. Sri Patanjali offers more information on the nature of subconscious impressions, since a yogi must overcome their influences in order to achieve the highest goal. We are told that they are as old as desire itself and are held together by ignorance, karma, the existence of the mind, and the impact of external events.

4. Once again, we come to the subject of the Seer and seen. This time, however, the particular aspect of the seen that interests Sri Patanjali is the mind. He wishes to ensure that we do not confuse the borrowed awareness of the mind with the awareness that is the Seer. When the distinction between the two is realized, the seeker experiences the pull of the Absolute. Like the sun evaporating dewdrops from the grass, the light of the Self evaporates ignorance.

5. The last five sutras explore dharmamegha samadhi, the final stage before nirbija samadhi. It is a state in which the only deep interest that remains for the seeker is merging with the Self. The activities of all karmas and the klesas (afflictions) have ceased, and what remains to be known is almost nothing.

Mother Nature (in the form of the gunas) now goes about her business of nudging the yogi out of the nest. Her work is done; the gunas no longer affect the yogi's mind. Finally, *"the power of pure consciousness settles in its own pure nature" (see sutra* 1.3).

What to Do

Review your sadhana: Is it regular? Where are your weaknesses? What can you do to address your weak areas?

Continue with your spiritual diary.

Revisit the subject of attachments. How have you done so far? What seems to be the most troublesome or persistent? Remember that overcoming attachments has a profound effect on your state of mind as well as your advancement in sadhana. Try to give a little more (time, energy, talent, money) for the benefit of others.

Don't ever give up. Continue with the path you have chosen. Countless others have succeeded. Why not you? It is not a matter of IQ but of purity of heart and persistence of will. All the joy, peace, and happiness that you have ever wanted, dreamed, or imagined—and much more—is in you *as* you. Don't wait, do it now, and discover that life can indeed be a supreme joy.

PADA FOUR

Study Guide

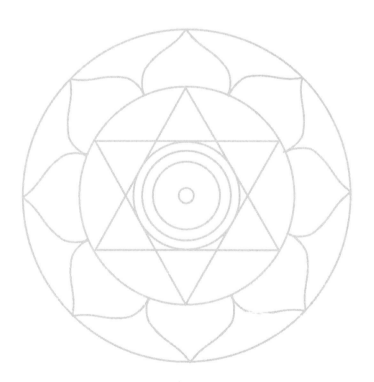

Study Guide

The following course of study, though nonsequential, follows a logical flow of thought and ensures that students incorporate practice into their study as soon as possible.

Track I presents the foundation teachings for all the subsequent sutras. After becoming familiar with this track, you can study the next five in any order you wish, although the sequence provided usually works well for most students.

It is not necessary to master a track before moving on, but it is best to not move ahead until there is at least a familiarity with the material in a track. If you wish to further your understanding of the sutras, you can start again from the beginning, perhaps substituting or adding a different commentary. Repeated readings are a great way to grow in understanding. See *Resources* at the end of this book for some suggestions for further study.

Those who are familiar with the sutras may prefer to study by topic. To proceed in this way, consult the *Sutra-by-Subject Index*, where sutras are grouped together by subject matter.

Track I: The Foundation

This track lays the foundation of Raja Yoga theory and engages the student in practice as soon as possible.

The two pillars that support all of the theories and practices of Raja Yoga are presented in this track: the first sixteen sutras of Pada One and the eight limbs of Raja Yoga that are the major topic of Pada Two.

Sutras 1.1–1.16

Introduction to the basic philosophy; practice and nonattachment are introduced.

Sutras 3.1–3.3

These sutras, which introduce meditation, are included at this point in order to facilitate and encourage the practice of meditation.

Sutras 1.30–1.41

These sutras cover the obstacles encountered in meditation and offer several possible objects of meditation to choose from; therefore the group nicely follows the sutras listed above. This group of sutras ends with our first exposure to a definition of samadhi, the superconscious state.

Sutras 2.28–2.45

The eight limbs are introduced. They reflect the central teachings and practices of Raja Yoga. In fact, many people know Sri Patanjali's work as *Ashtanga Yoga*, the eight-limbed Yoga. These eight limbs bring together the principles of nirodha, discriminative discernment, nonattachment, moral and ethical precepts, and the physical facets of Yoga—asana (posture) and pranayama (breath control).

The sutras of this group focus on the first two limbs: the moral and ethical precepts of Yoga, known as yama and niyama.

Sutras 2.46–2.55

We continue the exploration of the limbs of Yoga with asana, pranayama, and pratyahara (sense withdrawal). Their practice and benefits are introduced.

Sutras 2.1–2.12, 2.14–2.17, 2.24–2.26, *and* 2.28.

Since Track 1 emphasizes regularity in Yoga practice, it is important to become familiar with the obstacles that will be encountered and the method for their removal.

We are introduced to karma (the law of cause and effect) in sutra 2.14, and in sutra 2.26 we find the first sutra on viveka, discriminative discernment.

Sutra 2.26 and 2.28 bring us full circle back to the eight limbs by presenting the connection between the practice of the eight limbs and the discriminative insight necessary to remove ignorance

Track II: Meditation, Devotion, Obstacles
Sutras 1.23–1.29

This track discusses devotion as a viable means to Self-realization. It opens with sutras that describe Ishwara (the Creator) as "the Supreme Purusha (Self) free from afflictions and karmas."

Also introduced are mantras as meditation techniques.

At the end of this track, review sutra 1.30, on obstacles.

Track III: Samadhi
Sutras 1.17–1.22 and 1.42–1.51

This track describes the various samadhis (superconscious states).

Since this material is technical in nature, it has been placed here to allow students time to begin a personal practice and become familiar with the fundamental philosophical points.

The use of the *Sutras-by-Subject Index* can be especially helpful in studying this track. Before going on, review sutras 1.2 and 1.41.

Track IV: The Nature of the Seer and Seen
Sutras 2.18–2.27

In this section, Sri Patanjali teaches us that Nature needs to be understood for the Self to be realized. This track takes us on a journey of exploration where we discover the distinction between Nature (Prakriti) and the Seer (Purusha).

Track V: Development in Nirodha and the Siddhis
Sutras 3.4–3.55

This group of sutras begins by examining how nirodha (restraint of the mental modifications) is developed. It goes on to list the siddhis—the various accomplishments that can come as a result of Yoga practices.

Track VI: Freedom
Sutras 3.56–4.34

This track restates some of what has been covered before but in more depth. There are a number of sutras that discuss the topic of evolution. It also offers a breakdown of the seeker's experiences as he or she approaches Self-realization.

Appendix

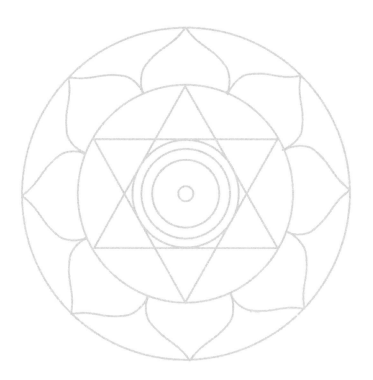

The Yoga Sutras
The Dualism of Classical Sankhya and
The Nondualism of Advaita Vedanta

The *Yoga Sutras* (referred to as "Classical Yoga" by scholars) and the philosophical systems of Classical Sankhya and Advaita Vedanta comprise three principle philosophical systems of the sacred traditions of India. Many influential schools of Yoga have adopted various aspects of Sankhya or Vedanta into the teachings of Classical Yoga, sometimes causing confusion among students of the *Yoga Sutras*. Following is a brief comparison.

According to Ishwara Krishna (c. 350 BCE), who systematized Sankhya Philosophy in his text, *Sankhya-Karika*, Classical Sankhya is a dualistic philosophy that states that there are two coexisting, eternal—but distinct—realities: Purusha (the principle of consciousness) and Prakriti (matter). There is an infinite number of eternal, omnipresent, and identical Purushas. Although preclassical Sankhya, influenced by the teachings of the Upanishads, taught a nondualistic theism, Classical Sankhya is atheistic. In Classical Sankhya, investigation into the nature of Reality relies on adherence to traditional doctrine, inference, and viveka (discriminative discernment).

Advaita (nondualistic) Vedanta, rooted in the Vedas and Upanishads, presents a different picture. There is only one eternal, omnipresent Reality. The names and forms that unawakened minds perceive around them are illusions seemingly projected by that Reality through the agency of ignorance. For Vedantins, Reality is comprised of one undivided, eternal Truth.

Although Sri Patanjali's sutras have much in common with Classical Sankhya, they differ in several important ways:

- Acceptance of Ishwara, the Lord. There are four instances in the sutras in which surrender to Ishwara is mentioned as a valid means of attaining enlightenment. Self-surrender is sufficient unto itself as a means of attaining Self-realization.
- Classical Yoga includes superconscious states (samadhi) as valid means for attaining knowledge in addition to doctrine, inference, and viveka.
- The *Yoga Sutras* do not speak explicitly of all the twenty-four categories of existence (*tattva*) listed in Sankhya philosophy:

Prakriti, buddhi, ahamkara, manas, the ten senses (five of action and five of knowledge), the five subtle elements, and the five material elements.

In regard to Vedanta, although Sri Patanjali does not explicitly speak of the oneness of Purusha and Prakriti, his philosophy does not overtly argue against it. Sri Patanjali teaches from a pragmatic viewpoint; he does not spend much time enumerating all the subtleties of philosophy, offering only as much theoretical guidance as is necessary to facilitate practice. What is clearly presented is the essential dualism of life experience:

- Individual consciousness: not intrinsic, but "borrowed" from the Purusha, the only sentient principle
- Sense objects: manifestations of Prakriti

Did Sri Patanjali see the Purusha and Prakriti as ultimately being one, as the nondualistic school of Vedanta believes, or separate, as Sankhya teaches? We do not know what Sri Patanjali would have said on this subject for certain, as the sutras do not go into it much. This uncertainty brings to mind a question asked of Lord Buddha just before he passed:

Two senior disciples came to the master to settle a philosophical disagreement: Is there a God or not? The disciple who believed that the teachings did not indicate the existence of a Supreme Being asked, "Revered master, kindly tell us once and for all: Is there a God?"

"I never said that there was," the enlightened one replied. At this the disciple smiled, believing he had correctly interpreted the teachings. After a pause, Lord Buddha added:

"But I never said there was not."

The Compassionate One would say no more on the subject.

Are Purusha and Prakriti ultimately one?

Here is one way to reconcile the views of Vedanta with the teachings of Sri Patanjali. Especially since the time of Vacaspati Mishra's influential commentary on the *Yoga Sutras* composed during the ninth century CE, the metaphor of individual consciousness arising due to the reflection of the Purusha on the buddhi has been used to represent the relationship of Prakriti to Purusha in the phenomenon of perception. Buddhi, the first and subtlest expression of Prakriti, is the mirror. Although this metaphor is a useful teaching device, it has limitations. The primary drawback is that the Purusha is neither a solid nor energy (like light) that can reflect onto a mirror. To understand more fully the subtlety of the relationship between Purusha and Prakriti, it will be useful to expand our understanding of "reflection." In a broader sense, "reflection" is "something that is a consequence of or arises from something else." For example, when examining a painting, we might observe that: The artist's work reflects the influences of her teacher. In this instance, the "reflection" is not a physical act—a bouncing back of light waves from a mirror-like object to a perceiver.

Maple syrup, maple cream, and maple candy all have mapleness as the essence of their taste. This being so, it is appropriate to say that the taste of maple is *reflected* in the syrup, cream, and candy. Their maple flavor is the consequence of the essential mapleness common to each form. Is this the way consciousness is reflected in the buddhi?

Could it be that the buddhi arises from Purusha?

At least one sutra (4.18) suggests this is so. In this sutra, Sri Patanjali refers to the Purusha as the prabhu of Prakriti. Commonly translated as "lord" or "master," prabhu is derived from the verb root, *bhu*, "to become," literally meaning "to be before." It is frequently applied to Brahman (the Absolute) as well as the deities Vishnu, Siva, and Indra. It is understandable how it came to mean "master." To be regarded as above or before anyone else implies a position of prominence and power. But to "be before" also suggests the role of a progenitor. Therefore, it seems appropriate to include in our understanding of *prabhu*, the suggestion that it is "the one who is the originator." Therefore it is what gives matter existence.

Three other sutras hint at a kinship between Purusha and Prakriti:

2.18: *"The seen (Prakriti)is of the nature of the gunas: illumination, activity, and inertia; and consists of the elements and sense organs, whose purpose is to provide both experiences and liberation to the Purusha."*

Prakriti is not simply undifferentiated matter; it is matter with purpose. In our common experience in life, we often observe that purpose precedes creation: "Necessity is the mother of invention."

2.21: *"The seen exists only for the sake of the Seer [Purusha]."*

The object of Prakriti's purpose is Purusha.

2.22: *"Although destroyed for him who has attained liberation, it (the seen) exists for others, being common to them."*

It is as if we are all having a common dream (a nightmare for some) of life. Upon awakening, all that was the dream universe vanishes. But for those who still dream, the dream reality continues.

If we combine these sutras with 4.18, we could produce a reasonable argument for the oneness of Purusha and Prakriti:

Purusha is the origin and Lord of Prakriti, which exists for the purpose of providing experiences and enlightenment. The seeming reality of Prakriti's existence as separate from Purusha ends with liberation. Consciousness and matter are then experienced as one.

Perhaps, the nature of Reality as viewed from the perspectives of the *Yoga Sutras* and Vedanta are not different after all.

Finally, when considering philosophical differences, keep in mind that all philosophies suffer from one huge drawback—they are words that try to explain experience. Words are analogies and should be treated as such when examining spiritual teachings. We can never look to words, no matter how precise or skillfully poetic, to describe adequately or take the place of experience.

Sutras-by-Subject Index

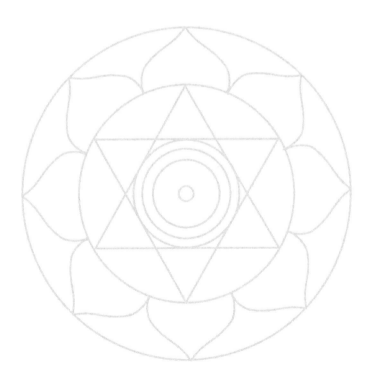

Sutras-by-Subject Index

This index can be used for the focused exploration of a major topic covered by the *Yoga Sutras* and for help in organizing Raja Yoga study groups. It can also be a useful tool in lesson-planning for Yoga teachers.

The sutras are arranged by topic with many appearing under more than one heading. Commentary is provided for major topics, for subjects that are not explicitly covered in the original text, and to clarify the reason a particular sutra is included under a specific topic.

Contents:
Ahamkara
Asmita
Avidya
Breath
Choice
Commitment/Dedication
Consciousness
Cravings/Greed/Desire
Discriminative Discernment
Ego
Enlightenment
Emotions
Everyday Yoga
Faith
God
Gunas (also see Prakriti; Nature)
Ignorance
Independence
Ishwara
Kaivalya
Karma
Knowledge
Mantra
Mind and Self, discrimination between
Meditation (also see Nirodha)
Nature

Nirodha (also see Meditation)
Nonattachment
Obstacles
Physical Aspects of Raja Yoga
Pleasure and Pain
Practice
Prakriti
Pranayama
Pratyaya
Purpose of Life
Purusha
Reincarnation
Relationships
Results of Practice
Sadhana
Samadhi
Samskaras (also see Vasanas)
Seer
Self
Self-realization
Spirit and Nature
True Identity
Union
Vairagya
Vasanas (also see Samskaras)
Viveka
Vritti
Yoga

A

Ahamkara, *see* E*go*

Asmita, *see* E*go*

Avidya, *see* I*gnorance*

B

Breath, *see* Pranayama

C

Choice

There is an age-old debate regarding the nature of an individual's free will versus Divine Will. If everything that happens is according to God's Will, what role, if any, does personal choice play? Sri Patanjali doesn't address this debate directly but he clearly recognizes that choice holds a central place in a seeker's spiritual life.

Take, for example, sutra 2.16. To state that pain can be avoided suggests that my chances of avoiding it are determined to a significant degree by my own actions (see Karma). Choice again surfaces with regard to picking an object for meditation.

How this free will relates to ignorance, karma, and Divine Will is a subject too involved for this work. But we can say this: satisfactory answers to some questions can come only through experience. Free will versus Divine Will is one of those questions.

1.39. *Or by meditating on anything one chooses that is elevating.*

2.16. *Pain that has not yet come is avoidable.*

2.44. *Through study comes communion with one's chosen deity.*

Commitment/Dedication

Success in Yoga requires clarity of purpose and firm resolve.

1.32. *The concentration on a single subject (or the use of one technique) is the best way to prevent the obstacles and their accompaniments. (See sutra 1.30)*

2.31. *These Great Vows (referring to yama, sutra 2.30) are universal, not limited by class, place, time, or circumstance.*

2.45. *By total surrender to Ishwara, samadhi is attained.*

Consciousness

Consciousness is another word for awareness. It is the ability to know or perceive. Here you will find sutras that discuss the nature of awareness, its relation to the senses and to the Purusha, and the reasons why the *Yoga Sutras* do not recognize the individual mind as having an independent consciousness of its own.

3.48. *Mastery over the sense organs is gained by samyama on the senses as they correlate to the process of perception, the essential nature of the senses, the ego-sense, and to their purpose.*

In the above sutra, the process of perception stands for consciousness.

4.4. *Individualized consciousness proceeds from the primary ego-sense.*

4.5. *Although the activities of the individualized minds may differ, one consciousness is the initiator of them all.*

4.6. *Of these (the different activities in the individual minds), what is born from meditation is without residue.*

4.15. *Due to differences in various minds, perception of even the same object may vary.*

4.17. *An object is known or unknown depending on whether or not the mind gets colored by it.*

4.19. *The mind-stuff is not self-luminous because it is an object of perception by the Purusha.*

4.20. *The mind-stuff cannot perceive both subject and object simultaneously (which proves it is not self-luminous).*

4.21. *If perception of one mind by another is postulated, we would have to assume an endless number of them, and the result would be confusion of memory.*

4.22. *The consciousness of the Purusha is unchangeable; by getting the reflection of it, the mind-stuff becomes conscious of the Self.*

4.23. *The mind-stuff, when colored by both Seer and seen, understands everything.*

4.24. *Though colored by countless subliminal traits (vasanas), the mind-stuff exists for the sake of another (the Purusha) because it can act only in association with It.*

4.34. *Thus the supreme state of Independence manifests, while the gunas reabsorb themselves into Prakriti, having no more purpose to serve the Purusha. Or, to look at it from another angle, the power of consciousness settles in its own nature.*

Craving/Greed/Desire

1.24. *Ishwara is the supreme Purusha, unaffected by any afflictions, actions, fruits of actions, or any inner impressions of desires.*

2.15. *To one of discrimination, everything is painful indeed, due to its consequences: the anxiety and fear over losing what is gained; the resulting impressions left in the mind to create renewed cravings; and the conflict among the activities of the gunas, which control the mind.*

2.27. *One's wisdom in the final stage is sevenfold.*

One experiences the end of 1) *desire to know anything more; 2) desire to stay away from any thing; 3) desire to gain anything new; 4) desire to do anything; 5) sorrow; 6) fear; 7) delusion.*

2.37. *To one established in nonstealing, all wealth comes.*

A very practical piece of advice for attaining financial security. Even some financial advisors suggest that the attitude of craving and anxious poverty actually prevents prosperity from coming to us. In part, this is because our attitude and decisions are based on fear, and fear clouds good judgment. In a sense, what this sutra really talks about is cultivating an attitude of non-craving; of security based on faith. Since we know that all Prakriti exists to serve Purusha, when we attune our lives—our motives, decisions, actions—to this truth, we will harmonize with the Divine Plan and be given all that we need to fulfill our part in it.

Another point is that wealth does not simply mean owning a large accumulation of money. Wealth includes such qualities as integrity, peace of mind, joy, meaning in life and faith. It is also the realization that we will be taken care of: *"Consider the lilies of the field. They neither sow nor reap, yet even Solomon in all his splendor was not arrayed as one of these"* (Matthew 6.28).

2.39. *To one established in nongreed, a thorough illumination of the how and why of one's birth comes.*

2.42. *By contentment, supreme joy is gained.*

Where there is craving, there can be no contentment and joy; and where there is contentment, there can be no craving.

2.54. *When the senses withdraw themselves from the objects and imitate, as it were, the nature of the mind-stuff, this is pratyahara.*

The mind that can withdraw its attention from sense-objects at will, will not be touched by the pangs of cravings. See also sutra 2.55, below.

2.55. *Then follows supreme mastery over the senses.*

3.52. *The yogi should neither accept nor smile with pride at the admiration of even the celestial beings, as there is the possibility of his getting caught again in the undesirable.*

Don't many people crave the admiration of others? How much more the temptation—the desire—for admiration from celestial beings?

4.9. *Vasanas, though separated (from their manifestation) by birth, place, or time, have an uninterrupted relationship (to each other and the individual) due to the seamlessness of subconscious memory and samskaras.*

Vasanas are often interpreted as subtle desires.

4.10. *Since the desire to live is eternal, vasanas are also beginningless.*

4.24. *Though colored by countless subliminal traits (vasanas), the mind-stuff exists for the sake of another (the Purusha) because it can act only in association with It.*

D

Discriminative Discernment, *see Viveka.*

E

Ego

2.3. *Ignorance, egoism, attachment, aversion, and clinging to bodily life are the five obstacles.*

2.6. *Egoism is the identification, as it were, of the power of the Seer (Purusha) with that of the instrument of seeing (body-mind).*

4.4. *Individualized consciousness proceeds from the primary ego-sense.*

4.5. *Although the activities of the individualized minds may differ, one consciousness is the initiator of them all.*

4.6. *Of these (the different activities in the individual minds), what is born from meditation is without residue.*

Enlightenment, *see Self-realization*

Emotions

Emotions belong to the mind, not the Self. They are reactions to external or internal stimuli that impact perceptions of our security and self-image. We fear, hate, or express anger at anything that threatens or belittles us, while we love and delight in that which makes us feel secure and good about ourselves.

Nowhere in the teachings of Yoga is it recommended that we suppress emotions. Emotions need to be acknowledged and understood. Sri Patanjali would probably not give an "A" to a student who did not acknowledge his or her emotions. But this does not mean that emotions should be indiscriminately welcomed into your mind.

Any emotion can be firmly rooted in ignorance, and if it is, it needs to be analyzed and transcended. That's why the thoughts that underlie our emotions are important factors to consider. Let's look at a few examples.

Sadness is not a pleasurable experience. It can be grounded in selfish attachment or an acute empathy for the pain of others. In the former case, it is not something to encourage, although it can teach us good lessons. Sadness can be a friend and teacher by pointing out where selfish expectations or attachments lie hidden. Once flushed into the open, these attachments can be gradually eliminated. On the other hand, if sadness is grounded in empathy, it can be a sign that compassion is growing. Pleasurable emotions—such as happiness—which we usually seek out in earnest, could be rooted in mean-spiritedness and ignorance. Would we regard someone who feels a joyful thrill over the suffering of an enemy as spiritually mature? That kind of happiness is not welcomed by the yogi, as it maintains the influence of ignorance on the mind.

There are some emotions that are reflections of the Self on a still, clear, selfless mind. Though still colored by the mind, these experiences are facsimiles of Divine attributes. Peace, selfless joy, unconditional love, and compassion are examples of this category of emotions. They are emotions without attachment, free from the taint of ignorance and egoism.

> 1.31. *Accompaniments to the mental distractions include distress, despair, trembling of the body, and disturbed breathing. (See sutra 1.30.)*
>
> 2.9. *Clinging to life, flowing by its own potency (due to past experience), exists even in the wise.*
>
> 2.15. *To one of discrimination, everything is painful indeed, due to its consequences: the anxiety and fear over losing what is gained; the resulting impressions left in the mind to create renewed cravings; and the conflict among the activities of the gunas, which control the mind.*

The above sutra offers good insight into the origin of emotions like fear, anxiety, psychological pain and cravings.

2.16. *Pain that has not yet come is avoidable.*

2.17. *The cause of that avoidable pain is the union of the Seer (Purusha) and seen (Prakriti).*

The following two sutras offer Sri Patanjali's primary method for dealing with emotions that are rooted ignorance.

2.33. *When disturbed by negative thoughts, opposite (positive) ones should be thought of. This is pratipaksha bhavana.*

2.34. *When negative thoughts or acts such as violence and so on are caused to be done, or even approved of, whether incited by greed, anger, or infatuation, whether indulged in with mild, medium, or extreme intensity, they are based on ignorance and bring certain pain. Reflecting thus is also pratipaksha bhavana.*

2.41. *Moreover (by the perfection in purity mentioned in sutra 2.40), one gains purity of sattwa, cheerfulness of mind, one-pointedness, mastery over the senses, and fitness for Self-realization.*

2.42. *By contentment, supreme joy is gained.*

3.24. *By samyama on friendliness and other such qualities, the power to transmit them is obtained.*

Everyday Yoga

There are important practices that do not require a special time or place to perform but are realized in the midst of life's daily activities. In fact, we need the experiences of everyday life to learn the lessons necessary for our growth.

1.33. *By cultivating attitudes of friendliness toward the happy, compassion for the unhappy, delight in the virtuous, and equanimity toward the nonvirtuous, the mind-stuff retains its undisturbed calmness.*

2.7. *Attachment is that which follows identification with pleasurable experiences.*

2.8. *Aversion is that which follows identification with painful experiences.*

2.29. *The eight limbs of Yoga are:*

    1. *yama – abstinence*

    2. *niyama – observance*

    3. *asana – posture*

    4. *pranayama – breath control*

    5. *pratyahara – sense withdrawal*

    6. *dharana – concentration*

    7. *dhyana – meditation*

    8. *samadhi – contemplation, absorption or super-conscious state*

SUTRAS-BY-SUBJECT

2.30. *Yama consists of nonviolence, truthfulness, nonstealing, continence, and nongreed.*

2.31. *These Great Vows are universal, not limited by class, place, time, or circumstance.*

2.32. *Niyama consists of purity, contentment, accepting but not causing pain, study and worship of God (self-surrender).*

2.43. *By austerity, impurities of body and senses are destroyed and occult powers gained.*

2.54. *When the senses withdraw themselves from the objects and imitate, as it were, the nature of the mind-stuff, this is pratyahara.*

In our daily endeavors, can we steer our mind away from objects and activities that distract us from our goals?

2.55. *Then follows supreme mastery over the senses.*

F

Faith

True, unshakable faith results from the deepening of our spiritual vision. It is not a matter of belief, no matter how strong, but rather of knowing. Faith is the antidote to fear, which is the primary emotional symptom of ignorance. As Sri Swami Satchidananda said, "Fear and faith do not go together." A precursor of faith is surrender.

1.20. *To the others, asamprajnata samadhi is preceded by faith, strength, mindfulness, (cognitive) samadhi, and discriminative insight.*

1.23. *Or (samadhi is attained) by devotion with total dedication to God (Ishwara).*

1.30. *Disease, dullness, doubt, carelessness, laziness, sensuality, false perception, failure to reach firm ground, and slipping from the ground gained—these distractions of the mind-stuff are the obstacles.*

2.32. *Niyama consists of purity, contentment, accepting but not causing pain, study and worship of God (self-surrender).*

The next six sutras are included in this section since they can help develop faith. They offer sound philosophical (and verifiable) proofs that there is a Higher Consciousness.

4.19. *The mind-stuff is not self-luminous because it is an object of perception by the Purusha.*

4.20. *The mind-stuff cannot perceive both subject and object simultaneously (which proves it is not self-luminous).*

4.21. *If perception of one mind by another is postulated, we would have to assume an endless number of them, and the result would be confusion of memory.*

4.22. *The consciousness of the Purusha is unchangeable; by getting the reflection of it, the mind-stuff becomes conscious of the Self.*

4.23. *The mind-stuff, when colored by both Seer and seen, understands everything.*

4.24. *Though colored by countless subliminal traits (vasanas), the mind-stuff exists for the sake of another (the Purusha) because it can act only in association with It.*

G

God, see Ishwara

Gunas (also see Prakriti)

2.15. *To one of discrimination, everything is painful indeed, due to its consequences: the anxiety and fear over losing what is gained; the resulting impressions left in the mind to create renewed cravings; and the conflict among the activities of the gunas, which control the mind.*

2.16. *Pain that has not yet come is avoidable.*

Though the above sutra doesn't speak about the gunas or Prakriti, it is the important lead-in to the following sutra, which does.

2.17. *The cause of that avoidable pain is the union of the Seer (Purusha) and seen (Prakriti).*

2.18. *The seen is of the nature of the gunas: illumination, activity, and inertia. It consists of the elements and sense organs, whose purpose is to provide both experiences and liberation to the Purusha.*

2.19: *The stages of the gunas are specific, nonspecific, defined, and undifferentiated.*

2.21 *The seen exists only for the sake of the Seer.*

2.22. *Although destroyed for him who has attained liberation, it (the seen) exists for others, being common to them.*

2.23. *The union of Owner (Purusha) and owned (Prakriti) causes the recognition of the nature and powers of them both.*

3.13. *By what has been said, the transformations of the form, characteristics, and condition of the elements and sense organs are explained.*

The above sutra refers to the sutras on development of nirodha, samadhi and one-pointedness. These sutras (3.9–3.12) discuss how the mind and Nature undergo the same process of change.

3.14. *The substratum (Prakriti) continues to exist, although by nature it goes through latent, uprising, and unmanifested phases.*

3.15. *The succession of these different phases is the cause of the differences in stages of evolution.*

3.45. *Mastery over the gross and subtle elements is gained by samyama on their essential nature, correlations, and purpose.*

3.49. *From that, the body gains the power to move as fast as the mind, the ability to function without the aid of the sense organs, and complete mastery over the primary cause (Prakriti).*

The "that" referred to in the above sutra is samyama on the power of perception, the ego-sense and the purpose of sense organs. (*See sutra* 3.48.)

4.2. *The transformation of one species into another is brought about by the inflow of nature.*

4.3. *Incidental events do not directly cause natural evolution; they just remove the obstacles as a farmer (removes the obstacles in a watercourse running to his field).*

4.12. *The past and future exist as the essential nature (of Prakriti) to manifest (perceptible) changes in an object's characteristics.*

4.13. *Whether manifested or subtle, these characteristics belong to the nature of the gunas.*

4.14. *The reality of things is due to the uniformity of the gunas' transformation.*

4.15. *Due to differences in various minds, perception of even the same object may vary.*

4.16. *Nor does an object's existence depend upon a single mind, for if it did, what would become of that object when that mind did not perceive it?*

4.17. *An object is known or unknown dependent on whether or not the mind gets colored by it.*

4.32. *Then (after dharmamegha samadhi) the gunas terminate their sequence of transformation because they have fulfilled their purpose.*

4.33. *The sequence (of transformation) and its counterpart, moments in time, can be recognized at the end of their transformations.*

4.34. *Thus the supreme state of Independence manifests, while the gunas reabsorb themselves into Prakriti, having no more purpose to serve the Purusha. Or, to look at it from another angle, the power of consciousness settles in its own nature.*

I

Ignorance

What is it, where does it originate, and how can we eliminate it?

2.3. *Ignorance, egoism, attachment, aversion, and clinging to bodily life are the five obstacles (klesas).*

2.4. *Ignorance is the field for the others mentioned after it, whether they be dormant, feeble, intercepted, or sustained.*

2.5. *Ignorance is regarding the impermanent as permanent, the impure as pure, the painful as pleasant, and the non-Self as the Self.*

2.9. *Clinging to life, flowing by its own potency (due to past experience), exists even in the wise.*

2.23. *The union of Owner (Purusha) and owned (Prakriti) causes the recognition of the nature and powers of them both.*

The above sutra is included since it is the lead-in for 2.24, which directly discusses ignorance.

2.24. *The cause of this union is ignorance.*

2.25. *Without this ignorance, no such union occurs. This is the independence of the Seer.*

2.26. *Uninterrupted discriminative discernment is the method for its removal.*

2.34. *When negative thoughts or acts such as violence and so on are caused to be done, or even approved of, whether incited by greed, anger, or infatuation, whether indulged in with mild, medium, or extreme intensity, they are based on ignorance and bring certain pain. Reflecting thus is also pratipaksha bhavana.*

4.30. *From that samadhi (dharmamegha samadhi) all afflictions (klesas) and karmas cease.*

Independence, *see Self-realization and Kaivalya*

Ishwara

1.23. *Or samadhi is attained by devotion with total dedication to God (Ishwara).*

1.24. *Ishwara is the supreme Purusha, unaffected by any afflictions, actions, fruits of actions, or any inner impressions of desires.*

1.25. *In Ishwara is the complete manifestation of the seed of omniscience.*

1.26. *Unconditioned by time, Ishwara is the teacher of even the most ancient teachers.*

1.27. *The expression of Ishwara is the mystic sound OM.*

2.1. Accepting pain as help for purification, study, and surrender to the Supreme Being (Ishwara) constitute Yoga in practice.

2.32. Niyama consists of purity, contentment, accepting but not causing pain, study and worship of (Ishwara) God (self-surrender).

2.45. By total surrender to Ishwara, samadhi is attained.

K

Kaivalya

Kaivalya is pure absolute awareness, completely unencumbered by ignorance, egoism, attachment, or aversion. It is the pure, eternal, unbounded power of seeing.

2.25. Without this ignorance, no such union occurs. This is the independence of the Seer.

3.51. By nonattachment even to that (all these siddhis), the seed of bondage is destroyed and thus follows Kaivalya (Independence).

3.56. When the tranquil mind attains purity equal to that of the Self, there is Absoluteness (kaivalya).

4.34. Thus the supreme state of Independence manifests, while the gunas reabsorb themselves into Prakriti, having no more purpose to serve the Purusha. Or, to look at it from another angle, the power of consciousness settles in its own nature.

Karma

1.24. Ishwara is the supreme Purusha, unaffected by any afflictions, actions, fruits of actions, or any inner impressions of desires.

2.12. The womb of karmas has its roots in these obstacles (the klesas of sutra 2.3), and the karmas bring experiences in the seen (present) or in the unseen (future) births.

2.13. With the existence of the root, there will also be fruits: the births of different species of life, their life spans, and experiences.

2.14. The karmas bear fruits of pleasure and pain caused by merit and demerit.

3.23. Karmas are of two kinds: quickly manifesting and slowly manifesting. By samyama on them, or on the portents of death, the knowledge of the time of death is obtained.

4.6. Of these (the different activities in the individual minds), what is born from meditation is without residue.

The residue spoken of in the above sutra refers to the remains of thoughts or actions—samskaras.

4.7. *The karma of the yogi is neither white (good) nor black (bad); for others there are three kinds (good, bad, and mixed).*

4.8. *From that (threefold karma) follows the manifestation of only those vasanas (subliminal traits) for which there are favorable conditions for producing their fruits.*

4.9. *Vasanas, though separated (from their manifestation) by birth, place, or time, have an uninterrupted relationship (to each other and the individual) due to the seamlessness of subconscious memory and samskaras.*

The above sutra is included since it expands nicely on the principles set forth in sutra 4.9, above.

4.30. *From that samadhi* (dharmamegha samadhi) *all afflictions and karmas cease.*

Knowledge

Here you will find sutras that discuss the knowledge of the Self, the levels of knowledge that the practitioner of Yoga will experience, and ways that insights can be attained.

1.7. *The sources of right knowledge are direct perception, inference, and authoritative testimony.*

1.47. *In the pure clarity of nirvichara samadhi, the supreme Self shines.*

1.48. *This is ritambhara prajna, the truth-bearing wisdom.*

1.49. *The purpose of this special wisdom is different from the insights gained by study of sacred tradition and inference.*

2.32. *Niyama consists of purity, contentment, accepting but not causing pain, study and worship of God (self-surrender).*

2.44. *Through study comes communion with one's chosen deity.*

3.5. *By mastery of samyama, knowledge born of intuitive insight shines forth.*

3.16. *By practicing samyama on the three stages of evolution comes knowledge of past and future.*

3.26. *By samyama on the light within, the knowledge of the subtle, hidden, and remote is obtained.* [Note: subtle as atoms, hidden as treasure, remote as far-distant lands.]

3.27. *By samyama on the sun, knowledge of the entire solar system is obtained.*

3.28. *By samyama on the moon comes knowledge of the stars' alignment.*

3.29. *By samyama on the pole star comes knowledge of the stars' movements.*

3.30. *By samyama on the navel plexus, knowledge of the body's constitution is obtained.*

3.31. By samyama on the pit of the throat, cessation of hunger and thirst is achieved.

3. 34. Or, in the knowledge that dawns by spontaneous intuition (through a life of purity), all the powers come by themselves.

3.35. By samyama on the heart, the knowledge of the mind-stuff is obtained.

3.36. The intellect (sattwa) and the Purusha are totally different, the intellect existing for the sake of the Purusha, while the Purusha exists for its own sake. Not distinguishing this is the cause of all experiences. By samyama on this distinction, knowledge of the Purusha is gained.

3.50. By recognition of the distinction between sattwa (the pure reflective aspect of the mind) and the Self, supremacy over all states and forms of existence (omnipotence) is gained, as is omniscience.

3.53. By samyama on single moments in sequence comes discriminative knowledge.

3.55. The transcendent discriminative knowledge that simultaneously comprehends all objects in all conditions is the intuitive knowledge (which brings liberation).

4.15. Due to differences in various minds, perception of even the same object may vary.

4.31. Then (due to dharmamegha samadhi) all the coverings and impurities of knowledge are totally removed. Because of the infinity of this knowledge, what remains to be known is almost nothing.

M

Mantra

1.27. The expression of Ishwara is the mystic sound OM.

1.28. To repeat it in a meditative way reveals its meaning.

1.29. From this practice, the awareness turns inward, and the distracting obstacles vanish.

4.1. Siddhis are born of practices performed in previous births, or by herbs, mantra repetition, asceticism, or samadhi.

Meditation (also see Nirodha)

This list includes the definition of meditation, tips on how to make the practice firmly grounded, and various suggestions for choosing a suitable object for meditation.

1.2. The restraint of the modifications of the mind-stuff is Yoga.

1.12. These mental modifications are restrained by practice and nonattachment.

1.13. *Of these two, effort toward steadiness is practice.*

1.14. *Practice becomes firmly grounded when well attended to for a long time, without break, and with enthusiasm.*

1.27. *The expression of Ishwara is the mystic sound OM.*

The above sutra serves as the lead-in for the two that follow.

1.28. *To repeat it in a meditative way reveals its meaning.*

1.29. *From this practice, the awareness turns inward, and the distracting obstacles vanish.*

1.32. *The concentration on a single subject (or the use of one technique) is the best way to prevent the obstacles and their accompaniments.*

1.35. *Or that (undisturbed calmness) is attained when the perception of a subtle sense object arises and holds the mind steady.*

1.36. *Or by concentrating on the supreme, ever-blissful Light within.*

1.37. *Or by concentrating on a great soul's mind which is totally freed from attachment to sense objects.*

1.38. *Or by concentrating on an insight had during dream or deep sleep.*

1.39. *Or by meditating on anything one chooses that is elevating.*

1.45. *The subtlety of possible objects of concentration ends only at the undifferentiated.*

2.11. *In the active state, they (the obstacles of 2.3) can be destroyed by meditation.*

2.29. *The eight limbs of Yoga are:*
   1. *yama – abstinence*
   2. *niyama – observance*
   3. *asana – posture*
   4. *pranayama – breath control*
   5. *pratyahara – sense withdrawal*
   6. *dharana – concentration*
   7. *dhyana – meditation*
   8. *samadhi – contemplation, absorption or super-conscious state*

2.33. *When disturbed by negative thoughts, opposite (positive) ones should be thought of. This is pratipaksha bhavana.*

2.33. *When disturbed by negative thoughts, opposite (positive) ones should be thought of. This is pratipaksha bhavana.*

Although this is usually given as advice for handling difficult situations in life, it also can be understood to be a fundamental technique for advancing in meditation. When applying this sutra to meditation, negative thoughts are any that distract our attention, and the opposing thought is the chosen object of meditation.

2.48. *Thereafter [after mastering asana], one is undisturbed by dualities.*

Discomfort of the body is one of the biggest obstacles in meditation. Good progress is made when the practitioner can forget the body and allow the focus to move more deeply within.

2.51. *There is a fourth kind of pranayama that occurs during concentration on an internal or external object.*

The above sutra is referring to breath retention that naturally occurs when the mind becomes very still.

2.53. *And the mind becomes fit for concentration.*

2.54. *When the senses withdraw themselves from the objects and imitate, as it were, the nature of the mind-stuff, this is pratyahara.*

2.55. *Then follows supreme mastery over the senses.*

To redirect the attention away from the objects that inhabit our ordinary consciousness, we need to learn to withdraw the senses, bring them within, and free the attention for more subtle explorations

3.1. *Dharana is the binding of the mind to one place, object, or idea.*

3.2. *Dhyana is the continuous flow of cognition toward that object.*

3.3. *Samadhi is the same meditation when the mind-stuff, as if devoid of its own form, reflects the object alone.*

Mind and Self, discrimination between

The ability to discriminate between the mind and the Atman is an attainment that leads to overcoming ignorance (*see sutras 4.25 and 4.26*). Here you will also find sutras that discuss the fundamental aspects and supports for the mind—the ego and intellect—as well as the relationship between Prakriti and Purusha.

2.6. *Egoism is the identification, as it were, of the power of the Seer (Purusha) with that of the instrument of seeing (body-mind).*

2.20. *The Seer is nothing but the power of seeing which, although pure, appears to see through the mind.*

2.21. *The seen exists only for the sake of the Seer.*

2.23. *The union of Owner (Purusha) and owned (Prakriti) causes the recognition of the nature and powers of them both.*

The mind is part of Prakriti.

3.36. The intellect (sattwa) and the Purusha are totally different, the intellect existing for the sake of the Purusha, while the Purusha exists for its own sake. Not distinguishing this is the cause of all experiences. By samyama on this distinction, knowledge of the Purusha is gained.

3.50. By recognition of the distinction between sattwa (the pure reflective aspect of the mind) and the Self, supremacy over all states and forms of existence (omnipotence) is gained, as is omniscience.

3.56. When the tranquil mind attains purity equal to that of the Self, there is Absoluteness.

4.18. The modifications of the mind-stuff are always known to the changeless Purusha, who is its lord.

4.19. The mind-stuff is not self-luminous because it is an object of perception by the Purusha.

4.20. The mind-stuff cannot perceive both subject and object simultaneously (which proves it is not self-luminous).

4.21. If perception of one mind by another is postulated, we would have to assume an endless number of them, and the result would be confusion of memory.

4.22. The consciousness of the Purusha is unchangeable; by getting the reflection of it, the mind-stuff becomes conscious of the Self.

4.23. The mind-stuff, when colored by both Seer and seen, understands everything.

4.24. Though colored by countless subliminal traits (vasanas), the mind-stuff exists for the sake of another (the Purusha) because it can act only in association with It.

4.25. To one who sees the distinction between the mind and the Atman, thoughts of the mind as Atman cease forever.

4.26. Then the mind-stuff is inclined toward discrimination and gravitates toward Absoluteness.

4.27. In between, distracting thoughts may arise due to past impressions.

4.28. They can be removed, as in the case of the obstacles explained before. (See sutras 2.10 and 2.11.)

N

Nature, see Gunas

Nirodha (also see Meditation)

1.2. The restraint of the modifications of the mind-stuff is Yoga.

1.12. These mental modifications are restrained by practice and nonattachment.

2.33. When disturbed by negative thoughts, opposite (positive) ones should be thought of. This is pratipaksha bhavana. (Also see comments on this sutra in the Meditation section.)

2.41. Moreover (by the practice of purity mentioned in sutra 2.32), one gains purity of sattwa, cheerfulness of mind, one-pointedness, mastery over the senses, and fitness for Self-realization.

2.54. When the senses withdraw themselves from the objects and imitate, as it were, the nature of the mind-stuff, this is pratyahara.

2.55. Then follows supreme mastery over the senses.

3.1. Dharana is the binding of the mind to one place, object, or idea.

3.2. Dhyana is the continuous flow of cognition toward that object.

3.3. Samadhi is the same meditation when the mind-stuff, as if devoid of its own form, reflects the object alone.

3.5. By the mastery of samyama (the practices of dharana, dhyana and samadhi all directed toward a single object), knowledge born of intuitive insight shines forth.

3.9. Impressions of externalization are subdued by the appearance of impressions of nirodha. As the mind begins to be permeated by moments of nirodha, there is development in nirodha.

3.10. The flow of nirodha parinama becomes steady through habit.

3.11. The mind-stuff transforms toward samadhi when distractedness dwindles and one-pointedness arises.

3.12. Then again, when the subsiding and arising images are identical, there is one-pointedness (ekagrata parinama).

Nonattachment

This list includes sutras that address both nonattachment and the root of attachment: ignorance.

1.12. These mental modifications are restrained by practice and nonattachment. See sutra 1.5, to review the five kinds of mental modifications.

1.15. Nonattachment is the manifestation of self-mastery in one who is free from craving for objects seen or heard about.

1.16. When there is nonthirst for even the gunas (constituents of Nature) due to realization of the Purusha, that is supreme nonattachment.

2.3. Ignorance, egoism, attachment, aversion, and clinging to bodily life are the five obstacles.

2.4. Ignorance is the field for the others mentioned after it, whether they be dormant, feeble, intercepted, or sustained.

2.7. *Attachment is that which follows identification with pleasurable experiences.*

2.8. *Aversion is that which follows identification with painful experiences.*

O

Obstacles

Although Sri Patanjali mentions obstacles only in sutras 1.30 and 2.3, additional sutras address various other impediments.

1.29. *From this practice, the awareness turns inward, and the distracting obstacles vanish.*

What is referred to in the above sutra is mantra repetition, mentioned in sutra 1.28. *To repeat it in a meditative way reveals its meaning.*

1.30. *Disease, dullness, doubt, carelessness, laziness, sensuality, false perception, failure to reach firm ground, and slipping from the ground gained—these distractions of the mind-stuff are the obstacles.*

1.31. *Accompaniments to the mental distractions include distress, despair, trembling of the body, and disturbed breathing.*

1.32. *The concentration on a single subject (or the use of one technique) is the best way to prevent the obstacles and their accompaniments.*

2.1. *Accepting pain as help for purification, study, and surrender to the Supreme Being constitute Yoga in practice.*

The above sutra is the lead-in for the one that follows.

2.2. *They help us minimize the obstacles and attain samadhi.*

2.3. *Ignorance, egoism, attachment, aversion, and clinging to bodily life are the five obstacles.*

2.4. *Ignorance is the field for the others mentioned after it, whether they be dormant, feeble, intercepted, or sustained.*

2.10. *In their subtle form, these obstacles can be destroyed by resolving them back into their original cause (the ego).*

2.11. *In the active state, they can be destroyed by meditation.*

2.12. *The womb of karmas has its roots in these obstacles, and the karmas bring experiences in the seen (present) or in the unseen (future) births.*

2.33. *When disturbed by negative thoughts, opposite (positive) ones should be thought of. This is pratipaksha bhavana.*

Pratipaksha bhavana is one of the best ways to overcome obstacles. See also the following sutra.

2.34. *When negative thoughts or acts such as violence and so on are caused to be done, or even approved of, whether incited by greed, anger, or infatuation, whether indulged in with mild, medium, or extreme intensity, they are based on ignorance and bring certain pain. Reflecting thus is also pratipaksha bhavana.*

2.40. *By purification, the body's protective impulses are awakened as well as a disinclination for detrimental contact with others.*

2.41. *Moreover, one gains purity of sattwa, cheerfulness of mind, one-pointedness, mastery over the senses, and fitness for Self-realization.*

In a way, purity of mind is the whole of spiritual life. With it, all obstacles vanish, without it, we remain in ignorance.

2.43. *By austerity, impurities of body and senses are destroyed and occult powers gained.*

In the above sutra, impurities are being considered as obstacles.

2.52. *As its result (of the practice of pranayama), the veil over the inner light is destroyed.*

The above sutra is primarily referring to the removal of tamas, which obstructs our experience of our inner light. This is one of two sutras that use the term "veil" to refer to an obstacle. The other one follows.

3.44. *(By virtue of samyama on ether) vritti activity that is external to the body is (experienced and) no longer inferred. This is the great bodilessness which destroys the veil over the light of the Self.*

4.3. *Incidental events do not directly cause natural evolution; they just remove the obstacles as a farmer (removes the obstacles in a watercourse running to his field).*

4.11. *The vasanas, being held together by cause, effect, basis, and support, disappear with the disappearance of these four.*

If we can remove vasanas—deep-seated, subconscious character traits—we will be well on our way to experiencing spiritual freedom.

P

Physical Aspects of Raja Yoga

Here you will find sutras that address such topics as the nature of the body, the importance of purifying it, and how it can be used to aid in the quest for Self-realization.

1.31. *Accompaniments to the mental distractions include distress, despair, trembling of the body, and disturbed breathing.*

The mental distractions are listed in sutra 1.30.

2.32. Niyama consists of purity, contentment, accepting but not causing pain, study and worship of God (self-surrender).

2.38. To one established in continence, vigor is gained.

2.40. By purification, the body's protective impulses are awakened as well as a disinclination for detrimental contact with others.

2.46. Asana is a steady, comfortable posture.

2.47. By lessening the natural tendency for restlessness and by meditating on the infinite, posture is mastered.

2.48. Thereafter, one is undisturbed by dualities.

2.49. That (firm posture) being acquired, the movements of inhalation and exhalation should be controlled. This is pranayama.

2.50. The modifications of the life-breath are external, internal, or stationary. They are to be regulated by space, time, and number and are either long or short.

2.51. There is a fourth kind of pranayama that occurs during concentration on an internal or external object.

3.25. By samyama on the strength of elephants and other such animals, their strength is obtained.

3.30. By samyama on the navel plexus, knowledge of the body's constitution is obtained.

3.31. By samyama on the pit of the throat, cessation of hunger and thirst is achieved.

3.32. By samyama on the kurma nadi (the tortoise-shaped nadi below the throat), motionlessness in the meditative posture is achieved.

3.40. By mastery over the udana nerve current (the upward-moving prana), one accomplishes levitation over water, swamps, thorns, and so on and can leave the body at will.

3.41. By mastery over the samana nerve current (the equalizing prana) comes radiance that surrounds the body.

3.42. By samyama on the relationship between ear and ether, supernormal hearing becomes possible.

3.43. By samyama on the relationship between the body and ether, lightness of cotton fiber is attained, and thus traveling through the ether becomes possible.

3.46. From that (mastery over the elements) comes attainment of anima and other siddhis, bodily perfection, and the nonobstruction of bodily functions by the influence of the elements.

The eight major siddhis alluded to are: anima (to become very small); mahima (to become very big); laghima (to become very light); garima (to become very heavy); prapati (to reach anywhere); prakamya (to achieve all one's desires); isatva (the ability to create anything); vasitva (the ability to command and control everything).

3.47. *Beauty, grace, strength, and adamantine hardness constitute bodily perfection.*

Pleasure and Pain

Our minds are habituated to either chasing after pleasure or trying to avoid pain. It is important to have a clear understanding of the nature and origins of these motivators. To experience the peace and joy of the Self, both craving for pleasure and aversion to pain need to be transcended.

1.5. *There are five kinds of mental modifications, which are either painful or painless.*

1.24. *Ishwara is the supreme Purusha, unaffected by any afflictions, actions, fruits of actions, or any inner impressions of desires.*

2.1. *Accepting pain as help for purification, study, and surrender to the Supreme Being constitute Yoga in practice.*

2.7. *Attachment is that which follows identification with pleasurable experiences.*

2.8. *Aversion is that which follows identification with painful experiences.*

2.13. *With the existence of the root, there will also be fruits: the births of different species of life, their life spans, and experiences.*

2.14. *The karmas bear fruits of pleasure and pain caused by merit and demerit.*

2.15. *To one of discrimination, everything is painful indeed, due to its consequences: the anxiety and fear over losing what is gained; the resulting impressions left in the mind to create renewed cravings; and the conflict among the activities of the gunas, which control the mind.*

2.16. *Pain that has not yet come is avoidable.*

2.17. *The cause of that avoidable pain is the union of the Seer (Purusha) and seen (Prakriti).*

2.48. *Thereafter (after mastering asana), one is undisturbed by dualities.*

The above sutra refers not only to remaining undisturbed during the practice of meditation, but at other times as well.

4.7. *The karma of the yogi is neither white (good) nor black (bad); for others there are three kinds (good, bad, and mixed).*

Practice

What follows is a list of the practices that are mentioned in the sutras. By reviewing this list, we can grasp the scope and depth of Raja Yoga techniques and methods. Because samadhi is a topic that is large and involved, most of the sutras that discuss samadhi are included under its own heading (see Samadhi).

1.2. *The restraint of the modifications of the mind-stuff is Yoga.*

1.7. *The sources of right knowledge are direct perception, inference, and authoritative testimony.*

1.12. *These mental modifications are restrained by practice and nonattachment.*

1.13. *Of these two, effort toward steadiness of mind is practice.*

1.14. *Practice becomes firmly grounded when well attended to for a long time, without break, and with enthusiasm.*

1.15. *Nonattachment is the manifestation of self-mastery in one who is free from craving for objects seen or heard about.*

Strictly speaking, the sutras list nonattachment as the complement to practice. In our daily life, the roots of attachments are discovered through such practices as mindfulness, study, and self-analysis. Seekers also seek strength and guidance for overcoming attachments through prayer and worship. In short, nonattachment is gained with the aid of a great deal of practice.

1.21. *To the keen and intent practitioner this (samadhi) comes very quickly.*

1.23. *Or (samadhi is attained) by devotion with total dedication to God (Ishwara).*

1.27. *The expression of Ishwara is the mystic sound OM.*

1.28. *To repeat it in a meditative way reveals its meaning.*

1.29. *From this practice, the awareness turns inward, and the distracting obstacles vanish.*

1.32. *The concentration on a single subject (or the use of one technique) is the best way to prevent the obstacles and their accompaniments.*

1.33. *By cultivating attitudes of friendliness toward the happy, compassion for the unhappy, delight in the virtuous, and equanimity toward the nonvirtuous, the mind-stuff retains its undisturbed calmness.*

1.34. *Or that calm is retained by the controlled exhalation or retention of the breath.*

1.35. Or that (undisturbed calmness) is attained when the perception of a subtle sense object arises and holds the mind steady.

1.36. Or by concentrating on the supreme, ever-blissful Light within.

1.37. Or by concentrating on a great soul's mind which is totally freed from attachment to sense objects.

1.38. Or by concentrating on an insight had during dream or deep sleep.

1.39. Or by meditating on anything one chooses that is elevating.

1.45. The subtlety of possible objects of concentration ends only at the undifferentiated.

2.1. Accepting pain as help for purification, study, and surrender to the Supreme Being constitute Yoga in practice.

2.2. They help us minimize the obstacles and attain samadhi.

2.10. In their subtle form, these obstacles can be destroyed by resolving them back into their original cause (the ego).

2.11. In the active state, they can be destroyed by meditation.

2.28. By the practice of the limbs of Yoga, the impurities dwindle away and there dawns the light of wisdom leading to discriminative discernment.

2.29. The eight limbs of Yoga are:

   1. *yama* – *abstinence*

   2. *niyama* – *observance*

   3. *asana* – *posture*

   4. *pranayama* – *breath control*

   5. *pratyahara* – *sense withdrawal*

   6. *dharana* – *concentration*

   7. *dhyana* – *meditation*

   8. *samadhi* – *contemplation, absorption or super-conscious state*

2.33. When disturbed by negative thoughts, opposite (positive) ones should be thought of. This is pratipaksha bhavana.

2.34. When negative thoughts or acts such as violence and so on are caused to be done, or even approved of, whether incited by greed, anger, or infatuation, whether indulged in with mild, medium, or extreme intensity, they are based on ignorance and bring certain pain. Reflecting thus is also pratipaksha bhavana.

2.45. By total surrender to Ishwara, samadhi is attained.

2.46. Asana is a steady, comfortable posture.

2.47. By lessening the natural tendency for restlessness and by meditating on the infinite, posture is mastered.

2.48. Thereafter, one is undisturbed by dualities.

2.49. That (firm posture) being acquired, the movements of inhalation and exhalation should be controlled. This is pranayama.

2.50. The modifications of the life-breath are external, internal, or stationary. They are to be regulated by space, time, and number and are either long or short.

2.51. There is a fourth kind of pranayama that occurs during concentration on an internal or external object.

2.54. When the senses withdraw themselves from the objects and imitate, as it were, the nature of the mind-stuff, this is pratyahara.

2.55. Then follows supreme mastery over the senses.

3.1. Dharana is the binding of the mind to one place, object, or idea.

3.2. Dhyana is the continuous flow of cognition toward that object.

3.3. Samadhi is the same meditation when the mind-stuff, as if devoid of its own form, reflects the object alone.

3.4. The practice of these three (dharana, dhyana, and samadhi) upon one object is called samyama.

3.5. By mastery of samyama, knowledge born of intuitive insight shines forth.

3.6. Its practice is accomplished in stages.

3.7. These three (dharana, dhyana and samadhi) are more internal than the preceding five limbs.

3.9. Impressions of externalization are subdued by the appearance of impressions of nirodha. As the mind begins to be permeated by moments of nirodha, there is development in nirodha.

3.10. The flow of nirodha parinama becomes steady through habit.

3.11. The mind-stuff transforms toward samadhi when distractedness dwindles and one-pointedness arises.

3.12. Then again, when the subsiding and arising images are identical, there is one-pointedness (ekagrata parinama).

3.16. By practicing samyama on the three stages of evolution comes knowledge of past and future.

3.17. A word, its meaning, and the idea behind it are normally confused because of superimposition upon one another. By samyama on the word (or sound) produced by any being, knowledge of its meaning is obtained.

3.18. By direct perception, through samyama, of one's mental impressions, knowledge of past births is obtained.

4.3. Incidental events do not directly cause natural evolution; they just remove the obstacles as a farmer (removes the obstacles in a watercourse running to his field).

After all the sutras on practice, Sri Patanjali reveals that they do not give us anything that we didn't have before. The truth is that peace, joy, and wisdom are within us as our True Identity.

Prakriti, *see Gunas*

Pranayama

1.34. Or that calm is retained by the controlled exhalation or retention of the breath.

2.29. The eight limbs of Yoga are:
1. *yama – abstinence*
2. *niyama – observance*
3. *asana – posture*
4. *pranayama – breath control*
5. *pratyahara – sense withdrawal*
6. *dharana – concentration*
7. *dhyana – meditation*
8. *samadhi – contemplation, absorption or super-conscious state*

2.49. That (firm posture) being acquired, the movements of inhalation and exhalation should be controlled. This is pranayama.

2.50. The modifications of the life-breath are external, internal, or stationary. They are to be regulated by space, time, and number and are either long or short.

2.51. There is a fourth kind of pranayama that occurs during concentration on an internal or external object.

2.52. As its result, the veil over the inner light is destroyed.

2.53. And the mind becomes fit for concentration.

Pratyaya

Pratyaya is a difficult word to translate. Sri Patanjali seems to use it mostly to refer to the immediate reaction of the mind to a stimulus, or to the mental impression that starts the process of vritti activity. Pratyaya is translated as "thought" or "thought wave" in sutras 1.10, 1.18, 1.19, and 4.27, "images" in sutra 3.12 and "idea" in sutra 3.17.

1.10. That mental modification which depends on the thought of nothingness is sleep.

1.18. Noncognitive (asamprajnata) samadhi occurs with the cessation of all conscious thought; only the subconscious impressions remain.

1.19. *Yogis who have not attained asamprajnata samadhi remain attached to Prakriti at the time of death due to the continued existence of thoughts of becoming.*

2.20. *The Seer is nothing but the power of seeing which, although pure, appears to see through the mind.*

Pratyaya is here translated by the phrase, "through the mind," since it is the presence of arising of thoughts that make the Seer appear to be perceiving through, and limited by, the mind.

3.2. *Dhyana is the continuous flow of cognition toward that object.*

Pratyaya in the above sutra refers to the state of meditation in which the attention is fixed on one thought. Use of the word pratyaya instead of vritti here suggests that vritti activity becomes diminished or weakened when the mind is in dhyana.

3.12. *Then again, when the subsiding and arising images are identical, there is one-pointedness (ekagrata parinama).*

3.17. *A word, its meaning, and the idea behind it are normally confused because of superimposition upon one another. By samyama on the word (or sound) produced by any being, knowledge of its meaning is obtained.*

3.36. *The intellect (sattwa) and the Purusha are totally different, the intellect existing for the sake of the Purusha, while the Purusha exists for its own sake. Not distinguishing this is the cause of all experiences. By samyama on this distinction, knowledge of the Purusha is gained.*

In the sutra above, "pratyaya" is not directly translated. Instead, it is described as that which constitutes or makes possible our experiences in the world. In other words, pratyayas are perceptions in which no distinction is made between the Purusha and the intellect.

4.27. *In between, distracting thoughts may arise due to past impressions.*

Purpose of Life

In a few simple sutras, we find an answer to the classic question: What is the purpose of life? The answer is practical and presents the world as not only helpful to our spiritual maturity but essential to it.

2.18. *The seen is of the nature of the gunas: illumination, activity, and inertia. It consists of the elements and sense organs, whose purpose is to provide both experiences and liberation to the Purusha.*

2.21. *The seen exists only for the sake of the Seer.*

4.24. *Though colored by countless subliminal traits (vasanas), the mind-stuff exists for the sake of another (the Purusha) because it can act only in association with It.*

Purusha

1.24. *Ishwara is the supreme Purusha, unaffected by any afflictions, actions, fruits of actions, or any inner impressions of desires.*

2.18. *The seen is of the nature of the gunas: illumination, activity, and inertia. It consists of the elements and sense organs, whose purpose is to provide both experiences and liberation to the Purusha.*

2.20. *The Seer is nothing but the power of seeing which, although pure, appears to see through the mind.*

2.25. *Without this ignorance, no such union occurs. This is the independence of the Seer.*

4.18. *The modifications of the mind-stuff are always known to the changeless Purusha, who is its lord.*

4.19. *The mind-stuff is not self-luminous because it is an object of perception by the Purusha.*

4.22. *The consciousness of the Purusha is unchangeable; by getting the reflection of it, the mind-stuff becomes conscious of the Self.*

4.23. *The mind-stuff, when colored by both Seer and seen, understands everything.*

4.24. *Though colored by countless subliminal traits (vasanas), the mind-stuff exists for the sake of another (the Purusha) because it can act only in association with It.*

R

Reincarnation

Most modern Western faith traditions either do not address or do not currently espouse the doctrine of reincarnation; therefore it is not well understood in the West.

There is good evidence that at least some sects of Judaism and early Christianity believed in this doctrine. In some cases, the reason it has been lost to these traditions may be as much political as philosophical.

There are some interesting biblical passages that strongly suggest reincarnation. There is an event in the Gospel of John in which one of the apostles, upon seeing a man blind from birth, asked Lord Jesus,

"Is this man's blindness due to his sins or the sins of his father?" (John 9.2). Considering that the man was born sightless, there would be no question of his blindness being the result of his own sins if there were not a belief in reincarnation.

The cosmic law of cause and effect exists universally or it does not. Therefore we have to apply it universally or ignore it altogether. It cannot be utilized only when convenient or comfortable. Physical death does not disable karma, because the functioning of karma is not limited to the gross physical level. When the body passes away, the soul moves on to experience karmas appropriate to past actions and the current state of existence. This may include experiences of heaven or hell. However, for the yogi both heaven and hell are temporary states of existence. Once that karma is purged, the individual takes on another physical body to continue experiencing his or her karma. The law of karma teaches us that no one "gets away with murder" and that good deeds do find their just rewards. Sooner or later, we will reap what we have sown.

Though the *Yoga Sutras* offer philosophical proofs for reincarnation, we are not asked simply to believe in it because Sri Patanjali says so; such blind faith is not in keeping with the spirit of his teachings. Reincarnation is an observable reality that can be experienced directly (see sutras 2.39 and 3.18).

2.9. *Clinging to life, flowing by its own potency (due to past experience), exists even in the wise.*

2.12. *The womb of karmas has its roots in these obstacles, and the karmas bring experiences in the seen (present) or in the unseen (future) births.*

2.13. *With the existence of the root, there will also be fruits: the births of different species of life, their life spans, and experiences.*

2.39. *To one established in nongreed, a thorough illumination of the how and why of one's birth comes.*

3.18. *By direct perception, through samyama, of one's mental impressions, knowledge of past births is obtained.*

4.1. *Siddhis are born of practices performed in previous births, or by herbs, mantra repetition, asceticism, or samadhi.*

Relationships

The *Yoga Sutras* do not directly address the subject of personal relationships. However, since there are certain factors common to all relationships, we can extrapolate helpful information from some of the sutras and apply it to our family, work, and romantic relationships.

1.33. *By cultivating attitudes of friendliness toward the happy, compassion for the unhappy, delight in the virtuous, and equanimity toward the non-virtuous, the mind-stuff retains its undisturbed calmness.*

Think of happy, unhappy, virtuous, and nonvirtuous as acts, not people, and you can see how this sutra would be of great benefit to any relationship. We remain calm while at the same time, others will feel supported.

2.30. *Yama consists of nonviolence, truthfulness, nonstealing, continence, and nongreed.*

This sutra contains much of practical use in our relationship to others.

2.33. *When disturbed by negative thoughts, opposite (positive) ones should be thought of. This is pratipaksha bhavana.*

All of us have our bad days, moody times, and anxieties. Often, we just unload our negativity on those around us. Here, we have a nice solution for keeping the peace.

2.34. *When negative thoughts or acts such as violence and so on are caused to be done, or even approved of, whether incited by greed, anger, or infatuation, whether indulged in with mild, medium, or extreme intensity, they are based on ignorance and bring certain pain. Reflecting thus is also pratipaksha bhavana.*

See the commentary for sutra 2.33 above.

2.35. *In the presence of one firmly established in nonviolence, all hostilities cease.*

Even before being perfectly established in this virtue, we will find that our spiritual work has produced a good measure of this benefit.

2.36. *To one established in truthfulness, actions and their results become subservient.*

3.24. *By samyama on friendliness and other such qualities, the power to transmit them is obtained.*

4.7. *The karma of the yogi is neither white (good) nor black (bad); for others there are three kinds (good, bad, and mixed).*

We all have faults and weaknesses. Most often, there is some selfishness even in a good act. And no person is totally evil. Some good is there, even if well hidden. Contemplating these truths makes us more compassionate and forgiving.

Results of Practice

1.16. When there is nonthirst for even the gunas (constituents of Nature) due to realization of the Purusha, that is supreme nonattachment.

1.21. To the keen and intent practitioner this (samadhi) comes very quickly.

1.22. The time necessary for success also depends on whether the practice is mild, moderate, or intense.

1.29. From this practice, the awareness turns inward, and the distracting obstacles vanish.

1.40. Gradually, one's mastery in concentration extends from the smallest particle to the greatest magnitude.

1.41. Just as the naturally pure crystal assumes shapes and colors of objects placed near it, so the yogi's mind, with its totally weakened modifications, becomes clear and balanced and attains the state devoid of differentiation between knower, knowable, and knowledge. This culmination of meditation is samadhi.

2.10. In their subtle form, these obstacles can be destroyed by resolving them back into their original cause (the ego).

2.11. In the active state, they can be destroyed by meditation.

2.35. In the presence of one firmly established in nonviolence, all hostilities cease.

2.36. To one established in truthfulness, actions and their results become subservient.

2.37. To one established in nonstealing, all wealth comes.

2.38. To one established in continence, vigor is gained.

2.39. To one established in nongreed, a thorough illumination of the how and why of one's birth comes.

2.40. By purification, the body's protective impulses are awakened as well as a disinclination for detrimental contact with others.

2.41. Moreover, one gains purity of sattwa, cheerfulness of mind, one-pointedness, mastery over the senses, and fitness for Self-realization.

2.43. By austerity, impurities of body and senses are destroyed and occult powers gained.

2.44. Through study comes communion with one's chosen deity.

2.45. By total surrender to Ishwara, samadhi is attained.

2.46. Asana is a steady, comfortable posture.

2.47. By lessening the natural tendency for restlessness and by meditating on the infinite, posture is mastered.

2.48. Thereafter, one is undisturbed by dualities.

2.51. There is a fourth kind of pranayama that occurs during concentration on an internal or external object.

2.52. As its result, the veil over the inner light is destroyed.

2.55. Then (after becoming established in pratyahara) follows supreme mastery over the senses.

3.5. By mastery of samyama, knowledge born of intuitive insight shines forth.

3.16. By practicing samyama on the three stages of evolution comes knowledge of past and future.

3.17. A word, its meaning, and the idea behind it are normally confused because of superimposition upon one another. By samyama on the word (or sound) produced by any being, knowledge of its meaning is obtained.

3.19. By samyama on the distinguishing signs of others' bodies knowledge of their mental images is obtained.

3.20. But this does not include the support in the person's mind (such as motive behind the thought, and so on), as that is not the object of the samyama.

3.21. By samyama on the form of one's body (and by) checking the power of perception by intercepting light from the eyes of the observer, the body becomes invisible.

3.22. In the same way, the disappearance of sound (and touch, taste, smell, and so on) is explained.

3.23. Karmas are of two kinds: quickly manifesting and slowly manifesting. By samyama on them, or on the portents of death, the knowledge of the time of death is obtained.

3.24. By samyama on friendliness and other such qualities, the power to transmit them is obtained.

3.25. By samyama on the strength of elephants and other such animals, their strength is obtained.

3.26. By samyama on the light within, the knowledge of the subtle, hidden, and remote is obtained. [Note: subtle as atoms, hidden as treasure, remote as far-distant lands.]

3.27. By samyama on the sun, knowledge of the entire solar system is obtained.

3.28. By samyama on the moon comes knowledge of the stars' alignment.

3.29. By samyama on the pole star comes knowledge of the stars' movements.

3.30. By samyama on the navel plexus, knowledge of the body's constitution is obtained.

3.31. By samyama on the pit of the throat, cessation of hunger and thirst is achieved.

3.32. By samyama on the kurma nadi (a tortoise-shaped nadi below the throat), motionlessness in the meditative posture is achieved.

3.33. By samyama on the light at the crown of the head (sahasrara chakra), visions of masters and adepts are obtained.

3.34. Or, in the knowledge that dawns by spontaneous intuition (through a life of purity), all the powers come by themselves.

3.35. By samyama on the heart, the knowledge of the mind-stuff is obtained.

3.36. The intellect (sattwa) and the Purusha are totally different, the intellect existing for the sake of the Purusha, while the Purusha exists for its own sake. Not distinguishing this is the cause of all experiences. By samyama on this distinction, knowledge of the Purusha is gained.

3.37. From this knowledge arises superphysical hearing, touching, seeing, tasting, and smelling through spontaneous intuition.

3.38. These (superphysical senses) are obstacles to (nirbija) samadhi but are siddhis in the externalized state.

3.39. By the loosening of the cause of bondage (to the body) and by knowledge of the channels of activity of the mind-stuff, entry into another body is possible.

3.40. By mastery over the udana nerve current (the upward-moving prana), one accomplishes levitation over water, swamps, thorns, and so on and can leave the body at will.

3.41. By mastery over the samana nerve current (the equalizing prana) comes radiance that surrounds the body.

3.42. By samyama on the relationship between ear and ether, supernormal hearing becomes possible.

3.43. By samyama on the relationship between the body and ether, lightness of cotton fiber is attained, and thus traveling through the ether becomes possible.

3.44. (By virtue of samyama on ether) vritti activity that is external to the body is (experienced and) no longer inferred. This is the great bodilessness which destroys the veil over the light of the Self.

3.45. Mastery over the gross and subtle elements is gained by samyama on their essential nature, correlations, and purpose.

3.46. From that (mastery over the elements) comes attainment of anima and other siddhis, bodily perfection, and the nonobstruction of bodily functions by the influence of the elements.

The eight major siddhis alluded to are: anima (to become very small); mahima (to become very big); laghima (to become very light); garima (to become very heavy); prapati (to reach anywhere); prakamya (to achieve all one's desires); isatva (the ability to create anything); vasitva (the ability to command and control everything).

3.48. *Mastery over the sense organs is gained by samyama on the senses as they correlate to the process of perception, the essential nature of the senses, the ego-sense, and to their purpose.*

3.49. *From that, the body gains the power to move as fast as the mind, the ability to function without the aid of the sense organs, and complete mastery over the primary cause (Prakriti).*

3.50. *By recognition of the distinction between sattwa (the pure reflective aspect of the mind) and the Self, supremacy over all states and forms of existence (omnipotence) is gained, as is omniscience.*

3.51. *By nonattachment even to that (all these siddhis), the seed of bondage is destroyed and thus follows Kaivalya (Independence).*

3.53. *By samyama on single moments in sequence comes discriminative knowledge.*

3.54. *Thus the indistinguishable differences between objects that are alike in species, characteristic marks, and positions become distinguishable.*

3.56. *When the tranquil mind attains purity equal to that of the Self, there is Absoluteness.*

4.1. *Siddhis are born of practices performed in previous births, or by herbs, mantra repetition, asceticism, or samadhi.*

4.34. *Thus the supreme state of Independence manifests, while the gunas reabsorb themselves into Prakriti, having no more purpose to serve the Purusha. Or, to look at it from another angle, the power of consciousness settles in its own nature.*

S

Sadhana, *see Practice*

Samadhi

Samadhi means to be completely absorbed; a merging of subject and object. It is the term used in the *Yoga Sutras* for superconscious states that result from attaining a clear, steady, one-pointed mind and nonattached attitude. A good general definition of samadhi is found in sutra 1.41:

Just as the naturally pure crystal assumes shapes and colors of objects placed near it, so the yogi's mind, with its totally weakened modifications, becomes clear and balanced and attains the state devoid of differentiation between knower, knowable, and knowledge. This culmination of meditation is samadhi.

The *Yoga Sutras* identify a number of samadhis that fall into four categories. They are, from most gross to most subtle:
Samprajnata (cognitive) samadhi:
- savitarka (with examination)
- nirvitarka (beyond examination)
- savichara (with insight)
- nirvichara (beyond insight)
- ananda (joy)
- asmita (pure I-am-ness)

Asamprajnata (noncognitive) samadhi
Dharmamegha samadhi (also considered a subcategory of asamprajnata samadhi)
Nirbija (seedless) samadhi

Samprajnata: Cognitive

The first category we encounter in the *Yoga Sutras* is samprajnata samadhi (cognitive samadhi). It is called "cognitive" because the mind holds its attention on an object (gross or subtle)—something that can be perceived. The samprajnata samadhis bring knowledge of the object of contemplation. The insight gained from these samadhis has a clarity, depth, breadth, and immediacy that is nothing like what we gain from ordinary thought processes. Sutra 1.17 lists four categories of samprajnata samadhi (also see sutras 1.42–1.44).

Sutra 1.17:
Vitarka (absorption on gross elements)
Vichara (absorption on subtle elements)
Ananda (absorption on pure, sattwic mind)
Asmita (absorption on the ego-sense)

The intention of sutra 1.17 is not only to present a description of the levels of samprajnata samadhi but to offer a breakdown of the broad categories of objects for meditation and contemplation: gross objects, subtle objects, the mind, and the ego-sense. Practitioners begin with the gross and, as their meditation deepens, naturally experience the other levels. This ultimately leads to the next major category of samadhi: asamprajnata.

Let's take a practical example that demonstrates how the mind moves through the four categories of objects in samprajnata samadhi. Suppose the object of meditation were a red rose.

Vitarka. In vitarka samadhi, the senses' perception of the flower is left behind for the inner impression—the image of a red rose on the mind. The mind's absorption on the rose begins a process of deep examination. However, in vitarka samadhi, the three facets involved in our usual understanding of gross objects—name, form, and ideas regarding the object—persist (see sutra 3.17). Also remaining, as with all the samprajnata samadhis, is the awareness of meditator, object of meditation, and act of meditating.

Vichara. The word vichara implies progressive movement. From examination of the gross aspects of an object, the mind penetrates the object more deeply to reflect on factors that brought the object into being and that constitute its subtle essence. This can include the subtle elements and such factors as time and space. In our example, as the meditation progresses, the mind naturally contemplates a subtle essence of the rose—perhaps its redness. Vichara samadhi provides direct insight into the principles of the evolution of matter as presented in sutra 3.13.

Ananda. As the mind becomes even more one-pointed and clear, the idea of redness evaporates and, in a natural progression, the mind probes the phenomenon of perception itself. The mind now focuses on the pure (sattwic) aspect of the mind. The pure mind is composed of the sattwa guna, whose nature is luminous, tranquil, and joyful; therefore the practitioner experiences joy (ananda).

Asmita. Finally, as the meditation naturally matures, the next object of examination is the ego-sense, the basis of individual perception.

The four stages of samprajnata samadhi can occur regardless of the (gross) object of meditation taken.

The next listing of samprajnata samadhis (see sutras 1.42–1.44) introduces us to a more detailed and technical examination of the vitarka and vichara samadhis:

Savitarka (absorption on gross elements)

Nirvitarka (absorption on gross elements without associated memories)

Savichara (absorption on subtle elements)

Nirvichara (absorption on subtle elements without associated memories)

Both vitarka samadhis are experienced with gross elements. The difference between them is that one is with (*sa*) and one beyond (*nir*) examination. In savitarka samadhi, this examination includes the influence of memories (name, learned characteristics, etc.) associated with the object of contemplation. In nirvitarka samadhi, since the examination of savitarka is completed, the object is known as it exists, independent of any memories and their attendant biases and colorations. The two vichara samadhis are explained in the same way, except the object of contemplation is a subtle element.

Nirvichara samadhi is referred to as *ritambhara prajna,* "truth-bearing" (see sutra 1.48). Since only the ego-sense remains and the samskaras of externalization are temporarily overcome by this experience, the yogi experiences the pure reflection of the Self on the mind. This state opens the practitioner to spontaneous and intuitive flashes of Self-knowledge. This experience is so powerful that it creates subconscious impressions of steady inner awareness—nirodha—that overcome the usual, day-to-day impressions that incline us toward externalization and distractedness (see sutras 1.50 and 3.9).

Yet in samprajnata samadhi, since the sense of individuality continues, the misidentification of the mental modifications as the Self persists.

Asamprajnata Samadhi: Noncognitive, or "The Samadhi That Is Not Samprajnata"

When even the ego-sense is transcended (at least temporarily), asamprajnata samadhi is attained. There are no objects in the conscious mind to contemplate; only the samskaras (subconscious impressions) remain in the mind. It is a state very close to complete freedom, but since subconscious impressions remain, there is still a chance that the practitioner can fall under the influence of ignorance if these "seeds" are activated by either external or internal stimuli (see sutra 1.18).

Dharmamegha Samadhi: "Cloud of Dharma" Samadhi

Understanding what Sri Patanjali meant by dharmamegha samadhi can be a little tricky.

The first problem is how to translate "dharma." It is a word with many important meanings, most of which fall into two categories:

- Virtue, law, duty, goal of life, and righteousness.
- Form, quality, or function. (You can find this usage of the word in sutras 3.13 and 4.12. In these instances, dharma is translated as form and characteristic.)

Understanding dharma as virtue leads to describing dharmamegha samadhi as an exalted state which occurs just prior to the highest samadhi (nirbija) and which confers on the practitioner the virtue of ending ignorance—the confusion between Self (Purusha) and Nature (Prakriti, specifically the individual body-mind) (see sutras 2.23–2.25).

Regarding dharma as form or quality also suggests that dharmamegha samadhi is the stage prior to complete enlightenment (nirbija samadhi), although the context is different. In this case, dharmamegha samadhi is the state in which the gunas (qualities of Nature) begin to evaporate for the practitioner. Dharmamegha samadhi is free from forms, characteristics, or functions. This interpretation of the term is supported by the subject matter of the sutras that surround sutra 4.29, which describe the gunas terminating their sequences of transformation for the practitioner and reabsorbing themselves into Prakriti. In sutra 4.34, this state is referred to as the "supreme state of Independence" (Kaivalya).

The two interpretations are not mutually exclusive. What we have here is the same experience—the "moments" before Self-realization in which all notions of the self and the universe dissolve—described from two different angles.

Dharmamegha samadhi is still sabija (with seed). For this reason, it may be understood as a subcategory of asamprajnata samadhi.

(see sutras 4.29–4.34, all of which are connected with this experience.)

Conditions that precede dharmamegha samadhi

Sutra 4.29 states that dharmamegha samadhi follows from two conditions:

A state of constant discriminative discernment (viveka) between the Spirit (Self, Purusha) and Nature (Prakriti). Discernment comes through practice. Recall that in sutra 2.28, we learned that discriminative discernment can be attained by the practice of the eight limbs of Yoga. We are told that in order to attain dharmamegha samadhi, our discernment must be "constant." This calls to mind sutra 1.13, "Of these two, effort toward steadiness is practice."

Complete nonattachment even to achieving the highest spiritual rewards. This describes the culmination of vairagya (nonattachment) (see sutra 1.16).

In other words, the two conditions required for the attainment of dharmamegha samadhi were set forth in sutra 1.12 ("These mental modifications are restrained by practice and nonattachment."). Dharmamegha samadhi represents the zenith of practice and nonattachment.

Nirbija Samadhi: Seedless Samadhi

Sutra 1.51 states it clearly: "With the stilling of even this impression, every impression is wiped out, and there is nirbija [seedless] samadhi." Nirbija samadhi is the state of complete enlightenment, Self-realization.

1.17. *Cognitive (samprajnata) samadhi (is associated with forms and) is attended by examination, insight, joy, and pure I-am-ness.*

1.18. *Noncognitive (asamprajnata) samadhi occurs with the cessation of all conscious thought; only the subconscious impressions remain.*

1.19. *Yogis who have not attained asamprajnata samadhi remain attached to Prakriti at the time of death due to the continued existence of thoughts of becoming.*

1.20. To the others, asamprajnata samadhi is preceded by faith, strength, mindfulness, (cognitive) samadhi, and discriminative insight.

1.21. To the keen and intent practitioner this (samadhi) comes very quickly.

1.22. The time necessary for success also depends on whether the practice is mild, moderate, or intense.

1.23. Or (samadhi is attained) by devotion with total dedication to God (Ishwara).

1.41. Just as the naturally pure crystal assumes shapes and colors of objects placed near it, so the yogi's mind, with its totally weakened modifications, becomes clear and balanced and attains the state devoid of differentiation between knower, knowable, and knowledge. This culmination of meditation is samadhi.

1.42. The samadhi in which an object, its name, and conceptual knowledge of it are mixed is called savitarka samadhi, the samadhi with examination.

1.43. When the subconscious is well purified of memories (regarding the object of contemplation), the mind appears to lose its own identity, and the object alone shines forth. This is nirvitarka samadhi, the samadhi beyond examination.

1.44. In the same way, savichara (with insight) and nirvichara (beyond insight) samadhis, which are practiced upon subtle objects, are explained.

1.45. The subtlety of possible objects of concentration ends only at the undifferentiated.

1.46. All these samadhis are sabija [with seed].

1.47. In the pure clarity of nirvichara samadhi, the supreme Self shines.

1.48. This is ritambhara prajna, the truth-bearing wisdom.

1.49. The purpose of this special wisdom is different from the insights gained by study of sacred tradition and inference.

1.50. Other impressions are overcome by the impression produced by this samadhi.

1.51. With the stilling of even this impression, every impression is wiped out and there is nirbija (seedless) samadhi.

2.22. Although destroyed for him who has attained liberation, it (the seen) exists for others, being common to them.

2.45. By total surrender to Ishwara, samadhi is attained.

3.3. Samadhi is the same meditation (referring to the seamless relationship between dharana and dhyana mentioned in sutras 3.1 & 3.2) when the mind-stuff, as if devoid of its own form, reflects the object alone.

3.4. *The practice of these three (dharana, dhyana, and samadhi) upon one object is called samyama.*

3.5. *By mastery of samyama, knowledge born of intuitive insight shines forth.*

3.6. *Its practice is accomplished in stages.*

3.7. *These three (dharana, dhyana and samadhi) are more internal than the preceding five limbs.*

3.8. *Even these three are external to the seedless samadhi.*

3.11. *The mind-stuff transforms toward samadhi when distractedness dwindles and one-pointedness arises.*

3.12. *Then again, when the subsiding and arising images are identical, there is one-pointedness (ekagrata parinama).*

3.51. *By nonattachment even to that (all these siddhis), the seed of bondage is destroyed and thus follows Kaivalya (Independence).*

3.56. *When the tranquil mind attains purity equal to that of the Self, there is Absoluteness.*

4.1. *Siddhis are born of practices performed in previous births, or by herbs, mantra repetition, asceticism, or samadhi.*

4.29. *The yogi, who has no self-interest in even the most exalted states, remains in a state of constant discriminative discernment called dharmamegha (cloud of dharma) samadhi.*

4.30. *From that samadhi (dharmamegha samadhi) all afflictions and karmas cease.*

4.34. *Thus the supreme state of Independence manifests, while the gunas reabsorb themselves into Prakriti, having no more purpose to serve the Purusha. Or, to look at it from another angle, the power of consciousness settles in its own nature.*

Samskaras (also see Vasanas)

Samskaras, subconscious impressions, hold an important place in Raja Yoga philosophy and practice because they exert a major influence on thought processes and perceptions.

1.18. *Noncognitive (asamprajnata) samadhi occurs with the cessation of all conscious thought; only the subconscious impressions remain.*

1.24. *Ishwara is the supreme Purusha, unaffected by any afflictions, actions, fruits of actions, or any inner impressions of desires.*

1.51. *With the stilling of even this impression, every impression is wiped out and there is nirbija (seedless) samadhi.*

2.15. To one of discrimination, everything is painful indeed, due to its consequences: the anxiety and fear over losing what is gained; the resulting impressions left in the mind to create renewed cravings; and the conflict among the activities of the gunas, which control the mind.

3.8. Even these three are external to the seedless samadhi (in which all impressions are wiped out)

3.9. Impressions of externalization are subdued by the appearance of impressions of nirodha. As the mind begins to be permeated by moments of nirodha, there is development in nirodha.

3.10. The flow of nirodha parinama becomes steady through habit.

3.18. By direct perception, through samyama, of one's mental impressions, knowledge of past births is obtained.

4.27. In between (when not making the distinction between mind and Atman), distracting thoughts may arise due to past impressions.

4.28. They can be removed, as in the case of the obstacles explained before.

Seer, *see Mind and Self, and Purusha*

Self, *see Mind and Self, and Purusha*

Self-realization

1.2. The restraint of the modifications of the mind-stuff is Yoga.

1.3. Then the Seer (Self) abides in Its own nature.

1.51. With the stilling of even this impression, every impression is wiped out and there is nirbija (seedless) samadhi.

2.22. Although destroyed for him who has attained liberation, it (the seen) exists for others, being common to them.

2.25. Without this ignorance, no such union (of Purusha and Prakriti) occurs. This is the independence of the Seer.

3.7. These three (dharana, dhyana and samadhi) are more internal than the preceding five limbs.

3.8. Even these three are external to the seedless samadhi.

3.55. The transcendent discriminative knowledge that simultaneously comprehends all objects in all conditions is the intuitive knowledge (which brings liberation).

3.56. When the tranquil mind attains purity equal to that of the Self, there is Absoluteness.

4.34. *Thus the supreme state of Independence manifests, while the gunas reabsorb themselves into Prakriti, having no more purpose to serve the Purusha. Or, to look at it from another angle, the power of consciousness settles in its own nature.*

Spirit and Nature

The spirit striving to break free from the limitations of matter highlights a basic dynamic of spiritual practice.

1.24. *Ishwara is the supreme Purusha, unaffected by any afflictions, actions, fruits of actions, or any inner impressions of desires.*

2.17. *The cause of that avoidable pain is the union of the Seer (Purusha) and seen (Prakriti).*

2.18. *The seen is of the nature of the gunas: illumination, activity, and inertia. It consists of the elements and sense organs, whose purpose is to provide both experiences and liberation to the Purusha.*

2.21. *The seen exists only for the sake of the Seer.*

2.22. *Although destroyed for him who has attained liberation, it (the seen) exists for others, being common to them.*

2.23. *The union of Owner (Purusha) and owned (Prakriti) causes the recognition of the nature and powers of them both.*

2.24. *The cause of this union is ignorance.*

2.25. *Without this ignorance, no such union occurs. This is the independence of the Seer.*

3.13. *By what has been said (in sutras 3.9–3.12) the transformations of the form, characteristics, and condition of the elements and sense organs are explained.*

4.2. *The transformation of one species into another is brought about by the inflow of nature.*

4.3. *Incidental events do not directly cause natural evolution; they just remove the obstacles as a farmer (removes the obstacles in a watercourse running to his field).*

4.18. *The modifications of the mind-stuff are always known to the changeless Purusha, who is its lord.*

T

True Identity, *see Mind and Self, and Purusha*

U

Union, *see Self-realization*

V

Vairagya, *see Nonattachment*

Vasanas (also see Samskaras)

Vasanas are a subset of samskaras. They are groups of related subconscious impressions that form the personality traits or tendencies that individuals carry with them throughout their lifetimes. Vasanas inhabit the subconscious mind, and because they induce a person to act, they are often regarded as subtle desires.

4.8. *From that (threefold karma) follows the manifestation of only those vasanas (subliminal traits) for which there are favorable conditions for producing their fruits.*

4.9. *Vasanas, though separated (from their manifestation) by birth, place, or time, have an uninterrupted relationship (to each other and the individual) due to the seamlessness of subconscious memory and samskaras.*

4.10. *Since the desire to live is eternal, vasanas are also beginningless.*

4.11. *The vasanas, being held together by cause, effect, basis, and support, disappear with the disappearance of these four.*

Viveka

1.20. *To the others, asamprajnata samadhi is preceded by faith, strength, mindfulness, (cognitive) samadhi, and discriminative insight.*

2.15. *To one of discrimination, everything is painful indeed, due to its consequences: the anxiety and fear over losing what is gained; the resulting impressions left in the mind to create renewed cravings; and the conflict among the activities of the gunas, which control the mind.*

2.26. *Uninterrupted discriminative discernment is the method for its (ignorance's) removal.*

2.28. *By the practice of the limbs of Yoga, the impurities dwindle away and there dawns the light of wisdom leading to discriminative discernment.*

3.53. *By samyama on single moments in sequence comes discriminative knowledge.*

3.54. *Thus the indistinguishable differences between objects that are alike in species, characteristic marks, and positions become distinguishable.*

3.55. *The transcendent discriminative knowledge that simultaneously comprehends all objects in all conditions is the intuitive knowledge (which brings liberation).*

4.25. *To one who sees the distinction between the mind and the Atman, thoughts of the mind as Atman cease forever.*

4.26. *Then the mind-stuff is inclined toward discrimination and gravitates toward Absoluteness.*

4.27. *In between, distracting thoughts may arise due to past impressions.*

4.29. *The yogi, who has no self-interest in even the most exalted states, remains in a state of constant discriminative discernment called dharmamegha (cloud of dharma) samadhi.*

Vrittis

Vrittis are usually translated as mental modifications or simply, modifications.

1.2. *The restraint of the modifications of the mind-stuff is Yoga.*

1.4. *At other times (the Self appears to) assume the forms of the mental modifications.*

1.5. *There are five kinds of mental modifications, which are either painful or painless.*

1.10. *That mental modification which depends on the thought of nothingness is sleep.*

1.41. *Just as the naturally pure crystal assumes shapes and colors of objects placed near it, so the yogi's mind, with its totally weakened modifications, becomes clear and balanced and attains the state devoid of differentiation between knower, knowable, and knowledge. This culmination of meditation is samadhi.*

2.11. *In the active state, the mental modifications can be destroyed by meditation.*

2.15. *To one of discrimination, everything is painful indeed, due to its consequences: the anxiety and fear over losing what is gained; the resulting impressions left in the mind to create renewed cravings; and the conflict among the activities of the gunas, which control the mind.*

In the above sutra, vritti is translated as "activities."

2.50. *The modifications of the life-breath are external, internal, or stationary. They are to be regulated by space, time, and number and are either long or short.*

3.44. (By virtue of samyama on ether) vritti activity that is external to the body is (experienced and) no longer inferred. This is the great bodilessness which destroys the veil over the light of the Self.

4.18. The modifications of the mind-stuff are always known to the changeless Purusha, who is its lord.

Y

Yoga, *see Self-realization*

Word-for-Word Sutra Dictionary

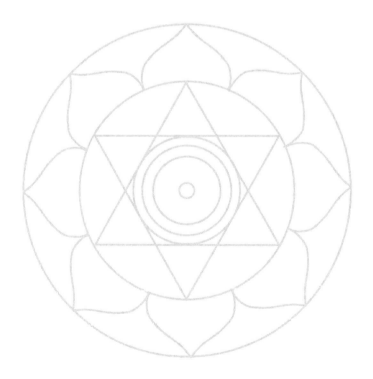

Word-for-word Yoga Sutras Dictionary

This section was assembled as an aid in preparing the commentary.

The sutra translations in this dictionary, as are those in the commentary, are based on *The Yoga Sutras of Patanjali*, by Sri Swami Satchidananda, although a number have been modified to varying degrees.

I did not use one of the standard methods for the transliteration of the Sanskrit terms. Instead, I have used a simplified system for easier reading.

The format is as follows:

- The sutra is rendered in English.
- Each word of the sutra is translated into English. Some words are translated literally, while others are given a more interpretive rendering or have commentary added in order to reflect the spirit and intent of the *Yoga Sutras*.
- The roots and the historical context of certain terms are presented when possible and noteworthy.

Pada One
Samadhi Pada: Portion on Absorption

1.1. Now, the exposition of Yoga.

Atha = now.

Usage of this term implies auspiciousness beginnings.

Yoga = to yoke; from the root, *yuj*.

In its spiritual usage, it originally referred to the control of the senses and harnessing the power of the mind toward the object of worship. This was later generalized to designate spiritual disciplines. The word is also used to refer to the union of the individual with the Absolute.

Anusasanam = exposition or instruction; from *sas* = to correct, restrain or teach + *anu* = after or with.

Use of this word implies that the exposition is on a subject that has been taught before.

1.2. The restraint of the modifications of the mind-stuff is Yoga.

Yogas = Yoga (*see sutra* 1.1).

Chitta = mind-stuff; from the verb root, *cit* = to perceive, observe, know.

In various philosophical systems of India, chitta has different meanings. For example, in Raja Yoga, the word is used to designate the mind (composed of manas, buddhi and ahamkara); in Advaita Vedanta, the subconscious.

Vritti = modifications; from *vrt* = to whirl, turn, revolve, go on, be conditioned by.

Vrittis describe the primary mental activity—the building of conceptions—which helps to create and maintain our sense of self-identity.

Nirodah = restraint; from *rudh* = to obstruct, restrict, arrest, avert, support + *nir* = down, into, back, within.

Nirodha is both a process and a state. The yogi needs to achieve nirodha on four basic levels of mental activity in order to attain Self-realization:

- Vrittis
- Presented thoughts (pratyaya, *see sutra* 1.10)
- Subconscious impressions (samskaras)
- Total nirodha, in which all mental activity comes to a standstill

In Buddhism, the word appears as the third of the Four Noble Truths and refers to the extinction (nirodha) of suffering (duhkha), the root of which is craving.

1.3. Then the Seer (Self) abides in Its own nature.

Tada = then.

Drastuh = Seer; from *drs* = to see.

> The Seer is the pure consciousness that comprehends all objects and events simultaneously. It is another way of referring to the Purusha.

Svarupe = in one's own nature; from *sva* = own or self + *rupa* = form, shape.

Avasthanam = abides; lit., to stand.

> State of consciousness, condition, state of experience, to remain.

1.4. At other times (the Self appears to) assume the forms of the mental modifications.

Vritti = modifications of the mind-stuff (*see sutra* 1.2).

Sarupyam = assumes the forms, conformity.

Itaratra = at other times, otherwise.

1.5. There are five kinds of mental modifications, which are either painful or painless.

Vrittayah = modifications (*see sutra* 1.2).

Panchatayyah = five kinds.

Klishta = painful, molested, afflicted, distressed, wearied, hurt, injured; from *klish* = to suffer, torment, cause pain, afflict.

> Klishta shares the same root with *klesa*, the "obstacles" of sutra 2.3, *"Ignorance, egoism, attachment, aversion and clinging to bodily life are the five obstacles."* Vrittis generated under the influence of the klesas bring pain.

Aklishta = painless.

1.6. They are right knowledge, misperception, conceptualization, sleep, and memory.

Pramana = right knowledge; from *ma* = to measure + *pra* = before or forward.

Viparyaya = misperception; from *i* = to go, flow or get about + *vi* = asunder or away + *pari* = around.

The sage Vyasa, who composed the *Yoga Bhashya*, the oldest known commentary on the *Yoga Sutras*, uses *viparyaya* interchangeably with *avidya* (ignorance). That is because he, along with other notable commentators (including Vicaspati Misra and Vijnana Biksu) understood ignorance to be the primary misperception (*see sutra 2.5 for a more detailed description*) because it makes possible all fundamental afflictions (*see sutra 2.3, the klesas*).

Vikalpa = conceptualization; from *klp* = to correspond, in accordance with, suitable to, well ordered + *vi* = asunder or away from, without.

Adherents of the philosophy of Saiva Siddhanta (a sect that worships Lord Shiva as the Absolute) recognize one allowable conceptualization: the thought "I am Shiva."

Nidra = sleep.

Smritayah = memory; from *smr* = to remember.

Smriti is also used to refer to the entire body of traditional sacred wisdom. It refers to that which is "remembered" by teachers as contrasted to *sruti*; that which is directly "heard" or revealed to the sages, saints and prophets.

1.7. The sources of right knowledge are direct perception, inference, and authoritative testimony.

Pratyaksha = direct perception; from *aks* = to reach, penetrate, embrace (*aks* also refers to the eyes or the sense of sight) + *prati* = in the direction of, in the presence of.

Pratyaksha is considered as a valid means of acquiring knowledge by all schools of philosophical thought in India.

Anumana = inference; from the verb root *ma* = to measure + *anu* = along or after.

Knowledge which is based on other previously known knowledge.

Agama = authoritative testimony; from *gam* = to go + *a* = toward; a source.

That which has come down from tradition.

Pramanani = sources of right knowledge, valid cognition (*see sutra 1.6*).

1.8. Misperception occurs when knowledge of something is not based on its true form.

Viparyayah = misperception (*see sutra 1.6*).

Mithyajnanam = false knowledge, not real, untrue, incorrect; from *mithya* = to conflict with or dispute + *jnana* = to know, knowledge.

Atadrupa = not on that form.

Pratishtham = based, settled in.

1.9. Knowledge that is based on language alone, independent of any external object, is conceptualization.

Sabdajnana = knowledge from words; from *sabda* = sound, words or language + *jnana* = knowledge, concept, idea.

Anupati = based on, follows; from *anu* = after + *pat* = to fall.

Vastu = reality; from *vas* = to live dwell, remain or abide.

Sunyo = without any.

Vikalpah = conceptualization (*see sutra* 1.6).

1.10. That mental modification which depends on the thought of nothingness is sleep.

Abhava = nothingness; from *bhu* = to become, exist + *a* = not.

Pratyaya = thought; from the verb root *i* = to go + *prati* = against, counter, in return, back.

In the *Yoga Sutras*, *pratyaya* is generally used to refer to the thought that instantly arises when the mind is impacted by an object of perception. As such, pratyayas form the content of vrittis. For example, if a birthday party can be likened to a vritti, then the guests, the cake, music and diversions are all pratyayas. Or, to take another example, the bit of sand that enters the oyster is a pratyaya. It irritates the oyster into making the pearl. The act of making the pearl represents vritti activity and the pearl itself can also be referred to as a vritti. In other words, while vritti refers to a fundamental mental *process*, pratyaya refers to the content of individual consciousness, including the insights (prajna) attained in all of the lower states of samadhi, which are not the result of virtti activity. This understanding of pratyaya is similar to one of the Buddhist uses of the word as a fundamental thought or idea.

Other views of pratyaya include: the total content of the mind at any moment, a cause, notion or idea. In Sankhya philosophy pratyaya is equivalent to the intellect or buddhi.

Alambana = support, depending on, resting on, based on.
Vrittir = modification of mind (*see sutra* 1.2).
Nidra = sleep.

1.11. Memory is the recollection of experienced objects.

Anubhuta = experienced, perceived, understood, apprehended.
Vishaya = objects.

Vishaya is anything that is experienced through the senses.
Asampramoshah = not forgotten.
Smritih = memory (*see* 1.6).

In the context of this sutra, smriti implies that the details of the past experience are accurately recalled. Nothing is added to or subtracted from that recollection. A smriti can include the object of experience, the subjective reaction to the experience or both.

1.12. These mental modifications are restrained by practice and nonattachment.

Abhyasa = practice; from *as* = to throw or apply oneself + *abhi* = toward.
Vairagyabhyam = nonattachment; from *vi* = without + *raj* = color, to be moved, excited, attracted.

Vairagya could also have its roots in, *vai* = not + *raj* = be attracted or excited
Tat = they.
Nirodhah = restrained (*see sutra* 1.2).

1.13. Of these two, effort toward steadiness is practice.

Tatra = of these.
Sthitau = steadiness; from *stha* = to stand.
Yatnah = effort; from *yat* = to marshal, to march in step, to be in line, to vie with.
Abhyasah = practice (*see sutra* 1.12).

1.14. Practice becomes firmly grounded when well attended to for a long time, without break, and with enthusiasm.

Sah = this.
Tu = and.
Dirgha = long.

Kala = time.

Nairantarya = without break, with nothing in between.

Satkara = enthusiasm; care, attention, devotion, sincerity, earnestness; from *sat* = right + *kr* = to do.

Satkara implies "to do right by," or in other words, to have the proper attitude towards.

Asevitah = well attended to, cultivated; from *sev* = to stay near, inhabit, honor.

Dridhabhumih = firm ground; from *drmh* = to fasten + *bhumih* = to become.

1.15. Nonattachment is the manifestation of self-mastery in one who is free from craving for objects seen or heard about.

Drishta = seen; from *drs* = to see.

Anusravika = heard; from *sru* = to hear.

Vishaya = object (*see sutra* 1.11).

Vitrishnasya = in one who is free from craving; from *vi* = without + *trs* = to be thirsty.

Vasikara = mastery; from *vas* = to will + *kr* = to make.

Samjna = manifestation, declaration, sign, acknowledgement, validation; from *jna* = to know.

Vairagyam = nonattachment (*see sutra* 1.12.)

1.16. When there is nonthirst for even the gunas (constituents of Nature) due to realization of the Purusha, that is supreme nonattachment.

Tat = that.

Param = supreme; from *para* = higher, supreme.

Purusha = Self, person, individual soul, cosmic person, pure Spirit, the eternal power of awareness, indwelling form of God. The root is uncertain. It may come from *puru* = a being connected with the sun.

A very similar idea in the tradition of Vedanta is referred to as atman.

Khyater = due to realization; from *khya* = to be known.

Guna = constituent of Nature; lit., strand or thread.

Vaitrishnyam = nonthirst (*see sutra* 1.15).

1.17. Cognitive (samprajnata) samadhi (is associated with forms and) is attended by examination, insight, joy, and pure I-am-ness.

Vitarka = examination, to ponder, think, discursive thought, cogitation, debate, logical argument, supposition, opinion, conjecture,
imagination; from *vi* = without, away + *tarka* = to reflect.

Examination was chosen in this text in order to contrast the knowledge
gained from this state to the usual mental processes of questioning,
comparing and contrasting. The word *examination* suggests to inspect
or to observe rather than to engage in a logical thought process in
order to arrive at understanding. In vitarka all details of the (gross)
object are revealed directly, intuitively and spontaneously.

Vichara = insight; from *vi* = without, way + *car* = to move.

Vichara is the next step deeper than vitarka. The word itself
implies a progressive movement away. In vichara samadhi, the
movement is away from the gross elements to the subtle elements
that are the support of the gross object. Vichara offers insights
into the causes of gross objects, the subtle elements and the
factors of space and time.

Ananda = joy.

Asmita = pure I-am-ness, egoism; the awareness of being distinct
from other beings and objects; from *asmi* = I am + *ta* = 'ness.'

Anugamat = attended by; lit., to go after, follow, observe.

Samprajnatah = cognitive; from *sam* = union, conjunction, complete-
ness, thoroughness + *prajna* = wisdom, knowledge, intelligence,
discrimination, judgment.

Samprajnata samadhi brings a thorough knowledge of the object
being contemplated.

1.18. Noncognitive (asamprajnata) samadhi occurs with the cessation of all conscious thought; only the subconscious impressions remain.

Virama = standstill; complete cessation, to stop, pause or cease.

Pratyaya = thoughts (*see sutra* 1.10).

Abhyasa = practice (*see sutra* 1.12).

Purvah = occurs (by the practice).

Samskara = impressions, subconscious impressions, subliminal
activators, conditioned memory responses; from *sam* = with + *kr* =
to do, make or cause.

Samskaras are deep-seated imprints left in the subconscious by experiences, which propel the mind into action. The *Yoga Sutras* discuss two basic categories of samskaras: those that lead toward the externalization of consciousness (vyutthana) and that maintain the influence of ignorance, and those that remove ignorance and lead toward nirodha.

Seshah = remain; from *sis* = to remain.

Anyah = the other.

1.19. Yogis who have not attained asamprajnata samadhi remain attached to Prakriti at the time of death due to the continued existence of thoughts of becoming.

Bhava = becoming, coming into existence, birth.

Pratyayah = thought, belief, presented idea, notion (*see sutra* 1.10).

Videha = bodiless, deceased.

The term also refers to celestial beings (gods).

Prakriti = Nature, unmanifest primary matter, from *pra* = forth + *kr* = to make, to do.

Other words that designate essentially the same principle are *avyakta* (unmanifest), *pradhana* (the originator, primordial matter), *drishya* (the Seen, that which is visible), *dharmin* (form holder, referring to a substance and its series of manifestations) and *alinga* (literally, without mark or sign; formless, undifferentiated, equilibrium of the gunas).

Prakriti is one, infinite and the source of the universe and all its objects—past, present and future. According to Sankhya and Classical Yoga, Prakriti has no consciousness of its own. Advaita Vedanta goes further, teaching that Prakriti is illusory (maya), not fundamentally real.

Prakriti and the gunas (sattwa, rajas and tamas) are closely related, but different philosophical schools have varying understandings of this relationship. For example, according to Advaita Vedanta, the gunas are characteristics of Prakriti, while in Sankhya, they are considered components of Prakriti.

Layanam = the act of sticking or clinging, to become attached, merged, absorbed, or dissolved.

1.20. To the others, asamprajnata samadhi is preceded by faith, strength, mindfulness, (cognitive) samadhi, and discriminative insight.

Sraddha = faith; from *srat* = to assure + *dha* = to put.

Virya = strength, energy, zeal, vigor, courage, heroism; from *vir* = to be powerful.

Smriti = mindfulness (*see sutra* 1.6).

Samadhi = (cognitive) samadhi; from *dha* = to hold + *a* + *sam* = together completely.

> In the *Yoga Sutras*, samadhi essentially refers to the integration or absorption of subject and object. The word *samapattih* is also used to designate the same experience. In this sutra, the samadhi referred to is samprajnata (cognitive) samadhi (*see sutra* 1.17).

Prajnapurvaka = discernment; from *prajna* = wisdom, knowledge, insight, intelligence, discrimination, judgment + *purvaka* = preceded by, conditioned or founded upon.

Prajnapurvaka is that which is based on, or preceded by, judgment or wisdom.

Itaresham = for the others.

1.21. To the keen and intent practitioner this (samadhi) comes very quickly.

Tivra = keen.

Samveganam = intent, intense ardor, desire for emancipation, violent agitation, excitement, flurry, high degree.

Asannah = near, close at hand, proximity; from *a* + *sad* = to sit.

> What is implied is that zeal in practice hastens the arrival of the experience of samadhi, in a sense, bringing it "near" to the practitioner.

1.22. The time necessary for success also depends on whether the practice is mild, moderate, or intense.

Mridu = mild.

Madhya = medium.

Adhimatratvat = intense; from *adhi* = above, over + *matra* = to measure.

> The roots of the word suggest an effort that is, "above the (usual) measure" made by most students.

Tato'pi = further.

Viseshah = differentiation, to distinguish, particularize, define.

This sutra is elaborating on factors that influence success in practice. In sutra 1.21, it was the personal intensity of the practitioner. In this sutra, it is the type of practices that are engaged in that determines the relative nearness (*see asannah, in sutra* 1.21) of success.

1.23. Or (samadhi is attained) by devotion with total dedication to God (Ishwara).

Ishwara = Supreme God, Lord, the Divine with form; from the verb root *is* = to rule, to own.

According to the *Yoga Sutras*, Ishwara is the Supreme Purusha, free from all afflictions and karmas; the teacher of even the most ancient teachers, who is designated by the mantra OM. In Advaita Vedanta, Ishwara is the Absolute (Brahman) as conditioned by ignorance or illusion.

Pranidhanat = dedicated devotion; from *pra* = before or in front + *ni* = down into or within + *dha* = place, put, hold.

Pranidhana, suggests: to bring within, to give priority before anything else. It refers to aligning one's own intent (personal will) to the wisdom of Ishwara (Divine Will).

In Buddhism, pranidhana is regarded as a vow and usually refers to the Boddisattva's vow of helping all beings attain liberation.

Va = or.

1.24. Ishwara is the supreme Purusha, unaffected by any afflictions, actions, fruits of actions, or any inner impressions of desires.

Klesa = afflictions; from *klis* = to be troubled, to suffer distress.

Karma = actions, cause and effect; rite; from *kr* = to do, act or make.

Karma includes physical, verbal and mental actions.

Vipaka = fruit of actions.

Vipaka implies a type of transformation, ripening, maturing, or consequence.

Asayair = impressions of desires; from *a* + *si* = to lie or rest.

In Yoga philosophy, asaya is the storehouse of impressions—the residue of previous actions - which lie stored in the subconscious and that bind the individual by impelling further action. (*See sutra* 2.12, "*karmasayah.*")

Aparamrishtah = unaffected by.

Purushaviseshah = supreme soul; from *purusha* = Self (*see sutra* 1.16) + *viseshah* (*see sutra* 1.22) = distinct .

Ishwara = God (*see sutra* 1.23).

1.25. In Ishwara is the complete manifestation of the seed of omniscience.

Tatra = in (Ishwara); lit., there.

Niratisayam = complete manifestation.

Sarvajna = omniscience; from *sarva* = all + *jna* = to know.

Bijam = seed.

1.26. Unconditioned by time, Ishwara is the teacher of even the most ancient teachers.

Sah = that, referring to Ishwara.

Purvesham = of the ancients; from *purva* = former.

Api = even.

Guru = teacher; from *gur* = to invoke or praise, to raise or lift up; the "weighty" or venerable one.

Scriptures such as the *Guru Gita* and the *Advaya-Taraka Upanishad* also state that the syllable, *gu* = darkness and *ru* = remover.

Kalena = by time.

Anavachchedat = unconditioned, not limited.

1.27. The expression of Ishwara is the mystic sound OM.

Tasya = that, referring to Ishwara (*see sutra* 1.23).

Vachakah = expression; from *vac* = to speak.

Pranavah = mystic sound OM, a pronouncement; from *pra* = to give, offer, bestow + *nu* = to praise or exult.

Sri Patanjali doesn't say what the sound is. Perhaps it was common knowledge that *pranavah* refers to the sacred syllable OM, a mantra used in India for thousands of years before his time.

If you would like other scriptural citations, you could refer to the *Mandukya Upanishad* which discusses the meaning of OM in detail.

1.28. To repeat it in a meditative way reveals its meaning.

Tat = that.

Japah = to repeat; from *jap* = to utter, whisper, mutter.

Tat = that.

Artha = meaning; purpose, aim, object of perception; from *arth* = to intend, to point out.

Bhavanam = meditation; from *bhu* = to become, exist, causing to be, effecting, producing, manifesting, displaying, contemplation, condition, inherent qualities of mind, feeling (in Bhakti Yoga).

Bhavanam is also understood as that cause of memory which arises from direct perception.

1.29. From this practice, the awareness turns inward, and the distracting obstacles vanish.

Tatah = from this.

Pratyak = inward, averted, to turn back; from *prati* = against, back + *ac* = to bend.

Chetana = awareness; from *chit* = consciousness.

Adhigamah = attainment, result, gain.

Api = also.

Antaraya = obstacles; from *antar* = go + *i* = between.

Abhavah = disappear.

Cha = and.

1.30. Disease, dullness, doubt, carelessness, laziness, sensuality, false perception, failure to reach firm ground, and slipping from the ground gained—these distractions of the mind-stuff are the obstacles.

Vyadhi = disease; from *a* = implying the contrary + *vi* = apart + *dha* = to have, hold.

Since *dha* implies stability and wholeness, *vyadhi* suggests that disease is anything that separates you from the experience of wholeness and that disrupts the stability or routine of your life.

Styana = dullness; from *styah* = to grow dense.

Samsaya = doubt.

Pramada = carelessness, heedless, negligent, indifferent, to neglect duty, to idle away time; from *mad* = intoxication.

Alasya = laziness.

Avirati = sensuality; from *ram* = to stop, dally.

Bhrantidarsana = false perception; from *bhranti* = to wander + *darsana* = vision.

Alabdhabhumikatva = failure to reach firm ground; from *alabdha* = not obtained + *bhumikatva* = groundedness, stage, place, basis.

Anavasthitatvani = slipping from the ground gained; from *stha* = to stand.

Chittavikshepah = distractions of the mind-stuff; from *chitta* = mind-stuff + *vikshepa* = shake, scatter, disperse.

Te = these.

Antarayah = obstacles.

1.31. Accompaniments to the mental distractions include distress, despair, trembling of the body, and disturbed breathing.

Duhkha = distress; from *dur* = bad + *kha* = state; or from *dus* = bad + *kha* = axle-hole.

The word translated as distress is *duhkha*, variously translated as pain, suffering, sorrow, or grief. But we can get a better, more vivid and instructive understanding of what dukha means in daily life by looking to the origin of the word. Literally translating as bad axle-hole, dukha suggests that we are driving a carriage with an axle-hole that is off-center, irregular and slightly too large. This off-center state of affairs would make our cart shake and wobble, giving us an uncomfortable and unsafe ride. Knowing this and wishing to avoid further pain, we scan the roadway for potholes. Sure enough, if we avoid the potholes, the ride is somewhat smoother. But we are still left with an unsteady ride that prolongs our feelings of unease and sorrow. Those who are wise look to see if there is something in their carriage that is at fault. Sooner or later, they find the bad axle-hole. They now know that in order to have a smooth, safe ride, it is not enough to be able to maneuver around potholes: they need to fix their carriage.

The road symbolizes life and the carriage is our body-mind. Duhkha is not simply a series of unpleasant experiences—potholes—that we inevitably encounter in life. It is the experience that there is something fundamentally misguided with our understanding and approach. That something, that which causes our suffering, is ignorance. Having lost our center (the Self), we are at the mercy of the pains that follow in the wake of ignorance. Buddhist translations of duhkha include imperfection, impermanence, emptiness, insubstantiality. Pleasurable experiences that are transitory are ultimately also duhkha, empty and unsatisfactory.

The Yoga Sutras mention duhkha seven times:

1.31: as an accompaniment to the mental distractions listed in 1.30.

1.33: compassion for those who experience duhkha.

2.5: one of the signs of ignorance, regarding that which brings duhkha as pleasant.

2.8: duhkha as the source of aversion.

2.15: all experiences based on ignorance bring certain duhkha.

2.16: duhkha that has not yet come is avoidable.

2.34: negative acts, regardless of motivation or intensity are based on ignorance and bring certain duhkha.

Daurmanasya = despair; from *dus* = bad + *man* = to think.

Angamejayatva = trembling of the body, restlessness; from *anga* = limb, body + *ejayatva* = tremble.

Svasa = (disturbed) inhalation.

Prasvasa = (disturbed) exhalation.

Vikshepa = mental distractions (*see sutra* 1.30).

Sahabhuvah = accompaniments; from *saha* = jointly + *bhu* = to become.

1.32. The concentration on a single subject (or the use of one technique) is the best way to prevent the obstacles and their accompaniments.

Tat = their, that.

Pratishedha = prevention, restrain, prohibit, disallow; from *prati* = counter + *sidh* = to ward off.

Artham = for, the purpose of (*see sutra* 1.28).

Eka = single.

Tattva = subject, reality, principle, the essence of anything; from *tat* = that; lit., "that-ness."

Tattva also refers to the elements in a system of philosophy.

Abhyasa = practice (*see sutra* 1.12).

1.33. By cultivating attitudes of friendliness toward the happy, compassion for the unhappy, delight in the virtuous, and equanimity toward the nonvirtuous, the mind-stuff retains its undisturbed calmness.

Maitri = friendliness.

Karuna = compassion.

Karuna is also understood as divine grace in certain philosophical schools.

Mudita = delight; from *mud* = to rejoice.

Upekshanam = equanimity; from *upa* = to go near, towards + *iksha* = to look at or on.

The roots of the word suggest, "to see clearly (accurately and objectively) by going near."

Sukha = happy; from *su* = well + *kha* = axle-hole (*see discussion of duhkha, sutra* 1.31).

Duhkha = unhappy (*see sutra* 1.31).

Punya = virtuous; from *pun* = to do good.

Apunya = non-virtuous (see *punya*, above).

Vishayanam = toward (experiences of).

Bhavanatah = by cultivating attitudes; from *bhu* = to become.

Chitta = mind-stuff (*see sutra* 1.2).

Prasadanam = undisturbed calmness, clarity, tranquility, a gift from God; from *pra* = to settle down, offer, grace + *sad* = to sit.

1.34. Or that calm is retained by the controlled exhalation or retention of the breath.

Panchchhardana = exhalation.

Vidharanabhyam = by retention.

Va = or.

Pranasya = of the breath; from *an* = to breathe + *pra* = forth.

1.35. Or that (undisturbed calmness) is attained when the perception of a subtle sense object arises and holds the mind steady.

Vishayavati = (subtle) sense object; from *vishaya* = sense-object (*see sutra* 1.11).

Although *vishaya* is literally translated simply as sense object, the adjective *subtle* has been added to help clarify the type of experience that is being referred to here.

Va = or.

Pravrittih = perception; from *pra* = forth + *vrt* = to turn.

Utpanna = arises.

Manasah = the mind.

Sthiti = steady; from *stha* = to stand (*see sutra* 1.13).

Nibandhani = holds, fixing, helpful in establishing, brings about; from *bandh* = to bind.

1.36. Or by concentrating on the supreme, ever-blissful Light within.

Visoka = blissful; from *vi* = not + *soka* = sorrow.

Va = or.

Jyotishmati = the supreme light; from *jyotish* = light + *mati* = having.

1.37. Or by concentrating on a great soul's mind which is totally freed from attachment to sense objects.

Vita = free from.

Raga = attachment; from *raj* = color, to be moved, excited, attracted.

Vishayam = for sense objects (*see sutra* 1.11).

Va = or.

Chittam = mind-stuff (*see sutra* 1.2).

1.38. Or by concentrating on an insight had during dream or deep sleep.

Svapna = dream.

Nidra = deep sleep.

Jnana = insights; from *jna* = to know.

Alambanam = resting on; concentrating; from *a* = hither, unto + *lamb* = depend, hang from, to hold or rest on.

Va = or.

1.39. Or by meditating on anything one chooses that is elevating.

Yatha = as.

Abhimata = per choice, dear, wished for, desired, allowed; from *abhi* = to, towards + *mati* (from *man*, to think).

Dhyanat = by meditating; from *dhyana* = meditation.

Va = or.

1.40. Gradually, one's mastery in concentration extends from the smallest particle to the greatest magnitude.

Paramanu = smallest particle; from *parama* = extreme, most + *anu* = smallest particle, minute, small.

Paramamahattva = greatest magnitude; from *parama* = greatest, most + *mahattva* = magnitude.

Anta = end.

Asya = of this (referring to the meditation techniques that preceded this sutra).

Vasikara = mastery (*see sutra* 1.15).

1.41. Just as the naturally pure crystal assumes shapes and colors of objects placed near it, so the yogi's mind, with its totally weakened modifications, becomes clear and balanced and attains the state devoid of differentiation between knower, knowable, and knowledge. This culmination of meditation is samadhi.

Kshina = totally weakened, waned or dwindled; from *kshi* = to decrease.

Vritter = modifications (*see sutra* 1.2).

Abhijatasya = naturally pure; from *abhi* = superior + *jan* = to be born.

Iva = like.

Maner = crystal, jewel.

Grahitri = knower; from *grah* = to seize.

Grahana = knowable.

Grahyeshu = knowledge.

Tatstha = similar; from *tad* = that + *stha* = to stand, abide; existing or being in.

The term literally means, "the mind abides like that;" like the object placed before the crystal.

Tadanjanata = assumes the shapes and colors; from *tad* = that + *anj* = applying ointment or pigment.

Samapattih = samadhi or balanced state, coming together, attainment, state of becoming one, complete engrossment; from *sam* = with + *pad* = to fall.

Samapattih is a synonym for samadhi, the mind's absorption into the object of contemplation.

1.42. The samadhi in which an object, its name, and conceptual knowledge of it are mixed is called savitarka samadhi, the samadhi with examination.

Tatra = there, in which case.

Sabda = sound, word, name (*see sutra* 1.9).

Artha = object, form, meaning (*see sutra* 1.28).

Jnana = knowledge, idea (*see sutra* 1.38).

Vikalpaih = conceptualization (*see sutra* 1.9.).

Samkirna = mixed.

Savitarka = with examination (*see sutra* 1.17), from *sa* = with + *vitarka* = observation, conjecture, reasoning, cogitation, speculation.

1.43. When the subconscious is well purified of memories (regarding the object of contemplation), the mind appears to lose its own identity, and the object alone shines forth. This is nirvitarka samadhi, the samadhi beyond examination.

Smriti = memory, content of the subconscious, remembered knowledge (*see sutra* 1.6).

In this sutra, smriti refers to notions regarding the object of contemplation that were previously constructed by vritti activity. The idea isn't that we lose our memory, but that the object is experienced as it is, without the distorting influence of memories that were formed under the influence of ignorance.

Parisuddhau = well purified; from *pari* = abundantly + *sudh* = to purify.

Svarupa = identity; from *sva* = own + *rupa* = form.

The essential nature of a thing; that which gives it its identity.

Sunya = empty, without any (*see sutra* 1.9.).

Here translated as "lose."

Iva = as it were.

Artha = object, form (*see sutra* 1.28).

Matra = only.

Nirbhasa = shining; from *bhas* = to be bright.

Nirvitarka = beyond examination; from *nir* = without + *tarka* = reasoning, cognition, debate, speculation.

In this context, the prefix *nir*, (without) suggests that the *tarka*, the examination of the gross object, is completed; it has reached its fulfillment. There is no more knowledge that can be gained regarding the object.

1.44. In the same way, savichara (with insight) and nirvichara (beyond insight) samadhis, which are practiced upon subtle objects, are explained.

Etaya = in the same way.

Eva = only.

Savichara = with insight; from *sa* = with + *chara* = reflection, investigation, mode of acting or proceeding (*see sutra* 1.17).

Nirvichara = beyond insight; from *nir* = without + *chara* (*see savichara
above*).

Use of the word *nirvichara* suggests that there are no more insights
to be gained regarding the subtle aspects of the object being
contemplated.

Cha = and.

Sukshma = subtle.

Vishaya = objects (*see sutra* 1.11).

Vyakhyata = are explained.

1.45. The subtlety of possible objects of concentration ends only at the undifferentiated.

Sukshma = subtle.

Vishayatvam = objects; from *vishaya*, object (*see sutra* 1.11).

Cha = and.

Alinga = undifferentiated; from *a* = without + *linga* = mark, sign, token,
emblem, characteristic (from *ling* = to paint).

Paryavasanam = end only at.

1.46. All these samadhis are sabija [with seed].

Ta = they.

Eva = all.

Sabijah = with seed.

Samadhih = contemplation (*see sutra* 1.20).

1.47. In the pure clarity of nirvichara samadhi, the supreme Self shines.

Nirvichara = beyond insight (*see sutra* 1.44).

Vaisaradye = pure clarity, experience, skill; from *vai* = used to express
emphasis or affirmation + *sarad* = autumnal sunshine, growing in
autumn, mature.

Adhyatma = supreme Self; from *adhi* = superior + *atma* = Self.

Prasadah = shines; from *pra* = filling, fulfilling + *sad* = to sit (especially at traditional rites of sacrificial worship), to wait for. The roots of the word suggest the fulfillment (*pra*) of attentive worship (from *sad* whose roots imply to patiently wait). Additional translations for *prasadah* include: to grow clear and bright, become placid and tranquil, to become distinct.

1.48. This is ritambhara prajna, the truth-bearing wisdom.

Ritambhara = absolute true; from *ritam* = truth + *bhara* = bearing.

Tatra = this is.

Prajna = wisdom, knowledge; from *jna* = to know.

1.49. The purpose of this special wisdom is different from the insights gained by study of sacred tradition and inference.

Sruta = sacred tradition or scripture; from *sru* = to hear.

Sruti refers to revealed knowledge of scripture and tradition. That which is taught orally; knowledge as *heard* and then transmitted by holy people. In Hinduism sruti traditionally refers to the Vedas and the Upanishads.

Anumana = inference (*see sutra* 1.7).

Prajnabhyam = than the insights (*see sutra* 1.48).

Anya = different.

Vishaya visesha = special insight; from *vishaya* = object (*see sutra* 1.11) + *visesha* = special or particular.

Arthatvat = purpose; from *artha* = purpose, utility, aim.

1.50. Other impressions are overcome by the impression produced by this samadhi.

Tad = that.

Jah = born of.

Samskarah = impression (*see sutra* 1.18).

Anya = other.

Samskara = impressions.

The impressions referred to here are those of *vyutthana*, externalization (*see sutra* 3.9).

Pratibandhi = overcome, to stop, exclude, cut off; from *prati* = in opposition to + *bandh* = to bind.

1.51. With the stilling of even this impression, every impression is wiped out and there is nirbija (seedless) samadhi.

Tasyapi = even this.

Nirodhe = restrained, stilled, ended, wiped out (*see sutra* 1.2).

Sarva = all.

Nirodhan = wiped out (*see sutra* 1.2).

Nirbijah = seedless.

Samadhih = samadhi (*see sutra* 1.20).

Pada Two
Sadhana Pada: Portion on Practice

2.1. Accepting pain as help for purification, study, and surrender to the Supreme Being constitute Yoga in practice.

Tapah = accepting pain as purification; from the verb root *tap* = to burn.

Svadhyaya = study; from *sva* = self + *adhi* = to go over, to go into.
Study is not mere intellectual exercise. Remember that originally, spiritual teachings in India were transmitted orally. Scriptures were memorized, recited, and meditated on as means of self- and Self-study. Therefore, study for the yogi is a contemplative affair, repeated acts performed in a meditative way, that take the practitioner to deeper and subtler levels of understanding.

Ishwara = Supreme Being (*see sutra* 1.23).

Pranidhanani = surrendering (*see sutra* 1.23).

Kriya = practice; from *kr*, to do.
In Saiva Siddhanta (a philosophy followed by devotees of Lord Siva, predominantly among the Tamil people of Sri Lanka and South India), kriya is a preparatory stage to liberation. Its goal is to attain nearness to God.

Yogah (*see sutra* 1.2).

2.2. They help us minimize obstacles and attain samadhi.

Samadhi = absorption (*see sutra* 1.20).

Bhavana = attain cultivate, realize, lead to, bring about; from *bhu* = to become.

Arthah = purpose, aim (*of the practices listed in sutra* 2.1).

Klesa = obstacles (*see sutra* 1.24).

Tanujaranarthah = minimize; from *tanu* = thinning, weakening, attenuating + *karana* = causing.

Cha = and.

2.3. Ignorance, egoism, attachment, aversion, and clinging to bodily life are the five obstacles.

Avidya = ignorance; from *vid* = to know + *a* = not.

Asmita = egoism (*see sutra* 1.17).

Raga = attachment (*see sutra* 1.12).

Dvesha = aversion; from *dvish* = to dislike.

Abhinivesah = clinging to bodily life, proneness, insistence on, obstinacy; from *abhi* = towards, into, upon + *vis* = to dwell, settle.

Klesah = obstacles (*see sutra* 1.24).

2.4. Ignorance is the field for the others mentioned after it, whether they be dormant, feeble, intercepted, or sustained.

Avidya = ignorance (*see sutra* 2.3).

Kshetram = field.

Uttaresham = for the others that follow.

Prasupta = dormant; from *pra* + *svap* = to sleep.

Tanu = feeble; from *tan* = to stretch out.

Vichchinna = intercepted; from the verb root *chid* = to break apart, cut asunder.

Udaranam = sustained; from *udara* = rousing, exalted, distinguished.

2.5. Ignorance is regarding the impermanent as permanent, the impure as pure, the painful as pleasant, and the non-Self as the Self.

Anitya = impermanent; from *a* = not + *nitya* = eternal.

Asuchi = impure; from *a* = not + *suchi* = pure.

Duhkha = painful (*see sutra* 1.31).

Anatmasu = non-Self; from *an* = not + *atman* = Self.

Nitya = permanent, eternal.

Suchi = pure.

Sukha = pleasant (*see sutra* 1.33).

Atma = Self; from the verb root *at* = to breathe; the verb root *ap* = to pervade or reach up to. The word could also be derived from *at* = to move.

Khyatir = regarding, seeing, identification, asserting, viewing; from *khya* = to be named, known, to declare.

Avidya = ignorance (*see sutra* 2.3).

2.6. Egoism is the identification, as it were, of the power of the Seer (Purusha) with that of the instrument of seeing (body-mind).

Drig = Seer; from *drsh* = to see.

Darsana = instrument of seeing; from *drsh* = to see.

Saktyor = powers; from *sak* = to be able.

Ekamata = identification; from *eka* = one + *atmata* = selfness.
Iva = as it were.
Asmita = egoism (*see sutra* 1.17).

2.7. Attachment is that which follows identification with pleasurable experiences.

Sukha = pleasure (*see sutra* 1.33).
Anusayi = follows with.
Ragah = attachment (*see sutra* 1.12).

2.8. Aversion is that which follows identification with painful experiences.

Duhkha = pain (*see sutra* 1.31).
Anusayi = follows with.
Dveshah = aversion (*see sutra* 2.3).

2.9. Clinging to life, flowing by its own potency (due to past experience), exists even in the wise.

Svarasa = by its own potency; from *sva* = own + *rasa* = inclination or
   taste.
   Rasa is often used to indicate the essence of something. It is
   derived from *ras* = to taste or relish. It is that element of
   something that gives it its characteristic taste.
      Use of this term here suggests that clinging to life persists
   because it has become self-perpetuating due to the mind's
   attachment to sense experiences. In other words, the mind has
   developed a taste (a liking and habit) for sense-based life in the
   world.
Vahi = flowing; from *vah* = to flow.
Vidusho'pi = even in the wise; from *vid* = to know.
Tatha = thus, so, in that way.
Rudha = exists; from *rudha* = rooted, established.
Abhinivesah = clinging to life (*see sutra* 2.3).

2.10. In their subtle form, these obstacles can be destroyed by resolving them back into their original cause (the ego).

Te = these.
Pratiprasava = resolving back into their cause; to return to the source.

Heyah = destroyed; from *ha* = to leave, desert, avoid or abandon.
Sukshman = subtle.

2.11. In the active state, they can be destroyed by meditation.

Dhyana = by meditation.
Heyas = destroyed (*see sutra* 2.10).
Tad = their.
Vrittayah = (active) modifications (*see sutra* 1.2).

2.12. The womb of karmas has its roots in these obstacles and the karmas bring experiences in the seen (present) or in the unseen (future) births.

Klesa = obstacles (*see sutra* 1.24).
Mulah = the root; from *mul* = to be rooted or firm.
Karmasayah = the womb of karmas; from karma = actions (*see sutra* 1.24) + *asayah* = reservoir.
Drishta = seen or present (*see sutra* 1.15).
Adrishta = unseen or future (*see sutra* 1.15).
Janma = births; from *jan* = to beget.
Vedaniyah = experienced; from *vid* = to know.

2.13. With the existence of the root, there will also be fruits: the births of different species of life, their life spans, and experiences.

Sati = with the existence; from *as* = to be.
Mule = of the root (*see sutra* 2.12).
Tad = its.
Vipakah = fruits (*see sutra* 1.24).
Jati = birth of a species of life; from *jan* = to beget.
Ayuh = their life span.
Bhogah = experiences, perceptions, experience appropriate return—pleasant and or unpleasant—for actions, the experience of sense-objects, worldly experience; from *bhuj* = to enjoy.

2.14. The karmas bear fruits of pleasure and pain caused by merit and demerit.

Te = they (the karmas).
Hlada = pleasure; from *hlad* = to bring delight, joy or to refresh.

Paritapa = pain; from *tap* = to burn.
    To feel distress or pain.
Phalah = fruits; from *phal* = to produce fruits, to ripen.
Punya = merit (*see sutra* 1.33).
Apunya = demerit (*see sutra* 1.33).
Hetutvat = cause; from *hetu* = impulse, motive, cause, reason for +
    tvat = made or composed by you.

2.15. To one of discrimination, everything is painful indeed, due to its consequences: the anxiety and fear over losing what is gained; the resulting impressions left in the mind to create renewed cravings; and the conflict among the activities of the gunas, which control the mind.

Parinama = consequences; from *pari* = around, fully, abundantly
    + *nam* = to bend or bow.
Tapa = anxiety and fear (*see sutra* 2.14).
Samskara = impressions (*see sutra* 1.18).
Duhkhair = pain.
    In this sutra, dukha refers to the suffering caused by renewed
    cravings (*see sutra* 1.31).
Guna = qualities of Nature.
    Not translated here (*see sutra* 1.16), but see 'vritti,' below.
Vritti = to whirl (*see sutra* 1.2).
    Translated here as *activities*, it refers to the constant struggle for
    dominance that takes place among the three gunas which control
    the mind.
Virodhat = conflict; from *rudh* = to stop.
Cha = and.
Duhkham = painful (*see sutra* 1.31).
Eva = indeed.
Sarvam = all.
Vivekinah = to one of discrimination; from *vic* = to separate (wheat
    from chaff) + *vi* = in parts, asunder.

2.16. Pain that has not yet come is avoidable.

Heyam = avoidable, to be overcome, eliminated (*see sutra* 2.10).
Duhkham = pain (*see sutra* 1.31).
Anagatam = not yet come; from *gam* = to go.

2.17. The cause of that avoidable pain is the union of the Seer (Purusha) and seen (Prakriti).

Drashtri = the Seer (*see sutra* 1.3).

Drisyayoh = the seen; from *drs* = to see.

Samyogah = union, true or complete union; from *yuj* = yoke + *sam* = together or with.

Heya = avoidable (*see sutra* 2.10).

Hetuh = cause (*see sutra* 2.14, '*hetutvat*').

2.18. The seen is of the nature of the gunas: illumination, activity, and inertia. It consists of the elements and sense organs, whose purpose is to provide both experiences and liberation to the Purusha.

Prakasa = illumination, to proclaim, reveal, to make visible, to cause to appear; from *pra* = forth + *kash* = to shine.

    Prakasa is a quality of the sattwa guna. It is the principle by which self-revelation is possible and also by which everything else is able to be known. The term is also used to refer to Pure Consciousness.

Kriya = activity (*see sutra* 2.1).

    Refers to *rajas* guna.

Sthiti = inertia (*see sutra* 1.13).

    Refers to the *tamas* guna.

Silam = nature, character, natural way of acting, tendency, habit, conduct.

Bhuta = elements; from *bhu* = to become, to be.

Indriya = sense organs; lit., pertaining to the God, Indra (meaning *ruler* or *chief*).

    Indra is the deity identified with strength, particularly the strength to grasp with the hands.

Atmakam = consists of, having the nature of, embodied by, exists in the form of.

Bhoga = experience (*see sutra* 2.13).

Apavarga = liberation; from *apa* = to take off + *vrij* = to turn, pull up, remove.

Artham = its purpose (*see sutra* 1.28).

Drisyam = the seen (*see sutra* 2.17).

2.19. The stages of the gunas are specific, nonspecific, defined, and undifferentiated.

Visesha = specific (*see sutra* 1.22).

Avisesha = non-specific (*see sutra* 1.22).

Lingamatra = defined; from *linga* = mark, characterized by + *matra* = an element, elementary matter, the full measure, only.

Alingani = undifferentiated, unindicated, unmanifest, without any distinguishing marks, without differentiating characteristics (*see lingamatra, above*).

Guna = qualities (*see sutra* 1.16).

Parvani = stages.

2.20. The Seer is nothing but the power of seeing which, although pure, appears to see through the mind.

Drashta = the Seer (*see sutra* 1.3).

Drisimatrah = the power of seeing; from *drish* = seeing + *matrah* = the totality, the full measure, only.

Suddho'pi = although pure; from *api* = although + *suddha* = pure.

Pratyaya = mind (*see sutra* 1.10).

Pratyaya, defined in sutra 1.10, as any stimulus that causes the mind-stuff to notice an object, is here rendered as *mind* and refers to all the various thoughts, notions and concepts that occur during the mind's functioning.

Anupasyah = appears as if seeing; from *anu* = after, alongside, near to, under, subordinate to, with + *pas* = to perceive, see, behold.

2.21. The seen exists only for the sake of the Seer.

Tad = that (the Seer).

Artha = for the purpose of, (*see sutra* 1.28).

Eva = only.

Drisyasya = the seen (Prakriti), (*see sutra* 2.17).

Atma = exists, existence.

2.22. Although destroyed for him who has attained liberation, it (the seen) exists for others, being common to them.

Kritartham = one whose goal has been fulfilled; from *krita* = done, accomplished + *artham* = purpose, goal (*see sutra* 1.28).

Prati = to him.

Nashtam = destroyed; from *nash* = to perish.
Api = even though.
Anashtam = not destroyed (*see nashtam, above*).
Tat = to the.
Anya = others.
Sadharanatvat = common.

2.23. The union of Owner (Purusha) and owned (Prakriti) causes the recognition of the nature and powers of them both.

Sva = owned, referring to Prakriti.
Svami = the Owner, referring to Purusha.
Saktyoh = of their powers (*see sutra* 2.6).
Svarupa = of the nature; from *sva* = own + *rupa* = form (*see sutra* 1.3).
Upalabdhi = recognition; from *upa* = towards + *labh* = to obtain.
Hetuh = cause (*see sutra* 2.14).
Samyogah = union (*see sutra* 2.17).

2.24. The cause of this union is ignorance.

Tasya = its.
Hetur = cause (*see sutra* 2.14).
Avidya = ignorance (*see sutra* 2.3).

2.25. Without this ignorance, no such union occurs. This is the independence of the Seer.

Tad = its (ignorance).
Abhavat = without, absence (*see sutra* 1.10).
Samyoga = union (*see sutra* 2.17).
Abhava = no such, is absent (*see sutra* 1.10).
Hanam = removal, absence.

This term refers to the *avoidable pain* of sutra 2.16 which, with the removal of ignorance, is now absent from the individual mind.

Tat = that.
Driseh = of the Seer (*see sutra* 1.3).
Kaivalyam = independence; from *kevala* = alone, one.

The use of the translation, *independence* should not be literally taken as the liberation of the Seer from bondage. The Seer is eternally free. The independence spoken of here is the power of the Seer abiding in its own nature (*see sutra* 1.3).

2.26. Uninterrupted discriminative discernment is the method for its removal.

Vivekakhyatih = discriminative discernment; from *viveka* = discernment (*see sutra* 2.15) + *khyati* = to be known.

Aviplava = uninterrupted; from *av* = to drive or impel, to animate + *plava* = to swim, float, hover, be inclined to, slope towards.
Aviplava suggests attaining a natural discernment rather than a forced practice. It is an unceasing inclination of the mind towards discrimination.

Hana = removal.

Upayah = method.

2.27. One's wisdom in the final stage is sevenfold.

Tashya = one's.

Saptadha = sevenfold.

Prantabhumih = in the final stage; from *pranta* = extreme edge, end + *bhumih* = stage.

Prajna = wisdom (*see sutra* 1.20).

2.28. By the practice of the limbs of Yoga, the impurities dwindle away and there dawns the light of wisdom leading to discriminative discernment.

Yoga = union (*see sutra* 1.1).

Anga = limbs, body.

Anushthanat = by the practice, acting in conformity to, doing, performance; from *anu* = alongside, with + *stha* = to stand.

Asuddhi = impurity (*see sutra* 2.20).

Kshaye = destruction or dwindling; from *kshi* = to destroy.

Jnana = knowledge (*see sutra* 1.38).

Diptih = light; from *dip* = to blaze, flare, shine, be luminous.

A = leads to.

Vivekakhyateh = discriminative discernment (*see sutra* 2.26).

2.29. The eight limbs of Yoga are:
1. **yama – abstinence**
2. **niyama – observance**
3. **asana – posture**
4. **pranayama – breath control**

5. **pratyahara – sense withdrawal**
6. **dharana – concentration**
7. **dhyana – meditation**
8. **samadhi – contemplation, absorption or super-conscious state**

Yama = abstinence, restraint, self-control, moral duty, any rule or observance; from *yam* = to rein, curb, bridle.

Niyama = observance; from *ni* = within + *yam*, see *yama*, above.
Niyama refers to any fixed rule or law, obligation; a lesser vow or observance dependent on external conditions, not as obligatory as *yama*.

Asana = posture; from *as* = to sit.

Pranayama = breath control; from *prana* = vital energy + *a* + *yam* = to restrain.

Pratyahara = withdrawal of the senses; lit., gathering towards oneself.

Dharana = concentration; from *dhr* = to hold or bear.

Dhyana = meditation (*see sutra* 1.39).

Samadhayah = contemplation, absorption or superconscious state (*see sutra* 1.20).

Ashta = eight.

Angani = limbs or part (*see sutra* 1.31).

2.30. Yama consists of nonviolence, truthfulness, nonstealing, continence, and nongreed.

Ahimsa = non-violence; from *himsa* = to injure + *a* = not.

Satya = truthfulness.

Asteya = non-stealing; from *shta* = to steal + *a* = not.

Brahmacharya = continence, dwelling or moving in Brahman; from *charya* = to move oneself + *brahman* (from *brih* = growth, expansion). In general, brahmacharya can refer to any code of conduct.

Aparigraha = non-greed; from *grah* = to grasp.

Yamah = abstinence (*see sutra* 2.29).

2.31. These Great Vows are universal, not limited by class, place, time, or circumstance.

Jati = class (*see sutra* 2.13).

Desa = place, position.

Kala = time (*see sutra* 1.14).

Samaya = circumstance; lit., coming together, agreement, occasion.

Anavachchhinnah = not limited by; lit., unseparated.

Sarvabhaumah = universal; from *sarva* = all + *bhauma* = stages.

Mahavratam = great vows; from *maha* = great + *vratam* = vow, command, law (from *vri* = to will).

2.32. Niyama consists of purity, contentment, accepting—but not causing—pain, study and worship of God (self-surrender).

Sauchat = purity; from *such* = clear, bright, luminous.

Samtosha = contentment; from *sam* = with + *tush* = to be satisfied.

Tapah = accepting pain and not causing pain (*see sutra* 2.1).

Svadhyaya = study (*see sutra* 2.1).

Ishwarapranidhanani = worship of God or self-surrender (*see sutra* 1.23).

Niyamah = observances (*see sutra* 2.29).

2.33. When disturbed by negative thoughts, opposite (positive) ones should be thought of. This is pratipaksha bhavana.

Vitarka = negative thoughts, unwholesome deliberations, thoughts obstructive to Yoga, perverse thoughts, improper thoughts, ideas that pervert the moral principles and observances, opposing beliefs.

This is the same word that used to describe a level of samadhi in sutra 1.17. However, in this instance the word is being used with reference to its other meanings.

Badhane = when disturbed by; from *badh* = to harass, attack, trouble.

Pratipaksha = opposite thoughts, an alternative; from *paksha* = flank or side.

Bhavanam = should be thought of (*see sutra* 1.28).

2.34. When negative thoughts or acts such as violence and so on are caused to be done, or even approved of, whether incited by greed, anger, or infatuation, whether indulged in with mild, medium, or extreme intensity, they are based on ignorance and bring certain pain. Reflecting thus is also pratipaksha bhavana.

Vitarka = negative thoughts.

Himsadayah = violence, etc.; from *himsa* = harming (*see sutra* 2.30) + *adayah* = etc. or beginning with.

Krita = done; from *kr* = to do.

Karita = caused to be done; from *kr* = to do.

Anumoditah = approved, to join in rejoicing, sympathize with, permit, sanction; from the verb root *mud* = to rejoice.

Lobha = greed; from *lubh* = to desire.

Krodha = anger; from the verb root *krudh* = to be angry.

Moha = infatuation; from the verb root *muh* = to become stupefied or deluded.

Moha means to be bewildered, perplexed, deluded, to go astray. It is delusion that leads to error. For Buddhists, it is an equivalent to darkness or ignorance.

Purvaka = proceeded by, arising from, accompanied by.

Mridu = mild.

Madhya = medium.

Adhimatrah = intense (*see sutra* 1.22).

Duhkha = pain (*see sutra* 1.31).

Ajnana = ignorance (*see sutra* 1.38).

Ananta = infinite; from *a* = not + *anta* = end.

Phalah = fruit (*see sutra* 2.14).

Iti = thus.

Pratipaksha = opposite thoughts (*see sutra* 2.33).

Bhavanam = should be thought of, contemplation (*see sutra* 1.28).

2.35. In the presence of one firmly established in nonviolence, all hostilities cease.

Ahimsa = non-violence (*see sutra* 2.30).

Pratishthayam = having established; from *pra* = on + *stha* = stand.

Tat = that.

Samnidhau = presence, to be in proximity; from the verb root *dha* = to put + *sanni* = to place together or near.

Vaira = hostility; from the verb root *vi* = to fall upon or attack.

Tyagah = cease; from *tyaj* = to abandon.

2.36. To one established in truthfulness, actions and their results become subservient.

Satya = truthfulness.

Pratishthayam = having established (*see sutra* 2.35).

Kriya = actions; from *kr* = to do.

Phala = fruits or results (*see sutra* 2.14).

Asrayatvam = become subservient; from *sri* = to rest on.

2.37. To one established in nonstealing, all wealth comes.

Asteya = non-stealing (*see sutra* 2.30).

Pratishthayam = having established (*see sutra* 2.35).

Sarva = all the.

Ratna = gems or wealth; from *ra* = to bestow.

Upasthanam = approaches or comes; from *upa* = near + *stha* = stand.

2.38. To one established in continence, vigor is gained.

Brahmacharya = continence (*see sutra* 2.30).

Pratishthayam = having established (*see sutra* 2.35).

Virya = vigor; from *vir* = to be powerful.

Labhah = gained; from *labh* = to obtain.

2.39. To one established in nongreed, a thorough illumination of the how and why of one's birth comes.

Aparigraha = non-greed (*see sutra* 2.30).

Sthairye = confirmed; from *shta* = to stand.

Janmakathamta = how and why of births; from *janma* = birth + *kathanta* = the why-ness, the nature of why.

Sambodha = thorough illumination; from *budh* = be awake, aware of, perceive + *sam* = thoroughness.

2.40. By purification, the body's protective impulses are awakened as well as a disinclination for detrimental contact with others.

Sauchat = by purification (*see sutra* 2.32).

Svanga = for one's own body; from *sva* = one's own + *anga* = limb or member.

Jugupsa = protective impulses.

Dictionaries generally give *disgust* as the main definition of *jugupsa*. However, translating *jugupsa* as disgust might mislead us to confuse it with aversion, a quality Sri Patanjali would have us overcome. But the word has an older, perhaps more relevant, meaning that might be clearer in the context of the *Yoga Sutras*: it can also be regarded as the invocation of a natural protective instinct.

Jugupsa is derived from *gup* = to protect. An earlier word derived from *gup* is *gopaya*, lit, the protector of the oblation of milk (from *gup* = to protect + *paya* = oblation of milk) In other words, gopaya is a cowherd or herdsman. A herdsman's primary responsibility is to protect the herd from harm. Someone, who by their mere presence or through action, would drive away—perhaps even kill, if necessary—predators.

A herdsman would likely not look fondly on predators that could harm the herd. We can understand how they might develop what might be understood as a kind of disgust for predators. It might be likened to how many vegetarians feel about eating meat. They do not consider meat to be a natural part of the human diet. To them, animal flesh is not regarded as a food item. The very idea of eating meat brings disgust: *dis* = which expresses reversal + *gustus* = taste; to not have a taste for.

Jugupsa as used by Buddhists means equanimity. Since there are several noteworthy parallels between key terms in used Buddhism and the *Yoga Sutras* (*nirodha* and *upeksha*, for example), it is not far-fetched that there is at least a hint of the Buddhistic view suggested in jugupsa's use in this sutra (whether or not Sri Patanjali was influenced by Buddhism). In this case, jugupsa might imply maintaining a healthy, "take-care-of-it-but-don't-get-attached-to-it" attitude toward the body.

Paraih = with others; from *para* = far, distant, opposite.

The word refers to the opposite shore of a river. Since the other side of a river would often be the location of another town, where customs and traditions might be different and whose reactions to contact unknown, it also implies something alien.

Asamsargah = cessation of contact; from *srj* = to emit or discharge + *sam* = with + *a* = not.

2.41. Moreover, one gains purity of sattwa, cheerfulness of mind, one-pointedness, mastery over the senses, and fitness for Self-realization.

Sattwasuddhi = purity of sattwa; from *sattwa* = being-ness, character, nature, illuminating + *suddhi* = purity (*see sutra* 2.20).

Saumanasya = cheerfulness of mind.

Ekagrya = one-pointedness; from *eka* = one + *agrya* = pointedness.

Indriyajaya = mastery of senses; from *indriya* (*see sutra* 2.18) = senses
+ *jaya* = mastery (from the verb root *ji* = to win).

Atmadarsana = realization of the Self; from *atman* = self (*see sutra* 2.5)
+ *darsana* = vision (*see sutra* 1.30).

Yogyatvani = fitness.

Cha = and.

2.42. By contentment, supreme joy is gained.

Samtoshat = by contentment (*see sutra* 2.32).

Anuttamah = supreme.

Sukha = joy (*see sutra* 1.33).

Labhah = gained (*see sutra* 2.38).

2.43. By austerity, impurities of body and senses are destroyed and occult powers gained.

Kaya = body.

Indriya = senses (*see sutra* 2.18).

Siddhi = occult powers, accomplishment, complete attainment, fulfillment. Any unusual skill, faculty, or capability; from *sidh* = to succeed or attain.

Asuddhi = impurities (*see sutra* 2.20).

Kshayat = due to destruction (*see sutra* 2.28).

Tapasah = austerities (*see sutra* 2.1).

2.44. Through study comes communion with one's chosen deity.

Svadhyayad = by study (*see sutra* 2.1).

In the sage Vyasa's commentary on sutra 2.1, he defines *svadhyaya* as, "either the repetition of such mantras as OM or the study of scriptures bearing upon Liberation."

Ishtadevata = chosen deity; from *ishta* = favorite, beloved (from *ish* = to desire) + *devata* = deity (from *div* = to shine).

Samprayogah = communion.

2.45. By total surrender to Ishwara, samadhi is attained.

Samadhi = contemplation (*see sutra* 1.20).

Siddhir = attainment (*see sutra* 2.43).

Isvarapranidhanat = by total surrender to God (*see sutra* 1.23).

2.46. Asana is a steady, comfortable posture.
Sthira = steady; from *stha* = to stand.
Sukham = comfortable (*see sutra* 1.33).
Asanam = posture (*see sutra* 2.29).

2.47. By lessening the natural tendency for restlessness and by meditating on the infinite, posture is mastered.
Prayatna = natural tendency for restlessness; from *yat* = to be active or effective.
Saithilya = by lessening; from *sithila* = loose, relaxed, untied, not rigid.
Ananta = infinite (*see sutra* 2.34).
Samapattibhyam = meditating on (*see sutra* 1.41).

2.48. Thereafter, one is undisturbed by dualities.
Tato = thereafter.
Dvandva = by the dualities; from *dva* = two.
Anabhighatah = undisturbed; from *a* = not + *abhi* = to, into, over, upon + *han* = strike, smite, destroy.

2.49. That (firm posture) being acquired, the movements of inhalation and exhalation should be controlled. This is pranayama.
Tasmin = that.
Sati = being acquired (*see sutra* 2.13).
Svasa = inhalation; from *svas* = to breathe.
Prasvasyor = and exhalation; from *svas* (to breathe) + *pra* = forth.
Gati = movements; from *gam* = to go.
Vicchedah = control (*see sutra* 2.4).
Pranayamah = pranayama (*see sutra* 2.29).

2.50. The modifications of the life-breath are external, internal, or stationary. They are to be regulated by space, time, and number and are either long or short.
Bahya = external; lit., being outside (of a door or house).
Abhyantara = internal; from *antar* = within, among.
Stambha = stationary; from *stambh* = to stop.
Vrittir = modifications (*see sutra* 1.2).
Desa = space.
Kala = time.

Samkhyabhih = and number; from *samkhya* = number.

Paridrishto = regulated (monitored and adjusted); from *drsh* = to see.

Dirgha = long.

Sukshmah = short, subtle.

2.51. There is a fourth kind of pranayama that occurs during concentration on an internal or external object.

Bahya = external (*see sutra* 2.50).

Abhyantara = internal (*see sutra* 2.50).

Vishaya = object (*see sutra* 1.11).

Akshepi = concentration, o throw down upon or towards (referring to the mind's attention); from *ksip* = to throw.

Chaturthah = the fourth; from *catur* = four.

2.52. As its result, the veil over the inner light is destroyed.

Tatah = as a result.

Kshiyate = destroyed; from *ksi* = to decrease.

Prakasa = light; from *kas* = to shine, be brilliant, to be visible.

Avaranam = veil; from *vr* = to cover + *a* = not.

2.53. And the mind becomes fit for concentration.

Dharanasu = for concentration (*see sutra* 2.29).

Cha = and.

Yogyata = becomes fit.

Manasah = mind.

2.54. When the senses withdraw themselves from the objects and imitate, as it were, the nature of the mind-stuff, this is pratyahara.

Sva = their own.

Vishaya = objects (*see sutra* 1.11).

Asamprayoga = withdrawal; from *a* = not + *sampra* = enter into completely + *yoga* = Union (*see sutra* 1.1).

Chitta-svarupa = nature of the mind-stuff; from *chitta* = consciousness (*see sutra* 1.2) + *svarupa* = own form, essential nature.

Anukara = imitate, to do afterwards, to following in doing, to equal, to adopt; from *kr* = to do.

Iva = as it were.

Indriyanam = senses (*see sutra* 2.18).

Pratyaharah = withdrawal of the senses; not translated here; (*see sutra* 2.29).

2.55. Then follows supreme mastery over the senses.

Tatah = thence.

Paranama vasyata = supreme mastery; from *para* = supreme + *vastya* = mastery.

Indriyanam = senses (*see sutra* 2.18).

Pada Three
Vibhuti Pada: Portion on Accomplishments

3.1. Dharana is the binding of the mind to one place, object, or idea.

Desabandhah = binding to one place; from *desa* = place (*see sutra* 2.31) + *bandhah* = bind.

Chittasya = of the mind (*see sutra* 1.2).

Dharana = concentration (*see sutra* 2.29).

3.2. Dhyana is the continuous flow of cognition toward that object.

Tatra = therein.

Pratyaya = cognition (of arising thoughts) (*see sutra* 1.10).

Ekatanata = continued flow; from *eka* = one + *tanata* = flow (from *tan* = reach, extend, spread).

Dhyanam = meditation (*see sutra* 1.39).

3.3. Samadhi is the same meditation when the mind-stuff, as if devoid of its own form, reflects the object alone.

Tad eva = that (referring to meditation or chitta) itself.

Arthamatra = the object alone; from *artha* = object (*see sutra* 1.28) + *matra* = alone.

Nirbhasam = shining (*see sutra* 1.43).

Svarupa = of its own form; from *sva* = own + *rupa* = form.

Sunyam = devoid of.

Iva = as if.

Samadhih = superconscious state, absorption (*see sutra* 1.20).

3.4. The practice of these three (dharana, dhyana, and samadhi) upon one object is called samyama.

Trayam = the three, group of three.

Ekatra = upon one object; from *eka* = one.

Samyama = constraint, perfect regulation, perfect discipline, the practice of dharana, dhyana and samadhi together; from *yam* = to restrain + *sam* = complete, full, perfect.

3.5. By mastery of samyama, knowledge born of intuitive insight shines forth.

Tat = from its.

Jayat = mastery (*see sutra* 2.41).

Prajnalokah = the light of knowledge; from *prajna* = intuitive insight or wisdom + *alokah* = brilliance, light, sight, looking, seeing, beholding.

3.6. Its practice is accomplished in stages.

Tasya = its.

Bhumishu = by stages; from *bhumi* = ground, earth, a place, a site.

As a metaphor, bhumishu suggests a step, degree or stage.

Viniyogah = practice.

3.7. These three (dharana, dhyana and samadhi) are more internal than the preceding five limbs.

Trayam = the three.

Antar = inner.

Angam = limb.

Purvebhyah = the preceding, previous.

3.8. Even these three are external to the seedless samadhi.

Tat api = even that.

Bahirangam = external; from *bahir* = external + *angam* = limb.

Nirbijasya = to the seedless; from *nir* = without + *bija* = seed.

3.9. Impressions of externalization are subdued by the appearance of impressions of nirodha. As the mind begins to be permeated by moments of nirodha, there is development in nirodha.

Vyutthana = externalization; from *ud* – implies separation or disjunction + *vi* = in two parts + *stha* = to stand.

Vyutthana is the predominant characteristic of ordinary consciousness in which the ego-sense is strengthened through the search for satisfaction in externals.

Since vyutthana is formed from impressions based on cognitions that are colored by avidya, they lead to the misperception of self-identity and the world.

In daily life vyutthana expresses as the desire to know and experience (and then either enjoy or avoid) sense objects, believing that they are separate from the self. Implied in this is the mistaken notion that permanent happiness can be attained by acquiring certain objects and experiences while avoiding others. In short, through lifetimes of repeating this same behavior, the mind becomes conditioned to look outside the Self for satisfaction.

Nirodha = (*see sutra* 1.2).

Samskarayoh = impressions (*see sutra* 1.18).

Abhibhava = subdued; from *abhi* = to, into, towards + *bhu* = to become.

Pradurbhavau = appear; from *pra* = before, in front + *dur* = door + *bhu* = to become.

Since *pradurbhavau* literally means "to be in front of the door," use of this term suggests images of nirodha as long awaited guests that have finally arrived and only need to be invited inside.

Nirodha = (*see sutra* 1.2).

Kshana = moment.

Chitta = mind (*see sutra* 1.2).

Anvayah = permeated; logical connection of cause and effect, conclusion, outcome, end product, connection, follows, associated, being linked or connected with.

The "cause" is the appearance of impressions of nirodha; the "effect" is a mind whose character is being changed. It is a mind that is no longer automatically influenced by impressions of externalization because it is beginning to be permeated by impressions of nirodha.

Nirodha = (*see sutra* 1.2).

Parinamah = transformation, evolution, change, ripening (*see sutra* 2.15).

3.10. When impressions of nirodha become strong and pervasive, the mind-stuff attains a calm flow of nirodha.

Tasya = its.

Prasanta = strong and pervasive; from *pra* = to go forth + *sam* = to stop, finish, come to an end, rest, be calm.

In this sutra *prasanta* implies the culmination of nirodha and could be understood as that which leads to rest or steadiness.

Vahita = flow, to be urged on, actuated by or caused to be born; from *vah* = bearing or carrying.

Samskarat = by habit (*see sutra* 1.18).

3.11. The mind-stuff transforms toward samadhi when distractedness dwindles and one-pointedness arises.

Sarvathata = distractedness; from *sarva* = all + *arthata* = sense object or intention (*see sutra* 1.28).

Ekagrata = one-pointedness (*see sutra* 2.41).

Kshaya = dwindling (of the former) (*see sutra* 2.28).

Udaya = arising (of the latter).

Chittasya = of the mind-stuff (*see sutra* 1.2).

Samadhi = (*see sutra* 1.20).

Parinamah = transforms (*see sutra* 2.15).

3.12. Then again, when the subsiding and arising images are identical, there is one-pointedness (ekagrata parinama).

Tatah = from that.

Punah = again.

Santa = subsiding (past); from *sam* = to stop, finish, come to an end, rest, be calm.

Udita = rising (present); from *ud* = to spring (as in water) + *i* = to go.

Tulya = identical; from *tul* = to compare by examining, to make equal.

Pratyaya = thought-waves (*see sutra* 1.10).

Chittasya = of the mind (*see sutra* 1.2).

Ekagrata = one-pointedness (*see sutra* 2.41).

3.13. By what has been said (in sutras 3.9–3.12) the transformations of the form, characteristics, and condition of the elements and sense organs are explained.

Etena = by this.

Bhuta = the elements (*see sutra* 2.18).

Indriyeshu = in the senses (*see sutra* 2.18).

Dharma = form; from *dhr* = to uphold, establish, support. Dharma translates literally as "that which holds together."

Dharma is the basis of order, whether physical social, moral or spiritual. The term is also used to refer to a mark, sign, token, attribute or quality.

Lakshanah = characteristics, to indicate or express indirectly; from *laksh* = to perceive or observe.

Lakshanah is the secondary meaning or characteristic of an object that is revealed over time.

Avasthah = condition; from *stha* = to stand.

Parinamah = transformations (*see sutra* 2.15).

Vyakhyatah = explained.

3.14. The substratum (Prakriti) continues to exist, although by nature it goes through latent, uprising, and unmanifested phases.

Santa = latent (past) (*see sutra* 3.12).

Udita = uprising (present) (*see sutra* 3.12).

Avyapadesya = unmanifest, indistinguishable, not to be determined or defined, uncertain, potential, indescribable; from the verb root, *dis* = to point out, show, exhibit.

Dharma = nature (*see sutra* 3.13).

Anupati = goes through (*see sutra* 1.9.).

Dharmi = substratum; that which has the essential characteristic (*see sutra* 3.13).

3.15. The succession of these different phases is the cause of the differences in stages of evolution.

Krama = succession; from *kram* = to stride.

Anyatvam = different (phases); from *anya* = different, opposed to, other.

Parinama = stage (in this sutra, referring to stages of evolution) (*see sutra* 2.15).

Anyatve = differences (*see above*).

Hetuh = cause (*see sutra* 2.14).

3.16. By practicing samyama on the three stages of evolution comes knowledge of past and future.

Parinama = stages; in this sutra, referring to stages of evolution (*see sutra* 2.15).

Traya = three.

Samyamad = by samyama (*see sutra* 3.4).

Atita = past; gone by; from *ati* = to pass by, elapse, to pass over + *i* = to go.

Anagata = future; from *an* + *a* + *gam* = to go = not yet come.

Jnanam = knowledge (*see sutra* 1.38).

3.17. A word, its meaning, and the idea behind it are normally confused because of superimposition upon one another. By samyama on the word (or sound) produced by any being, knowledge of its meaning is obtained.

Sabdha = word; from *sabd* = to make any noise or sound.

Artha = meaning (*see sutra* 1.28).

Pratyayanam = ideas (*see sutra* 1.10.)

Itaretara = among themselves; lit., one upon the other.

Adhyasat = because superimposed; from *adhi* = above, besides, over
+ *as* = to throw or cast.

Samkarah = mixed and confused; from *sam* = together with + *kr* =
to do.

Tat = their.

Pravibhaga = distinctions; from *pra* + *vi* = in two parts + *bhaj* =
to divide.

Samyamat = by samyama (*see sutra* 3.4).

Sarva = all.

Bhuta = living beings (*see sutra* 2.18).

Ruta = sound; from *ru* = to roar.

Jnanam = knowledge (*see sutra* 1.38).

3.18. By direct perception, through samyama, of one's mental impressions, knowledge of past births is obtained.

Samskara = mental impressions (*see sutra* 1.18).

Sakshat = direct; lit., *sa* = with + *aksha* = eye.

Karanat = perception, making, causing, perception; from *kr* = to do.

Purva = previous.

Jati = birth (*see sutra* 2.13).

Jnanam = knowledge (*see sutra* 1.38).

3.19. By samyama on the distinguishing signs (of others' bodies) knowledge of their mental images is obtained.

Pratayayasya = idea of distinction, cause, intention, ground of the
mind, cognitive process, notions, image occupying the mind (*see
sutra* 1.10).

Para = another; other.
Chitta = consciousness (*see sutra* 1.2).
Jnanam = knowledge (*see sutra* 1.38).

3.20. But this does not include the support in the person's mind (such as motive behind the thought, and so on), as that is not the object of the samyama.
Na = not.
Cha = and.
Tat = its, that.
Salambanam = the support (*see sutra* 1.10, *alambana*).
Tasya = its.
Avishayi = lit., which has no object (*see sutra* 1.11).
Bhuvatatvat = the nature or object of being.

3.21. By samyama on the form of one's body (and by) checking the power of perception by intercepting light from the eyes of the observer, the body becomes invisible.
Kayarupa = the body's form; from *kaya* = body + *rupa* = form.
Samyamat = by samyama (*see sutra* 3.4).
Tat = its.
Grahya = perception; lit., to be grasped.
Sakti = power (*see sutra* 2.6).
Stambhe = being checked (*see sutra* 2.50).
Chakshuh = eye.
Prakasa = light.
Asamprayoge = intercepting.
Antardhanam = invisible; from *antar* = within + *dha* = to put.

3.22. In the same way, the disappearance of sound (and touch, taste, smell, and so on) is explained.
Etena = by the same way.
Sabdadi = the sound, etc. (*see sutra* 3.17).
Antardhanam = disappearance (*see sutra* 3.21).
Uktam = is explained.

3.23. Karmas are of two kinds: quickly manifesting and slowly manifesting. By samyama on them, or on the portents of death, the knowledge of the time of death is obtained.

Sopakramam = quickly manifesting; from *sa* = with + *upa* = towards or near + *kram* = to step.

Nirupakramam = slow; from *nir* = without + *upa* = towards or near + *kram* = to step.

Cha = and.

Karma = actions (and their results).

Tat = over these.

Samyamat = by samyama (*see sutra* 3.4).

Aparanta = time of death; from *para* = other, extreme + *anta* = end.

Jnanam = knowledge (*see sutra* 1.38).

Arishtebhyo = on the portents.

Va = or.

3.24. By samyama on friendliness and other such qualities, the power (to transmit them) is obtained.

Maitri = friendliness.

Adishu = other such qualities.

Balani = powers; from *bala* = strength.

3.25. By samyama on the strength of elephants and other such animals, their strength is obtained.

Baleshu = on the strength (*see sutra* 3.24).

Hasti = elephant.

Bala = strength (*see sutra* 3.24).

Adini = others.

3.26. By samyama on the light within, the knowledge of the subtle, hidden, and remote is obtained. [Note: subtle as atoms, hidden as treasure, remote as far-distant lands.]

Pravritti – activity (*see sutra* 1.35).

Aloka = the light within (*see sutra* 3.5).

Nyasat = by samyama (*see sutra* 3.4). Nyasa is a synonym for samyama. It is derived from the verb root *as* = to sit + *ni* = down, back, into, in. It can be translated as, "to cast down or project," or "to throw upon."

Nyasa also refers to a ritual process which is used as a way of strengthening the experience of micro and macro-cosmic relationships. This sutra suggests this meaning since by meditating on the light within (the microcosm), remote aspects of the macrocosm that are subtle, hidden and remote are revealed.

Sukshma = subtle.

Vyavahita = hidden; from *a* + *va* + *dah* = to put = to conceal.

Viprakrishta = remote.

Jnanam = knowledge (*see sutra* 1.38).

3.27. By samyama on the sun, knowledge of the entire solar system is obtained.

Bhuvana = universe; from *bhu* = to become.

Jnanam = knowledge (*see sutra* 1.38).

Surye = on the sun; from *svar* = heaven.

Samyamat = by samyama (*see sutra* 3.4).

3.28. By samyama on the moon comes knowledge of the stars' alignment.

Chandre = on the moon.

Tara = of the stars.

Vyuha = arrangement, distribution, orderly arrangement of the parts of a whole; from *vyuh* = to array.

Jnanam = knowledge (*see sutra* 1.38).

3.29. By samyama on the pole star comes knowledge of the stars' movements.

Dhruve = on the pole star; from *dhruv* = firm or fixed.

Tat = their.

Gati = movements (*see sutra* 2.49).

Jnanam = knowledge (*see sutra* 1.38).

3.30. By samyama on the navel plexus, knowledge of the body's constitution is obtained.

Nabhi = navel, the navel or any navel-like cavity, the hub of a wheel, center, middle, rallying point; from *nabh* = an opening, fissure, spring.

Chakre = plexus, heel, orb, circle, multitude, army, circuit, district, province, domain.

Kaya = body, the trunk of a tree, the body of a lute.

Vyuha = arrangement (*see sutra* 3.28).

Jnanam = knowledge (*see sutra* 1.38).

3.31. By samyama on the pit of the throat, cessation of hunger and thirst is achieved.

Kantha = throat.

Kupe = on the pit; from *kupa* = hole, hollow, cave.

Kshut = hunger; from *kshudh* = to be hungry.

Pipsa = thirst; from *pa* = to drink.

Nivrittih = cessation; from *ni* = not + *vritti* = to whirl.

3.32. By samyama on the kurma nadi, motionlessness in the meditative posture is achieved.

Kurmanadyam = on the tortoise tube; from *kurma* = tortoise + *nadyam* = conduit, tube, channel, vein, artery.

Sthairyam = motionlessness (*see sutra* 2.39).

3.33. By samyama on the light at the crown of the head (sahasrara chakra), visions of masters and adepts are obtained.

Murdha = crown of the head.

Jyotishi = on the light; from *jyut* = to shine.

Siddha = masters and adepts; from *sidh* = to succeed, to attain, to be accomplished, fulfilled, to become perfect.

Darsanam = vision (*see sutra* 1.30).

3.34. Or, in the knowledge that dawns by spontaneous intuition (through a life of purity), all the powers come by themselves.

Pratibhad = spontaneous intuition:, a flash of illumination; from *bha* = light, brightness, splendor, to shine.

Pratibhad is that state of mind in which ever-new ideas burst forth into consciousness.

Va = or.

Sarvam = everything.

3.35. By samyama on the heart, the knowledge of the mind-stuff is obtained.

Hridaye = on the heart.

Chitta = mind-stuff (*see sutra* 1.2).

Samvit = the knowledge; from *sam* = thorough, complete + *vid* = to know.

3.36. The intellect (sattwa) and the Purusha are totally different, the intellect existing for the sake of the Purusha, while the Purusha exists for its own sake. Not distinguishing this is the cause of all experiences. By samyama on this distinction, knowledge of the Purusha is gained.

Sattwa = intellect, purity, buddhi, the guna of brightness or clarity, beingness (*see sutra* 2.41).

Purushayoh = and the Purusha (*see sutra* 1.16).

Atyanta = totally, absolute, endless, unbroken, perfect, perpetual.

Asamkirnayoh = different (*see sutra* 1.42).

Pratyaya = cognition (*see sutra* 1.10).

In this sutra, pratyaya suggests the typical state of cognition in which no distinction is made between the Purusha and the intellect. It is this that is the source of all experiences (*see bhoga below*).

Aviseshah = absence of distinction (*see sutra* 1.22).

Bhogah = worldly experiences of pleasure and pain (*see sutra* 2.13).

Para = another.

Arthat = for the sake of, purpose (*see sutra* 1.28).

Referring to the intellect existing for the sake of the Purusha.

Svartha = own sake; from *sva* = own or self + *artha* = interest, purpose.

Samyamat = by samyama (*see sutra* 3.4).

Purusha = Self (*see sutra* 1.16).

Jnanam = knowledge (*see sutra* 1.38).

3.37. From this knowledge arises superphysical hearing, touching, seeing, tasting, and smelling through spontaneous intuition.

Tatah = thence.

Pratibha = spontaneous intuition (*see sutra* 3.33).

Sravana = clairaudience; from *sru* = to hear.

Vedana = higher touch, sensation.

Adarsa = clairvoyance.

Asvada = higher taste; from *svad* = to taste.

Varta = higher smell.

Jayante = arises, occurs, are born, are produced; from *jan* = to beget.

3.38. These (superphysical senses) are obstacles to (nirbija) samadhi but are siddhis in the externalized state.

Te = these (siddhis).

Samadhav = for samadhi (*see sutra* 1.20).

Upasarga = obstacles.

Vyutthane = in the externalized state (*see sutra* 3.9).

Siddhayah = siddhis, powers (*see sutra* 2.43).

3.39. By the loosening of the cause of bondage (to the body) and by knowledge of the channels of activity of the mind-stuff, entry into another body is possible.

Bandha = bondage (*see sutra* 3.1).

Karana = cause; from *kr* = to do.

Saithilyat = by loosening (*see sutra* 2.47).

Prachara = channels of activity; from *pra* = forth + *char* = to go.

Samvedanat = by the knowledge; from *sam* = thorough, complete + *vid* = knowledge.

Cha = and.

Chittasya = of the mind-stuff (*see sutra* 1.2).

Parasarira = another body; from *para* = another or other + *sarira* = body.

Avesah = enter into; from *vis* = to enter.

3.40. By mastery over the udana nerve current (the upward-moving prana), one accomplishes levitation over water, swamps, thorns, and so on and can leave the body at will.

Udana = the nerve current of udana; from *ud* = up, upwards + *an* = to breathe.

Udana is the upward flow of prana.

Jayat = by mastery over (*see sutra* 2.41).

Jala = water.

Panka = swamp.

Kantaka = thorn.

Adishu = and others.

Asangah = unattached; from *a* = without + *sanga* = attachment.

Utkrantih = power to levitate; from *ud* = upward + *kram* = to step.

Cha = and.

3.41. By mastery over the samana nerve current (the equalizing prana) comes radiance to surround the body.

Samana = nerve current of samana.

Samana is the flow of prana that moves up to the navel.

Jayat = by the mastery over (*see sutra* 2.41).

Jvalanam = radiance; from *jval* = to blaze.

3.42. By samyama on the relationship between ear and ether, supernormal hearing becomes possible.

Srotra = ear; from *sru* = to hear.

Akasayoh = and ether; from *a* = not + *kas* = visible.

Sambandha = relationship; from *sam* = with + *bandh* = to bind.

Samyamat = by samyama (*see sutra* 3.4).

Divyam = divine; from *div* = to radiate.

Srotram = hearing (*as above*).

3.43. By samyama on the relationship between the body and ether, lightness of cotton fiber is attained, and thus traveling through the ether becomes possible.

Kaya = body.

Akasayoh = and ether (*see sutra* 3.42).

Sambandha = relationship (*see sutra* 3.42).

Samyamat = by samyama (*see sutra* 3.4).

Laghu = light.

Tula = cotton fiber.

Samapatteh = attainment (*see sutra* 1.41).

Cha = and.

Akasa = through ether (*see sutra* 3.42).

Gamanam = traveling, traversing, moving; from *gam* = to go.

3.44. (By virtue of samyama on ether) vritti activity that is external to the body is (experienced and) no longer inferred. This is the great bodilessness which destroys the veil over the light of the Self.

Bahir = external.

Akalpita = not inferred, not manufactured, not pretended, natural, genuine; from *a* = not + *kalpita* = made, fabricated, artificial, invented, inferred.

Vritter = vritti activity (*see sutra* 1.2).

Mahavideha = great bodilessness; from *maha* = great + *videha* = bodiless (*see sutra* 1.19).

Tatah = by that.

Prakasa = light (*see sutra* 2.18).

Avarana = veil (*see sutra* 2.52).

Kshayah = destruction (*see sutra* 2.28).

3.45. Mastery over the gross and subtle elements is gained by samyama on their essential nature, correlations, and purpose.

Sthula = gross.

Svarupa = essential nature; from *sva* = own + *rupa* = form.

Sukshma = subtle.

Anvaya = correlative (*see sutra* 3.9).

Arthavattva = purposefulness (*see sutra* 1.28).

Samyamat = by samyama (*see sutra* 3.4).

Bhuta = over elements (*see sutra* 2.18).

Jayah = mastery (*see sutra* 2.41).

3.46. From that (mastery over the elements) comes attainment of anima and other siddhis, bodily perfection, and the non-obstruction of bodily functions by the influence of the elements.

Note: The eight major siddhis alluded to are: *anima* (to become very small); *mahima* (to become very big); *laghima* (to become very light); *garima* (to become very heavy); *prapati* (to reach anywhere); *prakamya* (to achieve all one's desires); *isatva* (the ability to create anything); *vasitva* (the ability to command and control everything).

Tatah = from that, referring to the mastery over the elements gained by the samyama presented in the previous sutra.

Animadhi = anima and other siddhis; from *anima* = power to become minute + *adhi* = etc.

Pradurbhavah = attainment of (*see sutra* 3.9).

Kaya = body.

Sampad = perfection.

Tat = their.

Dharma = functions (*see sutra* 3.13).

Anabhighatah = non-obstruction (*see sutra* 2.48).

3.47. Beauty, grace, strength, and adamantine hardness constitute bodily perfection.

Rupa = beauty.

Lavanya = gracefulness, charm.

Bala = strength.

Vajrasamhananatvani = and adamantine hardness; from *vajra* = adamantine, hard + *samhananatvani* = firmness.

Kayasampat = perfection of the body; from *kaya* = body + *sampat* = perfection.

3.48. Mastery over the sense organs is gained by samyama on the senses as they correlate to the process of perception, the essential nature of the senses, the ego-sense, and to their purpose.

Grahana = to grasp, the act of perceiving.

Svarupa = essential nature.

Asmita = ego-sense (*see sutra* 1.17).

Anvaya = correlation (*see sutra* 3.9).

Arthavattva = purpose (*see sutra* 1.28).

Samyamat = by samyama (*see sutra* 3.4).

Indriya = senses (*see sutra* 2.18).

Jayah = mastery (*see sutra* 2.41).

3.49. From that, the body gains the power to move as fast as the mind, ability to function without the aid of the sense organs, and complete mastery over the primary cause (Prakriti).

Tato = thence.

Mano = mind.

Javitvam = fast movement.

Vikaranabhavah = ability to function without the aid of the senses; from *vikarana* = without organs + *bhavah* = condition, state.

Pradhana = primary cause.

Jayah = mastery (*see sutra* 2.41).

Cha = and.

3.50. By recognition of the distinction between sattwa (the pure reflective aspect of the mind) and the Self, supremacy over all states and forms of existence (omnipotence) is gained, as is omniscience.

Sattwa = essential purity, the basis of the principle of individual consciousness and perception (*see sutra* 2.41).

Purusha = Self (*see sutra* 1.16).

Anyatakhyatimatrasya = who recognizes the distinction between;
from *anyata* = distinction + *khyati* = vision (*see sutra* 1.16) + *matra* =
only, merely.

Sarva = all.

Bhava = states.

Adhishthartritvam = supremacy.

Sarvajnatritvam = omniscience; from *sarva* = all + *jnatritvam* = know-
ingness (from *jna* = to know).

Cha = and.

3.51. By nonattachment even to that (all these siddhis), the seed of bondage is destroyed and thus follows Kaivalya (Independence).

Tad = that.

Vairagyat = by nonattachment (*see sutra* 1.12).

Api = even.

Dosha bija = seed of bondage; from dosha (from *dush* = to be
impaired) + *bija* = seed.

Kshate = destroyed (*see sutra* 2.28).

Kaivalyam = independence (*see* 2.25).

3.52. The yogi should neither accept nor smile with pride at the admiration of even the celestial beings, as there is the possibility of his getting caught again in the undesirable.

Sthani = celestial, occupying a high position, high-placed, local
authority, the superphysical entity in charge of the world or plane;
from *stha* = to stand.

Upanimantrane = admiration.

Sanga = attachment.

Smaya = smile (with pride); from *smi* = to smile.

Akaranam = not doing, not accepting, not causing, not indulging;
from *a* = not + *kr* = to make.

Punah = again, renewed.

Anishta = undesirable; from *ish* = to desire.

Prasangat = possibility of getting caught; from *sanj* = to adhere to.

3.53. By samyama on single moments in sequence comes discriminative knowledge.

Kshana = (single) moments, instant.

Tat = its.

Kramayoh = in sequence (*see sutra* 3.15).

Samyamat = by samyama (*see sutra* 3.4).

Vivekajam = discriminative; from *viveka* = discrimination + *jam* = born (*see sutra* 2.15).

Jnanam = knowledge (*see sutra* 1.38).

3.54. Thus the indistinguishable differences between objects that are alike in species, characteristic marks, and positions become distinguishable.

Jati = species (*see sutra* 2.13).

Lakshana = characteristic marks (*see sutra* 3.13).

Desair = and position (*see sutra* 2.31).

Anyata = difference.

Anavacchedat = indistinguishable (*see sutra* 1.26).

Tulyayoh = the same (*see sutra* 3.12).

Tatah = thus (by the above described samyama).

Pratipattih = distinguishable.

3.55. The transcendent discriminative knowledge that simultaneously comprehends all objects in all conditions is the intuitive knowledge (which brings liberation).

Tarakam = transcendent, causing to cross beyond, deliverer; from *tr* = to traverse.

Sarva = all.

Vishayam = objects (*see sutra* 1.11).

Sarvatha = in all ways and/or conditions (*see vishayam below*).

Vishayam = objects (*see sutra* 1.11).

> In this sutra, *vishayam* and *sarvatha*, taken together refer to objects in all the different conditions that they pass through over time.

Akramam = without succession, simultaneous (*see sutra* 3.15).

Cha = and.

Iti = this.

Vivekajam = discriminative (*see sutra* 3.53).

Jnanam = knowledge (*see sutra* 1.38).

3.56. When the tranquil mind attains purity equal to that of the Self, there is Absoluteness.

Sattwa = tranquil mind (*see sutra* 2.41).

Purushayoh = and the Self (*see sutra* 1.16).

Suddhi = purity (*see sutra* 2.20).

Samye = equality; from *sama* = same.

Kaivalya = absoluteness (*see sutra* 2.25).

Pada Four
Kaivalya Pada: Portion on Absoluteness

4.1. Siddhis are born of practices performed in previous births, or by herbs, mantra repetition, asceticism, or samadhi.

Janma = birth (*see sutra* 2.12).

Aushadhi = herb.

Mantra = mantram; from *man* = to think + *tra* = that which protects.

Thought or intention expressed as sound, a prayer or song of praise, sacred text or speech, a sacred sound formula addressed to an individual deity. Mantras are also the hymns that make up the ritual portion of the Vedas (primarily in the Rig and Arthava Vedas).

Tapah = asceticism (*see sutra* 2.1).

Intensity in spiritual practice, austerities, mortification.

Samadhi = absorption (*see sutra* 1.20).

Jah = born.

Siddhayah = psychic powers (*see sutra* 2.43).

4.2. The transformation of one species into another is brought about by the inflow of nature.

Jatyantara = one species to another; from *jati* = species, category, birth + *antara* = other, another.

Parinamah = transformation (*see sutra* 2.15).

Prakriti = Nature (*see sutra* 1.19).

Apurat = by the inflow; lit., overflow; from *a* + *pr* = to fill.

4.3. Incidental events do not directly cause natural evolution; they just remove the obstacles as a farmer (removes the obstacles in a watercourse running to his field).

Nimittam = incidental events, cause, ground, motive, reason, to be the cause of anything; from *ni* = down, back, in, into, within + *ma* = to measure.

Aprayojakam = do not cause; from *yuj* = to yoke.

Prakritinam= natural evolution (*see sutra* 1.19).

This form of the word Prakriti refers to processes of Nature.

Varana = obstacles, rampart, mound; from *vr* = to choose.

In this context, varana can be referring to:
- Choice, in the sense of singling out the possibilities for the next stage in evolution.
- A wall or obstruction that is restraining the natural course of evolution.

Bhedah = remove; from *bhid* = to split.

Tu = but.

Tatah = from that.

Kshetrikavat = like a farmer; lit., farmer-like.

4.4. Individualized consciousness proceeds from the primary ego-sense.

Nirmana = individualized, to allocate, apportion, make, create; from *ma* = to measure.

In Buddhism, this term is used to refer to transformation.

Chittani = plural for consciousness (*see sutra* 1.2).

Asmita = ego-sense (*see sutra* 1.17).

Matrat = primary.

4.5. Although the activities of the individualized minds may differ, one consciousness is the initiator of them all.

Pravritti = activities (*see sutra* 1.35).

Bhede = differ.

Prayojakam = initiator (*see sutra* 4.3).

Chittam= mind-stuff (*see sutra* 1.2).

Ekam = one.

Anekesham = of them all.

4.6. Of these (the different activities in the individual minds), what is born from meditation is without residue.

Tatra = of these.

Dhyanajam = born of meditation.

Anasayam = without residue; from *an* + *asaya* = resting place.

In Yoga philosophy, anasayam refers to the storehouse of the fruits of previous actions which lie in the subconscious as impressions of merit or demerit.

4.7. The karma of the yogi is neither white (good) nor black (bad); for others there are three kinds (good, bad, and mixed).

Karma = actions (*see sutra* 1.24).

Asukla = neither white; from *suc* = to be bright.

Akrishnam = nor black; from *krishna* = black.

Yoginah = of the yogi.

Trividham = three kinds.

Itaresham = for others.

4.8. From that (threefold karma) follows the manifestation of only those vasanas (subliminal traits) for which there are favorable conditions for producing their fruits.

Tatah = from that.

Tat = their.

Vipaka = fruition (*see sutra* 1.24).

Anugunanam = favorable conditions, having similar qualities, congenial to, according or suitable to.

Eva = alone.

Abhivyaktih = manifestation, distinction.

Vasanam = subliminal trait; from *vas* = to abide, stay, dwell.

Vasanas are a subset of subconscious impressions (*samskaras*) that link together to form habit patterns or personality traits. The word is also used to refer to desire.

4.9. Vasanas, though separated (from their manifestation) by birth, place, or time, have an uninterrupted relationship (to each other and the individual) due to the seamlessness of subconscious memory and samskaras.

Jati = birth (*see sutra* 2.13).

Desa = place.

Kala = time.

Vyavahitanam = separated.

Api = though.

Anantaryam = unbroken relationship, immediate sequence or succession; absence of Interval.

Smriti = subconscious memory (*see sutra* 1.6).

Samskarayoh = impressions (*see sutra* 1.18).

Ekarupatvat = uniformity; from *eka* = one + *rupa* = form.

4.10. Since the desire to live is eternal, vasanas are also beginningless.

Tasam = they (the vasanas).

Anaditvam = beginningless.

Cha = and.

Asishah = desire to live.

Nityatvat = eternal.

4.11. The vasanas, being held together by cause, effect, basis, and support, disappear with the disappearance of these four.

Hetu = cause (*see sutra* 2.17).

Phala = effect (*see sutra* 2.14).

Asraya = basis (*see sutra* 2.36).

Alambanaih = support.

Samgrihitatvat = being held together; from *grah* = to grasp.

Esham = these.

Abhave = with the disappearance (*see sutra* 1.10).

Tat = they.

Abhavah = disappear (*see sutra* 1.10).

4.12. The past and future exist as the essential nature (of Prakriti) to manifest (perceptible) changes in an object's characteristics.

Atita = past (*see sutra* 3.16).

Anagatam = future (*see sutra* 2.16).

Svarupatah = essential nature; from *sva* = own + *rupa* = form.

Asti = exist; from *as* = to be.

Adhva = manifest; from *dhav* = to flow along.

Bhedat = changes (*see sutra* 4.3).

Dharmanam = characteristics (*see sutra* 3.13).

4.13. Whether manifested or subtle, these characteristics belong to the nature of the gunas.

Te = they (the characteristics).

Vyakta = manifest (*see sutra* 4.8).

Sukshmah = subtle.

Gunatmanah = nature of the gunas; from *guna* = primary constituents (*see sutra* 1.16) + *atman* = self; refering to the 'selfhood' or nature of the gunas.

4.14. The reality of things is due to the uniformity of the gunas' transformation.

Parinama = transformations (*see sutra* 2.15).

Ekatvat = due to the uniformity; from *eka* = one.

Vastu = things (*see sutra* 1.9).

Tattvam = reality (*see sutra* 1.32).

4.15. Due to differences in various minds, perception of even the same object may vary.

Vastu = objects (*see sutra* 1.9).

Samye = same (*see sutra* 3.56).

Chitta = minds (*see sutra* 1.2).

Bhedat = due to differences (*see sutra* 4.3).

Tayoh = their.

Vibhaktah = are different; from *bhaj* = to allot.

Panthah = ways (of perception); from *path* = to go, move, fly.

4.16. Nor does an object's existence depend upon a single mind, for if it did, what would become of that object when that mind did not perceive it?

Na = nor.

Cha = and.

Eka = a single.

Chitta = mind (*see sutra* 1.2).

Tantram = depend, essential part, framework, main point, characteristic feature; lit., a loom.

Vastu = object (*see sutra* 1.9).

Tat = their.

Apramanakam = not perceived, not provable, not a valid assessment,
not demonstrated, not cognized, not witnessed; from *a* = no or not
+ *pramana* = measure, scale, standard.

Tada = then.

Kim = what.

Syat = becomes; from *as* = to be.

4.17. An object is known or unknown dependent on whether or not the mind gets colored by it.

Tat = thus.

Uparaga = coloring, to tint, red color, inflammation, excitement, passion; from *raj* = to be excited.

The root is derived from the act of coloring or dyeing.

Apekshitvat = due to the need.

Chittasya = of the mind-stuff (*see sutra* 1.2).

Vastu = object (*see sutra* 1.9).

Jnata = known (*see sutra* 1.38).

Ajnatam = unknown (*see sutra* 1.38).

4.18. The modifications of the mind-stuff are always known to the changeless Purusha, who is its lord.

Sada = always.

Jnatah = known (*see sutra* 4.17).

Chitta = mind-stuff (*see sutra* 1.2).

Vrittayah = modifications (*see sutra* 1.2).

Tat = its.

Prabhoh = Lord; from *bhu* = to become + *pra* = forth.

Prabhu means: to come forth, originate from, to be before, surpass, to rule. It also has the meanings of: excelling, mighty, powerful, more powerful than.

Purushasya = of the Purusha (*see sutra* 1.16).

Aparinamitvat = due to changelessness; from *nam* = to bend + *a* = not.

4.19. The mind-stuff is not self-luminous because it is an object of perception by the Purusha.

Na = not.

Tat = it (the mind-stuff).

Svabhasam = self-luminous; from *sva* = self + *bhas* = to shine.

Drisyatvat = because of its perceptibility; from *drs* = to see.

Drisyatvat translated literally is seen-ness or seeable nature, in other words, something that can be perceived.

4.20. The mind-stuff cannot perceive both subject and object simultaneously (which proves it is not self-luminous).

Eka = one.

Samaye = time (*see sutra* 2.31).

Cha = and.

Ubhaye = both.

Anavadharanam = cannot perceive; from *dhr* = to hold.

4.21. If perception of one mind by another is postulated, we would have to assume an endless number of them, and the result would be confusion of memory.

Chittantara = another mind; from *chitta* = mind (*see sutra* 1.2) + *antara* = another (*see sutra* 4.2).

Drisye = perception (*see sutra* 2.17).

Buddhibuddheh = one mind perceiving another; lit., perceiver of perceivers.

From *buddhi* = perceiver (*budh* = to be aware) + *buddhi* = perceiver.

Atiprasangah = endlessness.

Smrittisamkarah = confusion of memory; from *smriti* = memory (*see sutra* 1.6) + *samkara* = confusion (*see sutra* 3.17).

Cha = and.

4.22. When the unchanging consciousness of the Purusha reflects on the mind-stuff, the function of cognition (buddhi) is experienced.

Chiteh = consciousness (*see sutra* 1.2).

Apratisamkramayah = unchanging, having nothing mixed in (referring to the Purusha); from *aprati* = without opponent, irresistible + *krama* = sequence, order, stage.

Tat = it (referring to the individual chitta).

Akarapattau = reflects; from *akara* = shape, form + *apattau* = upon the appearance, occurrence, assumes, arising.

Svabuddhi = cognition; from *sva* = own + *buddhi* = cognition (*see sutra* 4.21).

Samvedanam = experienced (*see sutra* 3.39).

4.23. The mind-stuff, when colored by both Seer and seen, understands everything.

Drashtri = the Seer (*see sutra* 1.3).

Drisya = the seen (*see sutra* 2.17).

Uparaktam = being colored (affected); from *raj* = to be colored.

Chittam = mind-stuff (*see sutra* 1.2).

Sarvartham = understands all; from *sarva* = all + *artha* = object (*see sutra* 1.28).

4.24. Though colored by countless subliminal traits (vasanas), the mind-stuff exists for the sake of another (the Purusha) because it can act only in association with It.

Tat = that.

Asamkhyeya = countless.

Vasanabhih = vasanas; subliminal traits (*see sutra* 4.8).

Chitram = colored, variegated, conspicuous, spotted, mottled, streaked.

Api = also.

Parartham = for another purpose; from *para* = other + *artha* = purpose (*see sutra* 1.28).

Samhatya = in association (with the Purusha).

Karitvat = acting; from *kr* = to do.

4.25. To one who sees the distinction between the mind and the Atman, thoughts of the mind as Atman cease forever.

Visesha = distinction (*see sutra* 1.22).

Darsina = of the seer.

Atmabhava = mind as Self; from *atma* = self (*see sutra* 2.5) + *bhava* = sense of (*see sutra* 3.9).

Atmabhava could also be understood as "sense of self."

Bhavana = thoughts.

Bhavana also means: produced by imagination or meditation; coming to be, producing or cultivating. It also can refer to a memory arising from direct perception and is used as a synonym for meditation.

Vinivrittih = ceases forever, to turn back, cease, desist, extinguish.

4.26. Then the mind-stuff is inclined toward discrimination and gravitates toward Absoluteness.

Tadahi = then.

Viveka = discrimination (*see sutra* 2.26).

Nimnam = inclines toward; from *nam* = to bend.

Kaivalya = absoluteness, independence (*see sutra* 2.25).

Pragbharam = gravitating toward; from *prak* = turned towards the front + *bhara* = mass, weight, burden, load.

Chittam = mind-stuff (*see sutra* 1.2).

4.27. In between, distracting thoughts may arise due to past impressions.

Tad = then.

Chidreshu = in between; from *chid* = to cut.

Pratyayantarani = arise distracting thoughts; from *pratyaya* = thoughts
(*see sutra* 1.10) + *antara* (*see sutra* 4.2) = other.

Samskarebhyah = from past impressions (*see sutra* 1.18).

4.28. They can be removed, as in the case of the obstacles explained before.

Hanam = removal.

Esham = of these, they (old impressions).

Klesavad = as in the case of obstacles (*see sutra* 1.24).

Uktam = has been said before.

4.29. The yogi, who has no self-interest in even the highest knowledge, remains in a state of constant discriminative discernment called dharmamegha (cloud of dharma) samadhi.

Prasamkhyane = the highest knowledge.

Prasamkhyane probably refers to dharmamegha samadhi, a state that
was suggested in sutra 4.26.

Api = even.

Akusidasya = no self interest; from *a* = not + *kusidaysa* = usurious.
Usury refers to the practice of lending money at an unreasonably high
interest rate. In the context of this sutra, akusidasya can be understood
as someone who is not interested in personal profit from their actions.

Sarvatha = constant (*see sutra* 3.55).

Vivekakhyateh = discriminative discernment; from *viveka* (*see sutra*
2.26) = discernment + *khyateh* = vision (*see sutra* 1.16).

Dharmameghah = cloud of dharma; from *dharma* = that which holds
together (*see sutra* 3.13) + *megha* = cloud (from *mih* = to make water).

Samadhi = samadhi; absorption (*see sutra* 1.20).

4.30. From that samadhi all afflictions and karmas cease.

Tatah = from that (samadhi).

Klesa = affliction (*see sutra* 1.24).

Karma = action (*see sutra* 1.24).

Nivrittih = cessation (*see sutra* 3.31).

4.31. Then all the coverings and impurities of knowledge are totally removed. Because of the infinity of this knowledge, what remains to be known is almost nothing.

Tada = then.

Sarva = all.

Avarana = coverings (*see sutra* 2.52).

Malapetasya = removal of impurities; from *mala* = impurities, imperfections, sediment + *apetasya* = removed.

Jnanasya = of knowledge (*see sutra* 1.38).

Anantyat = because of the infinity; from *anta* = end.

Jneyam = to be known (*see sutra* 1.38).

Alpam = very little.

4.32. Then the gunas terminate their sequence of transformation because they have fulfilled their purpose.

Tatah = then.

Kritarthanam = having fulfilled their purpose (*see sutra* 2.22).

Parinama = transformations (*see sutra* 2.15).

Krama = sequence (*see sutra* 3.15).

Samaptih = terminate.

Gunanam = gunas (*see sutra* 1.16).

4.33. The sequence (of transformation) and its counterpart, moments in time, can be recognized at the end of their transformations.

Kshana = moments in time.

Pratyogi = counterpart; from *prati* = towards or near + *yogi* = to join (from *yuj*).

Parinama = transformation (*see sutra* 2.15).

Aparanta = end.

Nigrahyah = recognized; from *grah* = to grasp.

Kramah = sequence (*see sutra* 3.15).

4.34. Thus the supreme state of Independence manifests, while the gunas reabsorb themselves into Prakriti, having no more purpose to serve the Purusha. Or, to look at it from another angle, the power of consciousness settles in its own nature.

Purusha = Self (*see sutra* 1.16).

Artha = purpose (*see sutra* 1.28).

Sunyanam = devoid, having no more (*see sutra* 1.9).

Gunanam = of the gunas (*see sutra* 1.16).

Pratiprasavah = reabsorb (*see sutra* 2.10).

Kaivalyam = absoluteness, independence (*see sutra* 2.25).

Svarupa = in its own nature.

Pratishtha = settles in (*see sutra* 1.8).

Va = or.

Chitisakteh = power of consciousness; from *citi* = consciousness (*see sutra* 1.2) + *sakti* = power (*see sutra* 2.6).

Iti = thus.

Continuous Translation

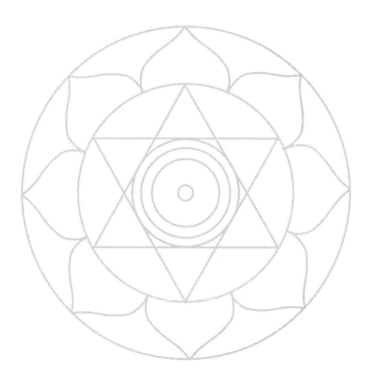

Pada One
Samadhi Pada: Portion on Absorption

1.1. Now, the exposition of Yoga.

1.2. The restraint of the modifications of the mind-stuff is Yoga.

1.3. Then the Seer (Self) abides in Its own nature.

1.4. At other times (the Self appears to) assume the forms of the mental modifications.

1.5. There are five kinds of mental modifications, which are either painful or painless.

1.6. They are right knowledge, misperception, conceptualization, sleep, and memory.

1.7. The sources of right knowledge are direct perception, inference, and authoritative testimony.

1.8. Misperception occurs when knowledge of something is not based on its true form.

1.9. Knowledge that is based on language alone, independent of any external object, is conceptualization.

1.10. That mental modification which depends on the thought of nothingness is sleep.

1.11. Memory is the recollection of experienced objects.

1.12. These mental modifications are restrained by practice and nonattachment.

1.13. Of these two, effort toward steadiness is practice.

1.14. Practice becomes firmly grounded when well attended to for a long time, without break, and with enthusiasm.

1.15. Nonattachment is the manifestation of self-mastery in one who is free from craving for objects seen or heard about.

1.16. When there is nonthirst for even the gunas (constituents of Nature) due to realization of the Purusha, that is supreme nonattachment.

1.17. Cognitive (samprajnata) samadhi (is associated with forms and) is attended by examination, insight, joy, and pure I-am-ness.

1.18. Noncognitive (asamprajnata) samadhi occurs with the cessation of all conscious thought; only the subconscious impressions remain.

1.19. Yogis who have not attained asamprajnata samadhi remain attached to Prakriti at the time of death due to the continued existence of thoughts of becoming.

1.20. To the others, asamprajnata samadhi is preceded by faith, strength, mindfulness, (cognitive) samadhi, and discriminative insight.

1.21. To the keen and intent practitioner this samadhi comes very quickly.

1.22. The time necessary for success also depends on whether the practice is mild, moderate, or intense.

1.23. Or samadhi is attained by devotion with total dedication to God (Ishwara).

1.24. Ishwara is the supreme Purusha, unaffected by any afflictions, actions, fruits of actions, or any inner impressions of desires.

1.25. In Ishwara is the complete manifestation of the seed of omniscience.

1.26. Unconditioned by time, Ishwara is the teacher of even the most ancient teachers.

1.27. The expression of Ishwara is the mystic sound OM.

1.28. To repeat it in a meditative way reveals its meaning.

1.29. From this practice, the awareness turns inward, and the distracting obstacles vanish.

1.30. Disease, dullness, doubt, carelessness, laziness, sensuality, false perception, failure to reach firm ground, and slipping from the ground gained—these distractions of the mind-stuff are the obstacles.

1.31. Accompaniments to the mental distractions include distress, despair, trembling of the body, and disturbed breathing.

1.32. The concentration on a single subject (or the use of one technique) is the best way to prevent the obstacles and their accompaniments.

1.33. By cultivating attitudes of friendliness toward the happy, compassion for the unhappy, delight in the virtuous, and equanimity toward the nonvirtuous, the mind-stuff retains its undisturbed calmness.

1.34. Or that calm is retained by the controlled exhalation or retention of the breath.

1.35. Or that (undisturbed calmness) is attained when the perception of a subtle sense object arises and holds the mind steady.

1.36. Or by concentrating on the supreme, ever-blissful Light within.

1.37. Or by concentrating on a great soul's mind which is totally freed from attachment to sense objects.

1.38. Or by concentrating on an insight had during dream or deep sleep.

1.39. Or by meditating on anything one chooses that is elevating.

1.40. Gradually one's mastery in concentration extends from the smallest particle to the greatest magnitude.

1.41. Just as the naturally pure crystal assumes shapes and colors of objects placed near it, so the yogi's mind, with its totally weakened modifications, becomes clear and balanced and attains the state devoid of differentiation between knower, knowable, and knowledge. This culmination of meditation is samadhi.

1.42. The samadhi in which an object, its name, and conceptual knowledge of it are mixed is called savitarka samadhi, the samadhi with examination.

1.43. When the subconscious is well purified of memories (regarding the object of contemplation), the mind appears to lose its own identity, and the object alone shines forth. This is nirvitarka samadhi, the samadhi beyond examination.

1.44. In the same way, savichara (with insight) and nirvichara (beyond insight) samadhis, which are practiced upon subtle objects, are explained.

1.45. The subtlety of possible objects of concentration ends only at the undifferentiated.

1.46. All these samadhis are sabija [with seed].

1.47. In the pure clarity of nirvichara samadhi, the supreme Self shines.

1.48. This is ritambhara prajna [the truth-bearing wisdom].

1.49. The purpose of this special wisdom is different from the insights gained by study of sacred tradition and inference.

1.50. Other impressions are overcome by the impression produced by this samadhi.

1.51. With the stilling of even this impression, every impression is wiped out, and there is nirbija [seedless] samadhi.

Pada Two
Sadhana Pada: Portion on Practice

2.1. Accepting pain as help for purification, study, and surrender to the Supreme Being constitute Yoga in practice.

2.2. They help us minimize the obstacles and attain samadhi.

2.3. Ignorance, egoism, attachment, aversion, and clinging to bodily life are the five obstacles.

2.4. Ignorance is the field for the others mentioned after it, whether they be dormant, feeble, intercepted, or sustained.

2.5. Ignorance is regarding the impermanent as permanent, the impure as pure, the painful as pleasant, and the non-Self as the Self.

2.6. Egoism is the identification, as it were, of the power of the Seer (Purusha) with that of the instrument of seeing.

2.7. Attachment is that which follows identification with pleasurable experiences.

2.8. Aversion is that which follows identification with painful experiences.

2.9. Clinging to life, flowing by its own potency (due to past experience), exists even in the wise.

2.10. In their subtle form, these obstacles can be destroyed by resolving them back into their original cause (the ego).

2.11. In the active state, they can be destroyed by meditation.

2.12. The womb of karmas has its roots in these obstacles, and the karmas bring experiences in the seen (present) or in the unseen (future) births.

2.13. With the existence of the root, there will also be fruits: the births of different species of life, their life spans, and experiences.

2.14. The karmas bear fruits of pleasure and pain caused by merit and demerit.

2.15. To one of discrimination, everything is painful indeed, due to its consequences: the anxiety and fear over losing what is gained; the resulting impressions left in the mind to create renewed cravings; and the conflict among the activities of the gunas, which control the mind.

2.16. Pain that has not yet come is avoidable.

2.17. The cause of that avoidable pain is the union of the Seer (Purusha) and seen (Prakriti).

2.18. The seen is of the nature of the gunas: illumination, activity, and inertia. It consists of the elements and sense organs, whose purpose is to provide both experiences and liberation to the Purusha.

2.19. The stages of the gunas are specific, nonspecific, defined, and undifferentiated.

2.20. The Seer is nothing but the power of seeing which, although pure, appears to see through the mind.

2.21. The seen exists only for the sake of the Seer.

2.22. Although destroyed for him who has attained liberation, it (the seen) exists for others, being common to them.

2.23. The union of Owner (Purusha) and owned (Prakriti) causes the recognition of the nature and powers of them both.

2.24. The cause of this union is ignorance.

2.25. Without this ignorance, no such union occurs. This is the independence of the Seer.

2.26. Uninterrupted discriminative discernment is the method for its removal.

2.27. One's wisdom in the final stage is sevenfold.

2.28. By the practice of the limbs of Yoga, the impurities dwindle away and there dawns the light of wisdom leading to discriminative discernment.

2.29. The eight limbs of Yoga are:
yama—abstinence
niyama—observance
asana—posture
pranayama—breath control
pratyahara—sense withdrawal
dharana—concentration
dhyana—meditation
samadhi—contemplation, absorption, or superconscious state

2.30. Yama consists of nonviolence, truthfulness, nonstealing, continence, and nongreed.

2.31. These Great Vows are universal, not limited by class, place, time, or circumstance.

2.32. Niyama consists of purity, contentment, accepting but not causing pain, study, and worship of God (self-surrender).

2.33. When disturbed by negative thoughts, opposite (positive) ones should be thought of. This is pratipaksha bhavana.

2.34. When negative thoughts or acts such as violence and so on are caused to be done, or even approved of, whether incited by greed, anger, or infatuation, whether indulged in with mild, medium, or extreme intensity, they are based on ignorance and bring certain pain. Reflecting thus is also pratipaksha bhavana.

2.35. In the presence of one firmly established in nonviolence, all hostilities cease.

2.36. To one established in truthfulness, actions and their results become subservient.

2.37. To one established in nonstealing, all wealth comes.

2.38. To one established in continence, vigor is gained.

2.39. To one established in nongreed, a thorough illumination of the how and why of one's birth comes.

2.40. By purification, the body's protective impulses are awakened, as well as a disinclination for detrimental contact with others.

2.41. Moreover, one gains purity of sattwa, cheerfulness of mind, one-pointedness, mastery over the senses, and fitness for Self-realization.

2.42. By contentment, supreme joy is gained.

2.43. By austerity, impurities of body and senses are destroyed and occult powers gained.

2.44. Through study comes communion with one's chosen deity.

2.45. By total surrender to Ishwara, samadhi is attained.

2.46. Asana is a steady, comfortable posture.

2.47. By lessening the natural tendency for restlessness and by meditating on the infinite, posture is mastered.

2.48. Thereafter, one is undisturbed by dualities.

2.49. That (firm posture) being acquired, the movements of inhalation and exhalation should be controlled. This Is pranayama.

2.50. The modifications of the life-breath are external, internal, or stationary. They are to be regulated by space, time, and number and are either long or short.

2.51. There is a fourth kind of pranayama that occurs during concentration on an internal or external object.

2.52. As its result, the veil over the inner light is destroyed.

2.53. And the mind becomes fit for concentration.

2.54. When the senses withdraw themselves from the objects and imitate, as it were, the nature of the mind-stuff, this is pratyahara.

2.55. Then follows supreme mastery over the senses.

Pada Three
Vibhuti Pada: Portion on Accomplishments

3.1. Dharana is the binding of the mind to one place, object, or idea.

3.2. Dhyana is the continuous flow of cognition toward that object.

3.3. Samadhi is the same meditation when the mind-stuff, as if devoid of its own form, reflects the object alone.

3.4. The practice of these three (dharana, dhyana, and samadhi) upon one object is called samyama.

3.5. By mastery of samyama, knowledge born of intuitive insight shines forth.

3.6. Its practice is accomplished in stages.

3.7. These three (dharana, dhyana and samadhi) are more internal than the preceding five limbs.

3.8. Even these three are external to the seedless samadhi.

3.9. Impressions of externalization are subdued by the appearance of impressions of nirodha. As the mind begins to be permeated by moments of nirodha, there is development in nirodha.

3.10. When impressions of nirodha become strong and pervasive, the mind-stuff attains a calm flow of nirodha.

3.11. The mind-stuff transforms toward samadhi when distractedness dwindles and one-pointedness arises.

3.12. Then again, when the subsiding and arising images are identical, there is one-pointedness (ekagrata parinama).

3.13. By what has been said (in sutras 3.9–3.12) the transformations of the form, characteristics, and condition of the elements and sense organs are explained.

3.14. The substratum (Prakriti) continues to exist, although by nature it goes through latent, uprising, and unmanifested phases.

3.15. The succession of these different phases is the cause of the differences in stages of evolution

3.16. By practicing samyama on the three stages of evolution comes knowledge of past and future.

3.17. A word, its meaning, and the idea behind it are normally confused because of superimposition upon one another. By samyama on the word (or sound) produced by any being, knowledge of its meaning is obtained.

CONTINUOUS TRANSLATION

3.18. By direct perception, through samyama, of one's mental impressions, knowledge of past births is obtained.

3.19. By samyama on the distinguishing signs of others' bodies, knowledge of their mental images is obtained.

3.20. But this does not include the support in the person's mind (such as motive behind the thought, and so on), as that is not the object of the samyama.

3.21. By samyama on the form of one's body (and by) checking the power of perception by intercepting light from the eyes of the observer, the body becomes invisible.

3.22. In the same way, the disappearance of sound (and touch, taste, smell, and so on) is explained.

3.23. Karmas are of two kinds: quickly manifesting and slowly manifesting. By samyama on them or on the portents of death, the knowledge of the time of death is obtained.

3.24. By samyama on friendliness and other such qualities, the power to transmit them is obtained.

3.25. By samyama on the strength of elephants and other such animals, their strength is obtained.

3.26. By samyama on the light within, the knowledge of the subtle, hidden, and remote is obtained. [Note: subtle as atoms, hidden as treasure, remote as far-distant lands.]

3.27. By samyama on the sun, knowledge of the entire solar system is obtained.

3.28. By samyama on the moon comes knowledge of the stars' alignment.

3.29. By samyama on the pole star comes knowledge of the stars' movements.

3.30. By samyama on the navel plexus, knowledge of the body's constitution is obtained.

3.31. By samyama on the pit of the throat, cessation of hunger and thirst is achieved.

3.32. By samyama on the kurma nadi, motionlessness in the meditative posture is achieved.

3.33. By samyama on the light at the crown of the head (sahasrara chakra), visions of masters and adepts are obtained.

3.34. Or, in the knowledge that dawns by spontaneous intuition (through a life of purity), all the powers come by themselves.

3.35. By samyama on the heart, the knowledge of the mind-stuff is obtained.

3.36. The intellect (sattwa) and the Purusha are totally different, the intellect existing for the sake of the Purusha, while the Purusha exists for its own sake. Not distinguishing this is the cause of all experiences. By samyama on this distinction, knowledge of the Purusha is gained.

3.37. From this knowledge arises superphysical hearing, touching, seeing, tasting, and smelling through spontaneous intuition.

3.38. These (superphysical senses) are obstacles to (nirbija) samadhi but are siddhis in the externalized state.

3.39. By the loosening of the cause of bondage (to the body) and by knowledge of the channels of activity of the mind-stuff, entry into another body is possible.

3.40. By mastery over the udana nerve current (the upward-moving prana), one accomplishes levitation over water, swamps, thorns, and so on and can leave the body at will.

3.41. By mastery over the samana nerve current (the equalizing prana) comes radiance that surrounds the body.

3.42. By samyama on the relationship between ear and ether, supernormal hearing becomes possible.

3.43. By samyama on the relationship between the body and ether, lightness of cotton fiber is attained, and thus traveling through the ether becomes possible.

3.44. (By virtue of samyama on ether) vritti activity that is external to the body is (experienced and) no longer inferred. This is the great bodilessness which destroys the veil over the light of the Self.

3.45. Mastery over the gross and subtle elements is gained by samyama on their essential nature, correlations, and purpose.

3.46. From that (mastery over the elements) comes attainment of anima and other siddhis, bodily perfection, and the non-obstruction of bodily functions by the influence of the elements.

3.47. Beauty, grace, strength, and adamantine hardness constitute bodily perfection.

3.48. Mastery over the sense organs is gained by samyama on the senses as they correlate to the process of perception, the essential nature of the senses, the ego-sense, and to their purpose.

3.49. From that, the body gains the power to move as fast as the mind, the ability to function without the aid of the sense organs, and complete mastery over the primary cause (Prakriti).

3.50. By recognition of the distinction between sattwa (the pure reflective aspect of the mind) and the Self, supremacy over all states and forms of existence (omnipotence) is gained, as is omniscience.

3.51. By nonattachment even to that (all these siddhis), the seed of bondage is destroyed and thus follows Kaivalya (Independence).

3.52. The yogi should neither accept nor smile with pride at the admiration of even the celestial beings, as there is the possibility of his getting caught again in the undesirable.

3.53. By samyama on single moments in sequence comes discriminative knowledge.

3.54. Thus the indistinguishable differences between objects that are alike in species, characteristic marks, and positions become distinguishable.

3.55. The transcendent discriminative knowledge that simultaneously comprehends all objects in all conditions is the intuitive knowledge (which brings liberation).

3.56. When the tranquil mind attains purity equal to that of the Self, there is Absoluteness.

Pada Four
Kaivalya Pada: Portion on Absoluteness

4.1. Siddhis are born of practices performed in previous births, or by herbs, mantra repetition, asceticism, or samadhi.

4.2. The transformation of one species into another is brought about by the inflow of nature.

4.3. Incidental events do not directly cause natural evolution; they just remove the obstacles as a farmer (removes the obstacles in a watercourse running to his field).

4.4. Individualized consciousness proceeds from the primary ego-sense.

4.5. Although the activities of the individualized minds may differ, one consciousness is the initiator of them all.

4.6. Of these (the different activities in the individual minds), what is born from meditation is without residue.

4.7. The karma of the yogi is neither white (good) nor black (bad); for others there are three kinds (good, bad, and mixed).

4.8. From that (threefold karma) follows the manifestation of only those vasanas (subliminal traits) for which there are favorable conditions for producing their fruits.

4.9. Vasanas, though separated (from their manifestation) by birth, place, or time, have an uninterrupted relationship (to each other and the individual) due to the seamlessness of subconscious memory and samskaras.

4.10. Since the desire to live is eternal, vasanas are also beginningless.

4.11. The vasanas, being held together by cause, effect, basis, and support, disappear with the disappearance of these four.

4.12. The past and future exist as the essential nature (of Prakriti) to manifest (perceptible) changes in an object's characteristics.

4.13. Whether manifested or subtle, these characteristics belong to the nature of the gunas.

4.14. The reality of things is due to the uniformity of the gunas' transformation.

4.15. Due to differences in various minds, perception of even the same object may vary.

4.16. Nor does an object's existence depend upon a single mind, for if it did, what would become of that object when that mind did not perceive it?

4.17. An object is known or unknown depending on whether or not the mind gets colored by it.

4.18. The modifications of the mind-stuff are always known to the changeless Purusha, who is its lord.

4.19. The mind-stuff is not self-luminous because it is an object of perception by the Purusha.

4.20. The mind-stuff cannot perceive both subject and object simultaneously (which proves it is not self-luminous).

4.21. If perception of one mind by another is postulated, we would have to assume an endless number of them, and the result would be confusion of memory.

4.22. When the unchanging consciousness of the Purusha reflects on the mind-stuff, the function of cognition (buddhi) becomes possible.

4.23. The mind-stuff, when colored by both Seer and seen, understands everything.

4.24. Though colored by countless subliminal traits (vasanas), the mind-stuff exists for the sake of another (the Purusha) because it can act only in association with It.

4.25. To one who sees the distinction between the mind and the Atman, thoughts of the mind as Atman cease forever.

4.26. Then the mind-stuff is inclined toward discrimination and gravitates toward Absoluteness.

4.27. In between, distracting thoughts may arise due to past impressions.

4.28. They can be removed, as in the case of the obstacles explained before.

4.29. The yogi, who has no self-interest in even the most exalted states, remains in a state of constant discriminative discernment called dharmamegha (cloud of dharma) samadhi.

4.30. From that samadhi all afflictions and karmas cease.

4.31. Then all the coverings and impurities of knowledge are totally removed. Because of the infinity of this knowledge, what remains to be known is almost nothing.

4.32. Then the gunas terminate their sequence of transformation because they have fulfilled their purpose.

4.33. The sequence (of transformation) and its counterpart, moments in time, can be recognized at the end of their transformations.

4.34. Thus the supreme state of Independence manifests, while the gunas reabsorb themselves into Prakriti, having no more purpose to serve the Purusha. Or, to look at it from another angle, the power of consciousness settles in its own nature.

Glossary of Sanskrit Terms

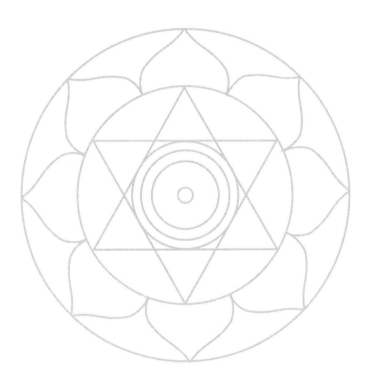

Glossary of Sanskrit Terms

This glossary contains definitions for some common terms used in and around the science of Yoga. Sanskrit terms that appear in the *Yoga Sutras* are cross-referenced to pertinent sutras.

Several key terms, such as *Ishwara* and *moksha* include the definitions from different philosophical schools. They are included to help explain differences in their use by various authors or scriptures; differences whose impact is usually on a philosophical rather than practical level.

Also included in this glossary are pertinent quotes that provide a little extra clarity and inspiration.

A

abhinivesha – Clinging to bodily life, the will to live. Abhinivesha is rooted in ignorance of our True Identity as the immortal Purusha. (*See sutras 2.3 and 2.9.*)

abhyasa – Practice, continuous endeavor, vigilance, exercise, repetition, exertion; lit., to apply oneself toward. (*See sutras* 1.12-1.14.)

"Every aspiration may indeed be achieved if one remembers to keep the goal ever before the mind" (The Thirukkural).

advaita – Nondualism, monism. Advaita regards Reality as one and indivisible; beyond pairs of opposites, such as hot/cold, up/down, male/female, good/bad.

agami karma – Karma unfolding in the present. (*See sutra 2.12.*)

ahamkara – Egoism, ego feeling, the sense of self-identity; lit., the I-maker. (*See sutra 2.6.*)

ahimsa – Non-injury. One of the yamas. (*See sutras 2.30 and 2.35.*)

"The code of the pure in heart is not to return hurt for angry hurt" (The Thirukkural).

akasha – Ether, space; lit., the not visible. The subtlest of the five elements, it is the all-pervasive and dynamic ground of other elements.

anagata – That which is not yet come (referring to the silence beyond the OM vibration), belonging to the future.

anahata – The unstruck, the continuous inner humming vibration, the heart chakra.

ananda – Bliss.

"Happiness is the natural life of man" (Thomas Aquinas).

apana – Energy descending from the navel pit within the human body. Its sphere of influence is the abdominal region and it is responsible for the excretion of wastes. It is the downward moving prana.

aparigraha – Nongreed, nonhoarding, nonacceptance of gifts. It is one of the yamas. (*See sutra 2.39.*) Aparigraha is also one of the five *mahavratam* (great vows) of the Jain religion; the other four are the same as the remaining four principles of yama.

"Of no avail is keenness of intellect or wide knowledge if greed seizes us and leads us to folly" (The Thirukkural).

apunya – Nonvirtuous; wicked.

asana – The third limb of the eight limbs of Raja Yoga. A steady comfortable posture for meditation. Most of the thousands of different bending and stretching postures utilized in Hatha Yoga to enhance health and well-being are also referred to as asanas.

Ashtanga Yoga – Refers to the eight limbs of Raja Yoga: yama, niyama, asana, pranayama, pratyahara, dharana, dhyana, samadhi. (*See sutra* 2.29.)

Atman – The Self or Brahman when regarded as abiding within the individual.

B

bhakti – Devotion; lit., to partake of, to turn to.

Bhakti Yoga – The Yoga of devotion to any name and form of the Divine.

"Bhakti is not mere emotionalism, but is the turning of the will as well as the intellect towards the Divine. It is supreme love of God. It leads to immortality or God-realization" (Sri Swami Sivananda).

Bhagavad Gita – A Hindu scripture, a portion of the great epic the *Mahabharata* composed perhaps 2400 years ago, in which Lord Krishna instructs his disciple Arjuna in the various aspects of Yoga.

bhuvanam – Universe.

bijam – Seed, source.

Brahma – God as creator of the universe. One of the Hindu trinity which also includes Lord Vishnu and Lord Siva.

brahmacharya – Continence; lit. the path that leads to Brahman, or moving in Brahman. One of the yamas. (*See sutra* 2.38.) Also, a code of conduct referring to someone who studies the Vedas. It can also refer to the stage of life of a celibate student of religious studies. Practically speaking, it means to have moderation in all things.

brahmamuhurta – The two-hour period before sunrise (roughly between four and six a.m.) that is especially conducive to meditation.

Brahman – The unmanifest supreme consciousness or God; the Absolute; lit. greater than the greatest.) In Vedanta, it refers to the Absolute Reality and is regarded as that which is beyond differences. It is considered *nirguna*, beyond nature, that which cannot be conceptualized. Brahman is pure absolute existence, knowledge and bliss. It is considered as the only absolute reality, whereas the created universe is but an appearance.

buddhi – Intellect, discriminative faculty of the mind, understanding, reason. From the root *budh* to enlighten, to know. (*See mahat.*)

C

chakra – One of the subtle nerve centers along the spine; lit., wheel.

chit – To perceive, observe; to know.

chitta – Mind-stuff. While in the *Yoga Sutras*, chitta refers to the mind-stuff, in the nondualistic school of Vedanta (Advaita Vedanta) it refers to the subconscious.

D

darshana – The insight, vision or experience of a divine or enlightened being; any philosophical school. Yoga is traditionally considered one of six orthodox darshanas (philosophies) in India.

deva – Celestial being, controller of an aspect of nature.

dharana – Concentration, the practice of continually refocusing the mind on the object of meditation. The sixth of the eight limbs of Raja Yoga. (*See sutras* 2.29 *and* 3.1.)

"As you gain control of your mind with the help of your higher Self, then your mind and ego become your allies. But the uncontrolled mind behaves as an enemy" (Bhagavad Gita 6.6).

dharma – Duty, righteousness, religion, virtue, characteristics, law, justice, universal law; lit., that which holds together. It is the foundation of all order: religious, social and moral. Sri Swami Sivananda Maharaj defines dharma as that which brings harmony. In general there are two classifications of dharma: that which is common to all, and that which is specific to a particular class or stage of life. It has been further broken down as follows:

- *varna ashrama dharma*: one's specific duty according to class and stage of life
- *sanatana dharma*: the Eternal Truth (the more accurate name for what is now commonly called Hinduism)
- *swadharma*: one's one duty as dictated by inborn talents, traits, etc. One's purpose in this life
- *apad dharma*: duties prescribed in times of adversity
- *yuga dharma*: the laws and codes of conduct appropriate to one's era in time
- *sadharana dharma*: the general obligations of common duties incumbent on everyone

In Buddhism, dharma is often used to refer to cosmic order, natural law, the teachings of Lord Buddha, codes of conduct, objects, facts, or ideas.

"Keep the mind free from non-virtuous thoughts. This is the whole of dharma. All else is only of the nature of sound and show" (The Thirukkural).

dhyana – Meditation, the steady focus of the mind's attention on the object of meditation. The seventh of the eight limbs of the Raja Yoga.

"Little by little your mind becomes one-pointed and still and you can focus on the Self without thinking of anything else" (Bhagavad Gita, 6.25).

duhkha – Suffering, pain, sorrow, grief.

"You can advance farther in grace in one hour during this time of affliction than in many days during a time of consolation" (John Eudes).

"Suffering is a short pain and a long joy" (Blessed Henry Suso).

dvesha – Dislike, aversion.

E

ekagrata – One-pointedness of mind. (*See sutras* 3.11 *and* 3.12.)

ekam – One; Reality. Ekam is the term used in the well-known phrase from the Upanishads, *"Ekam sat, vipraha bahudha vadanti," "The Truth is one (ekam); seers express it in many ways."* This principle is the basis of the nondualistic Advaita Vedanta philosophy which proclaims that although we see many names and forms, they are all manifestations of the One Absolute Reality.

G

guna – Quality, attribute, characteristic; lit., strand or thread. One of the three qualities of nature: sattwa, rajas and tamas; or balance, activity and inertia. (*See sutras* 1.16, 2.15, 2.19, 4.13 *and* 4.34.)

guru – A spiritual guide or teacher; lit., the weighty or venerable one. The Guru Gita and the Advaya-Taraka Upanishad also state that the syllable, *gu* = darkness and *ru* = remover. The sage Shankaracharya described a guru as one whose mind is steadfast in the highest reality; who has a pure tranquil mind; and who has directly experienced identity with Brahman. Although it is understood that God is the true and only guru, the human guru acts as a conduit for the Divine teachings, grace and guidance.

guru-parampara – The lineage of teachers; the uninterrupted succession of teachers. In sutra 1.26, Ishwara is referred to as *"the teacher of even the most ancient teachers."*

H

hatha – Ha = sun; *tha* = moon. Analogous the yang and yin, ha and tha are symbolic of the interplay of the polarities of masculine and feminine, activity and rest, hot and cold, and so on, that exist within each individual and in Nature.

Hatha Yoga – The physical branch of Yoga practice. It includes postures (*asanas*), breathing techniques (*pranayama*), seals (*mudras*), locks (*bandhas*) and cleansing practices (*kriyas*). Though known for its ability to bring health, flexibility and relaxation, its ultimate objectives are the purification of the *nadis* (subtle nerve pathways) and uniting of the outgoing and incoming (or upward and downward) flows of prana. When the flow of prana is balanced and harmonious, the mind becomes still and tranquil and ready for the subtler practices of concentration, meditation and samadhi. Hatha Yoga helps return the body to its natural state of health and ease.

himsa – Injury, violence.

I

ida – The subtle *nadi* (nerve current) that flows through the left nostril. It has the effect of cooling the system as opposed to pingala, the heating nadi on the right.

indriya – Sense organ. It can refer to either the external physical organ or the inner organ of perception. (*See sutras* 2.18, 2.41, 2.43, 2.54, 2.55, 3.13 *and* 3.48.)

Integral Yoga – The principles and practices of the six major branches of Yoga: Hatha, Jnana, Bhakti, Karma, Japa, and Raja, as taught by Sri Swami Satchidananda. The mix and emphasis of the practices is dependent on the taste, natural inclinations and temperament of the individual.

"The goal of Integral Yoga is to have an easeful body, a peaceful mind and a useful life" (Sri Swami Satchidananda).

ishta devata – One's chosen deity. There is only one absolute God with the various deities being manifestations or representing aspects of that one Reality. In Hinduism and Yoga, seekers are free to choose whichever form is most meaningful to them for veneration and worship.

Ishwara – Lord, God, the Divine with form, the Supreme Cosmic Soul; from the verb root *ish* = to rule, to own.

There are several meanings for this term:

- The Supreme ruler and Controller; both transcendent and immanent.
- According to Advaita Vedanta, Ishwara is the Absolute (Brahman) as seen from within ignorance or illusion.
- The material and efficient cause of the world.
- According to Sri Patanjali: the Supreme Purusha, unaffected by afflictions, karmas or desires, the omniscient teacher of all teachers, expressed by the mantra OM. (*See sutras* 1.24 – 1.27.)

Ishwara pranidhanam – Worship of God or self-surrender. One of the principles of Sri Patanjali's kriya yoga and one of the principles of niyama. (*See sutras* 1.23, 2.1, 2.32 *and* 2.45.)

"And you shall love the Lord thy God with all your heart, and with all your soul and with all your might" (Deuteronomy 6.5).

J

japa – Repetition or recitation, usually of a mantra or name of God.

Japa Yoga – Science of mantra repetition. The repetition could be out loud, with lip movement only or mentally; or as a writing meditation (*likhita japa*). (*See sutras* 1.27 – 1.29.)

"Japa purifies the heart. Japa steadies the mind. Japa makes one fearless. Japa removes delusion. Japa gives supreme peace. Japa gives health, wealth, strength and long life. Japa brings God-consciousness" (Sri Swami Sivananda).

jaya – Victory, mastery. (*See sutras* 2.41, 3.5, 3.40, 3.45, 3.48, 3.49.)

jiva(tman) – Individual soul. According to Sankhya philosophy, *jivas* (souls) are infinite in number, conscious and eternal. There is neither birth nor death for the jiva. According to Advaita Vedanta, the jiva is a blending of the Self and not-Self due to an incorrect identification of the Self with the body-mind.

jivanmukta – Liberated living soul. Liberation results from the discrimination between the spirit and Nature and the ultimate dissolution of ignorance (*avidya*).

A jivanmukta, *"has double consciousness. He enjoys the bliss of Brahman. He also has the experience of this world"* (Sri Swami Sivananda).

jnanam – Wisdom of the Self; knowledge, idea. The word is often used to refer to insights gained from meditation and samadhi.

Jnana Yoga – Yoga of Self-inquiry, knowledge and study. It is characterized by contemplation on the true nature of the Self, the constant effort to discriminate between what is real (permanent and unchanging) and what is unreal (that which changes).

jyoti – Illumination, effulgence, light.

K

kaivalya – Absolute freedom, independence, isolation, liberation. (*See sutras* 2.25, 3.51, 3.56, 4.26 *and* 4.34.)

kala – Time.

karma – The universal law of action and reaction; cause and effect. It is of four classes (*see sutra* 1.7.) according to the effects the actions produce.
- white = happiness
- black = unhappiness
- black & white (mixed) = a mix of happiness and sorrow

- neither black nor white = actions – like those of the yogi – which transcend karma, leaving the individual free

Karma can also be classified as follows:
- *Sanjita* – all the accumulated actions from previous births awaiting another lifetime to bear fruit
- *Prarabdha* – karmas manifesting in the present birth
- *Agami* – karmas currently being created

(*See sutras* 1.24, 2.12, 2.13, 3.23, 4.7 *and* 4.30.)

Karma Yoga – Performing actions as selfless service without attachment to the results, performance of one's duties without selfish expectation, actions performed for the joy of serving.

"*Live for the sake of others. Spend a little time every day for your own health and peace and then share it with everyone*" (Sri Swami Satchidananda).

karmasaya – Womb, or bag, of karmas. The karmasaya is the storehouse of past karmas waiting for the proper time and environment to come to fruition.

karuna – Mercy, compassion.

"*Diverse are the teachings of the religions of the world, but in all will be found that compassion is that which confers spiritual deliverance. Hold on to it*" (The Thirukkural).

klesa – Misery, root obstruction. (*See sutra* 2.3.) In Indian scriptural literature, klesas are also referred to as *viparyaya* or error (*see sutra* 1.8).

kriya – Action, practices. According to Sri Patanjali, it comprises the three preliminary steps in Yoga (tapas, svadhyaya, and Ishwara pranidhanam, or austerity, study and self-surrender). (*See sutra* 2.1.) The word also is used to refer to the cleansing practices of Hatha Yoga.

kumbhaka – Breath retention. It could be voluntary as part of the practice of pranayama (as in the breathing practices of Hatha Yoga) or occurring naturally in deep meditative states (in which case it is referred to as *kevala kumbhaka*).

kundalini – The primordial energy, lit., the coiled energy, stored at the base of the spine in the *muladhara chakra* of every individual. When awakened naturally through the one-pointed attentiveness and purification of selfishness, it begins to move upward within the subtle central channel (*sushumna*) of the spine, piercing and enlivening the chakras and initiating a total rejuvenation and spiritual evolution of the entire being. Because a forced, premature awakening of this energy can result in undesirable consequences, it is compared to a cobra that must be handled with great care.

M

mahat – Great (in space, time, quality or degree). Also a synonym for *buddhi*, the discriminative faculty of the mind. According to Sankhya philosophy, it is the cosmic aspect of the intellect and the first expression of Prakriti. From, mahat, the ego evolves. Mahat is also used as a term of respect and reverence for evolved spiritual individuals.

maharishi – Great sage. It is from *maha* = great + *drsh* = to see. Therefore, maharishi literally means, *great seer*; the one who has seen (experienced) spiritual truths.

mahavratam – Great vows. In the *Yoga Sutras*, it refers to the principles of yama. The same five vows are central to the Jain religion and are considered as essential to gain liberation from the bondage of cause and effect (karma). (*See sutra* 2.31.)

maitri – Friendliness. A virtue to be cultivated in Yoga, it is also one of the fundamental principles cherished by all Buddhas and Bodhisattvas (awakened ones). (*See sutras* 1.33 *and* 3.24.)

"The triple service of friendship is to take the friend out of the wrong path, to lead him into the right path and to share in his misfortune" (The Thirukkural).

manas – Mind, from the root *man*, to think. This important term has several variations in meaning according to different schools of traditional thought. It emerges from the pure (*sattwic*) aspect of ego (*ahamkara*) and is regarded as the inner organ (*antahkarana*). As such, it receives and arranges input from the senses and conveys it to the buddhi.

mantra – A sound formula used for meditation, a sacred word or phrase of great spiritual significance and power, scriptural hymns; lit., a thought that protects. (*See sutra* 1.27.)

"A mantra is divinity encased within a sound-structure. It is divine power or Daivi Shakti manifesting in a sound-body" (Sri Swami Sivananda). The Bible also teaches the significance and power of sound: *"In the beginning was the word, and the word was with God, and the word was God"* (John 1.1).

maya – Illusion, the principle of appearance, the mysterious power of creation. It has several shades of meaning:

- The force or quality that persuades us to misperceive the unreal as real, the temporary as permanent, the painful as pleasurable, the non-Self as the Self and the unconditioned Absolute as having attributes. (See *sutra 2.5, which though not using the word maya, presents ignorance as having the same power. In fact, the sage Shankaracharya used the terms maya and avidya interchangeably.*)
- According to Advaita Vedanta, it is the beginningless cause which brings about the illusory manifestation of the universe. It is not ultimately real and cannot function without Brahman. Maya is how the one reality can appear as many. Because it is illusory, it has significance only on the relative level.

mudra – Sign, seal or symbol. In Hatha Yoga, it is a posture, or a gesture or movement of the hands, which holds or directs the prana within. Many deities and saints are depicted performing mudras which grant benediction.

N

nada – Sound, the sound heard in deep meditation. The first vibration out of which all creation manifests. Sound is the first manifestation of the Absolute Brahman and is represented by the crescent shape in the Sanskrit script for OM.

nadi – Subtle channels of energy flow in the body. There are 72,000 such conduits of vital energy in the body. The most important are *ida, pingala* and *sushumna*. Ida functions as the cooling, receptive parasympathetic nervous system-like activities and is associated with the left nostril. Pingala's activities bring more movement, heat and sympathetic nervous system-like functions and are associated with the right nostril. The *sushumna* is associated with the hollow in the center of the spinal cord and is the channel through which the awakened kundalini energy moves in its journey from chakra to chakra until it reaches the crown of the head (*sahasrara*). The *Yoga Sutras* only mention *kurma nadi* (tortoise-shaped nadi) whose primary function is to bring stability to the body and mind. (*See sutra* 3.32.)

nirbija – Without seed. Nirbija samadhi is the highest spiritual state since both conscious thought and samaskaras (subconscious or seed impressions) are rendered inactive and transcended. (*See sutras* 1.51 *and* 3.8.)

nirodha – To still or restrain; cessation. From the verb root *rudh* = to obstruct, restrict, arrest, avert + *ni* = down or into, it refers to both the process and attainment of stilling all activities of the mind (which obscure the experience of the Purusha). Traditionally, it is said to be applied on four levels: *vritti, pratyaya, samskara* and *sarva*. These four levels describe increasingly more complete and deeper attainments of nirodha.

- Vrittis – modifications of the mind-stuff; movements or currents of thought; thought processes.
- Pratyaya – notions, beliefs; the thoughts that immediately arise in the mind when it is stimulated by an object.
- Samskara – subconscious impressions.
- Sarva – a complete cessation of all mental activity.

(*See sutras* 1.2, 1.12, 1.51 [*in which nirodha is translated as "wiped out"*] *and* 3.9.)

Sri Swami Vivekananda says the following regarding nirodha: "*The chitta is always trying to get back to its natural pure state, but the organs draw it out. To restrain it, to check this outward tendency, and to start it on the return journey to the Essence of Intelligence is the first step in yoga, because only in this way can the chitta get into its proper state.*"

nirvana – To extinguish, blow out. In Buddhist teachings, it refers to the state of liberation. It has also been referred to as unborn, unconditional, unchanging, indescribable, a state of nonattachment to either being or non-being; the state of absolute freedom.

nirvichara – Samadhi that is beyond insight. (*See sutras* 1.44 *and* 1.47.)

nirvikalpa – A term used in Vedanta for the samadhi that is without thought or imagination. It is analagous to asamprajnata samadhi in the *Yoga Sutras*.

nirvitarka – Samadhi that is beyond examination. (*See sutra* 1.43.)

niyama – Observance (the second of the eight limbs of Yoga). (*See sutras 2.32 and 2.40-45.*)

O

OM – The cosmic sound vibration which is the source of, and includes, all other sounds and vibrations. OM is the absolute Brahman as sound and the foundation of all mantras. It is composed of the letters A, U, and M, which respectively represent creation, evolution and dissolution, or the waking, dreaming and dreamless sleep states. Beyond these states is a fourth, the *anahata* or unrepeated. (*See sutra 1.27, in which the word "pranava", or humming, is equivalent to OM.*)

ojas – A subtle energy that enlivens the body and mind. It is accumulated in many ways but is particularly associated with the preservation of sexual energy. Poor diet, overwork, anger, stress and worry deplete ojas, while the opposite conditions increase it. When ojas becomes chronically low, it leads to degenerative disease and premature aging. Although ojas is present throughout the body, it is especially associated with the heart.

P

pada – A one-fourth portion. Each of the four sections of the *Yoga Sutras* is referred to as a pada.

pancha indriyam – The five senses.

Parabrahman – The supreme unmanifest consciousness or God.

param – Highest, supreme

Patanjali – The sage who compiled the *Yoga Sutras*. He is often referred to as the "Father of Yoga." Some identify him as also the author of the *Mahabhashya*, an important Sanskrit grammatical text, which dates to the second century B.C. E. There are also other works attributed to an author(s) named Patanjali, including texts on medicine.

In popular tradition, Sri Patanjali is considered an incarnation of the mythical serpent *Ananta* (or *Sesha*), on whom Lord Vishnu rests before the beginning of a new cycle of creation. Symbolically, snakes were said to be the guardians of esoteric teachings and *Ananta*, as Lord of the snakes, presided over them all. *Ananta* took on human form as Patanjali for the benefit of humanity.

In another version, Patanjali is said to have fallen from the sky as a newborn serpent into the hands of his mother as she was offering water in worship of the sun. She called him Patanjali from *pata* (meaning both serpent and fallen) and *anjali* (referring to hands cupped in worship).

pingala – A subtle nerve current that flows to the right nostril and is heating in its effect.

prakasha – Illumination, radiance, light, sattwa. (*See sutras* 2.18, 2.52, 3.21 *and* 3.44.)

Prakriti – Primordial Nature. In Sankhya philosophy it is one of the two fundamental categories of existence, the other being Purusha. Although Prakriti is active, consciousness is not intrinsic to its nature. In Advaita Vedanta, Prakriti is a principle of illusion (maya) and is therefore not real.

prana – The vital energy, life breath, life force. Though one, prana is divided into five major categories according to its functions:
- *prana*: rising upwards
- *apana*: moving downwards. Governs the abdomen and excretory functions
- *vyana*: governs circulation of blood
- *samana*: the force that equalizes; also responsible for the digestive process. (*See sutra* 3.41.)
- *udana*: directs vital currents upwards (*See sutra* 3.40.)

pranava – OM, the basic hum of the vibration of the universe. (*See* "OM" *and sutra* 1.27.)

pranayama – The practice of controlling the vital force, usually through control of the breath. The fourth of the eight limbs of Raja Yoga. (*See sutras* 2.49 - 2.53.)

pranidhanam – Total dedication, self-surrender. (*See sutras* 1.23, 2.1, 2.32 *and* 2.45.) In Buddhism, pranidhanam is taken to mean a vow and usually refers to the Boddisattva's vow of helping all beings attain liberation.

prarabdha karma – The karma which has caused one's present birth.

prasadam – Consecrated food offering, grace, tranquility.

pratipaksha bhavanam – Practice of substituting positive thought forms for disturbing, negative ones. (*See sutras 2.33 and 2.34.*)

pratyahara – Sense control, withdrawal of the senses from their objects (the fifth of the eight limbs of the *Yoga Sutras*). (*See sutras 2.54 and 2.55.*)

pratyaya – Thought, notion, idea. In the context of the *Yoga Sutras*, pratyaya is generally used to refer to the thought that instantly arises when the mind is impacted by an object of perception. As such, pratyayas form the content of vrittis. While vritti refers to a fundamental mental process, pratyaya refers to the content of individual consciousness, including the insights (*prajna*) attained in all of the lower states of samadhi, which are not the result of virtti activity. In Sankhya philosophy pratyaya is equivalent to the intellect or buddhi. (*See sutras 1.10, 1.18, 1.19, 2.20, 3.2, 3.12, 3.17, 3.36 and 4.27.*)

puja – Worship service.

punya – Virtuous, meritorious. (*See sutras 1.33 & 2.14.*)

Purusha – The divine Self which abides in all beings; individual soul. Depending on the context, texts might use "Purusha" to refer to the individual soul or to the Absolute God. In Sankhya philosophy, Purusha along with Prakriti constitute the two basic categories of creation. It is pure consciousness which is unchanging, eternal and pure. The *Yoga Sutras* also use the word "Seer" (*see sutras 2.17, 2.20, 2.21, and 2.25*) and "Owner" (*see sutra 2.23*), to refer to the same reality. According to Advaita Vedanta, Purusha is One and is the eternal witness of all there is. (*See sutras 1.16, 1.24; 3.36, 3.50, 3.56; 4.18 and 4.34.*)

R

raga – Attachment, liking, desire. (*See sutras 1.37, 2.3 and 2.7.*)

raja – King.

Raja Yoga –Royal Yoga; another name by which the *Yoga Sutras of Patanjali* are known. Sri Swami Satchidananda writes in the preface to his commentary on the *Yoga Sutras*: "*It is a practical handbook. Every time you pick it up you can absorb more for your growth. Let us slowly try to understand more; and, what little we understand, let us try to practice. Practice is the most important factor in Yoga.*"

rajas – Activity, restlessness (one of the three gunas).

S

sa-ananda samadhi – Samadhi in which the sattwic mind is experienced. (*See sutra* 1.17.)

sa-asmita samadhi – Samadhi in which the ego alone is experienced. (*See sutra* 1.17.)

sabda – Sound, word or name.

sabija – With seed.

sadhana – Spiritual practices, usually formal, but also refers to the cultivation of mindfulness and proper attitudes in life.

"You must have interest and liking in your sadhana. You must understand well the technique and benefits of sadhana" (Sri Swami Sivananda).

sahasrara chakra – The thousand-petaled lotus; the subtle center of consciousness at the crown of the head, where the awareness and energy go in the higher samadhis.

shakti, Shakti – Energy, power, capacity, the kundalini force; the divine cosmic energy which creates, evolves and dissolves the universe. As a proper name, *Shakti* is used to designate the consort of Lord Siva or the Divine Mother in general.

samadhi – Contemplation, superconscious state, absorption (the eighth and final limb of the eight limbs listed in the *Yoga Sutras*); lit., to hold together completely. Samadhi can refer to any of several states in which the mind is (to a greater or lesser degree) absorbed in a state of union with the object of meditation. It is beyond all thought, untouched by speech or words. It is the experience of unwavering stillness and awareness and leads to intuitive wisdom. (*See sutras* 1.17, 1.18; 1.41-1.51, 2.29, 3.3, 3.11 *and* 4.29.)

samapatti – Coming together, meeting. A synonym for samadhi.

samprajnata – Cognitive samadhi in which information or understanding is gained intuitively. (*See sutra* 1.17.)

samsara – The continuing rounds of birth, death and rebirth.

samskara – Latent, subconscious impression; innate tendency due to past actions. (*See sutras* 1.18, 1.50, 2.15, 3.9, 3.18, 4.9 *and* 4.27.)

samyama – The combined practice of dharana, dhyana and samadhi upon one object. (*See sutras* 3.4, 3.16 – 3.33, 3.35, 3.36, 3.42 – 3.45, 3.48 *and* 3.53.)

samyoga – Connection, contact, perfect union. (*See sutras* 2.17, 2.23 *and* 2.25.)

sanjita karma – Karma awaiting a future birth to bear fruit.

santosha – Contentment (one of the principles of niyama). (*See sutras* 2.32 & 2.42.)

sat – Existence or Truth

Satchidananda, Swami (1914-2002) – world-renowned Yoga Master and founder-spiritual head of the Integral Yoga Institutes and Satchidananda Ashrams.

He is the inspiration behind the building of the LOTUS (Light Of Truth Universal Shrine). Located at Satchidananda Ashram-Yogaville in Buckingham, Virginia, the LOTUS is a sanctuary dedicated to the One Truth that illumines all faiths.

sattwa – Purity, balanced state (one of the three gunas). (*See sutras* 2.41, 3.50 *and* 3.56.)

satya – Truth, truthfulness (one of the principles of yama). (*See sutras* 2.30 *and* 2.36.)

"Truthfulness is attained if one's speech is such that it harms no being in the world" (The Thirukkural).

saucha – Purity (one of the principles of niyama). (*See sutras* 2.40 *and* 2.41.)

savichara samadhi – Samadhi with insight. (*See sutra* 1.17.)

savitarka samadhi – Samadhi with examination. (*See sutras* 1.17 *and* 1.42.)

siddha – An accomplished one, a term often associated with one who has attained supernatural powers.

siddhi – Accomplishment, the term used to refer to the extraordinary powers listed in Pada Three of the *Yoga Sutras*. (*See sutras* 2.43, 3.38 *and* 4.1.)

shanti – Peace.

Sivananda, Swami (1887-1963) – The great sage of the Himalayas, founder of the Divine Life Society; author of over 300 books on Yoga and spiritual life, Guru of Sri Swami Satchidananda and many other respected Yoga teachers.

shraddha – Faith. (*See sutra* 1.20.)

"For if you had faith even as small as a tiny mustard seed, you could say to this mountain, 'Move!' and it would go far away. Nothing would be impossible" (Matthew 17.20).

Sri – Eminent or illustrious. A prefix placed before names of scriptures and great women and men to show respect or reverence; a name of the Goddess of Divine Wealth.

sukha –Happy, pleasant, agreeable. (*See sutras* 1.33, 2.5, 2.7, 2.42 *and* 2.46.)

sutra – Aphorism; lit., thread.

"A sutra is an aphorism with minimum words and maximum sense" (Sri Swami Sivananda).

svadhyaya – Study, scriptural study, study of the self and the Self. One of the niyamas. (*See sutras* 2.1, 2.32 *and* 2.44.)

"Books are infinite in number, and time is short; therefore the secret of knowledge is to take only what is essential. Take what is essential and try to live up to it" (Sri Swami Vivekananda).

swami – In the Hindu tradition, a renunciate or monk; a member of the Holy Order of Sannyas.

T

tamas – Inertia, dullness (one of the three gunas).

tanmatra – Subtle essence, energy or potential that gives rise to material elements. According to Sankhya philosophy, they evolve from the tamasic aspect of the ego principle. The five elements derived from the tanmatras are as follows:

- sound – ether
- touch – air
- sight – fire
- taste – water
- smell – earth

Tantra Yoga – Practices that use rituals, yantras and mantras to experience the union of Siva and Shakti (the masculine and feminine, or positive and negative forces) within the individual. The practices offer detailed explanations of the knowledge of mantras and the essence of things (see *tatwa*). From *tan* = do in detail + *tra* = to protect, tantric practices are believed to have protective powers for its practitioners.

tapas – Lit., to burn. Spiritual austerity; purificatory action, accepting but not causing pain (one of the niyamas). (*See sutras* 2.1, 2.32, *and* 2.43.)

tatwa – From *tat* = that + *tvam* = ness, or *"thatness,"* tatwa is the essence of anything; its essential being. The word also refers to the fundamentals of a philosophical system.

tejas – Illumination, fire, splendor (especially spiritual), brilliance.

tyaga – The renunciation of the selfish ego or the dedication of the fruits of actions to God or humanity. (*See sutra* 2.35, *in which tyaga is translated as "cease."*)

"Tyagat shantir anantaram; The dedicated ever enjoy Supreme Peace" (Bhagavad Gita, 12.12).

U

Upanishads – Lit., to devotedly sit close. The final portion of each of the Vedas which teaches the principles of the nondualistic Advaita Vedanta philosophy. The essential teaching of the Upanishads is that the Self of an individual is the same as Brahman, the Absolute. Therefore, the goal of spiritual life is presented as the realization of Brahman as one's True Identity or Self. There are ten principle Upanishads: *Isha, Kena, Katha, Prasna, Mundaka, Mandukya, Taittiriya, Aitareya, Chandogya,* and *Brihadaranyaka.*

V

vairagya – Dispassion, nonattachment. (*See sutras* 1.12, 1.15, 1.16 *and* 3.51.)

vasana – A subset of samskaras (subconscious impressions) that link together to form habit patterns or personality traits. They are regarded as the immediate cause of rebirth and in some philosophical schools, associated with subtle desires.

Vedanta – The culmination or end objective of knowledge; the final experience resulting from the study of the Vedas. There are two subdivisions of this philosophical school: complete, and qualified nondualism.

Vedas – The primary revealed wisdom scriptures of Hinduism (Rig, Sama, Yajur, and Atharva).

vidya – Knowledge, learning.

vikalpa – Conceptualization. (*See sutras 1.6 and 1.9.*)

viparyaya – Misperception. (*See sutras 1.6 and 1.8.*)

virya – Vital energy, strength. Traditionally, it is one of the attributes attributed to Ishwara. In Buddhism, it is regarded as one of six important virtues.

viveka – Discriminative discernment; discrimination between the Real and the unreal, the permanent and impermanent and the Self and the non-Self. A state of continuous discrimination between that which changes and that which does not. (*See sutras 2.26, 2.28, 3.53, 3.55, 4.26, and 4.29.*)

"A discriminating mind is the greatest of possessions. Without it, all other possessions will come to nothing" (The Thirukkural).

Vivekananda, Swami (1862-1902) – A disciple of Sri Ramakrishna and one of the founders of the Ramakrishna Order. He is a classic commentator of the *Yoga Sutras* and the first Hindu monk to come to America (1893). His teachings remain a central influence in Yoga and spirituality today.

vrittis – Modification or fluctuation of the mind-stuff in which the mind seeks to find meaning by linking together related pieces of information. According to Advaita Vedanta, vritti activity serves as the connecting link between knower (subject) and known (object) and is what makes knowledge of things within creation possible.

Vyasa ("arranger or compiler") – The name of several great sages of Hinduism. Vyasa's commentary on the *Yoga Sutras* is the oldest in existence, dating from the fifth century, C.E. He is also said to have compiled the four Vedas, the Mahabharata, the Bhagavad Gita and the Puranas. Though tradition has it that all these scriptures were compiled by one Vyasa, it is not likely due to the large span of years involved. One reason for this could be that Vyasa was more of a title than a name.

vyutthana – Externalization of individual consciousness. It is the predominant characteristic of ordinary consciousness. Vyutthana implies the desire to know the nature of sense objects, believing that they are separate from the self. It also suggests the desire for gaining satisfaction or permanent happiness from the knowledge of those objects. (*See sutra* 3.9.)

Y

yama – Abstinence (the first of the eight limbs of Raja Yoga). (*See sutra* 2.30.)

Yoga – Union of the individual with the Absolute; any course that makes for such union; a tranquil and clear state of mind under all conditions.

Resources

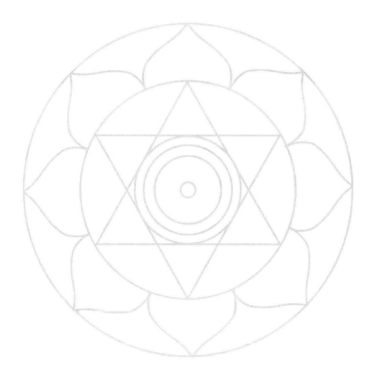

Resources

Dictionaries and Encyclopedias:

A *Concise Dictionary of Indian Philosophy*, John Grimes, State University of New York Press, 1996.

Sanskrit English Dictionary, Arthur A. Macdonell, Award Publishing House, 1979.

Yoga–Vedanta Dictionary, Sri Swami Sivananda, Yoga Vedanta Forest Academy. (No publication date listed.)

A *Sanskrit–English Dictionary*, Monier-Williams, Sir Monier. Searchable Digital Facsimile Edition. The Bkaktivedanata Book Trust, 2002.

The Practical Sanskrit—English Dictionary, Web edition, 2000.

Capellar's Sanskrit—English Dictionary, Web edition, 1891.

Hinduism's Lexicon, Web edition, 2002.

A *Classical Dictionary of Hindu Mythology and Religion: Geography, History and Literature*, John Dowson, D.K. Printworld Ltd., 2000.

The Shambhala Encyclopedia of Yoga, Georg Feurstein, Shambhala Publications, 1997.

A *Dictionary of Sanskrit Names*, Integral Yoga Institute, Integral Yoga Publications, 1989.

Translations and Commentaries of the Yoga Sutras:

The Yoga Sutras of Patanjali, Sri Swami Satchidananda, Integral Yoga Publications, 1990.

The Yoga Sutra Workbook: The Certainty of Freedom, Vyaas Houston, American Sanskrit Institute, 1995.

The Yoga-Sutra of Patanjali, Georg Feuerstein, Inner Traditions International, 1979.

Yoga Sutras, Ramamurti S. Mishra, Anchor Books, 1973.

Kriya Yoga Sutras of Patanjali and the Siddhas, Marshall Govindan, Kriya Yoga Publications, 2000.

The Science of Yoga, L.K. Taimni, The Theosophical Publishing House, 1961.

Yoga-Darshana:Sutras of Patanjali with Bhasya of Vyasa, Ganganatha Jha, Asian Humanities Press, 2002.

The Yoga-Sutra of Patanjali, Chip Hartranft, Shambhala Publicatons, Inc., 2003.

The Yoga Sutras of Patanjali: A Study Guide for Book I, Samadhi Pada, Baba Hari Dass, Sri Rama Publishing, 1999.

The Integrity of the Yoga Darsana, Ian Whicher, State University of New York Press, 1998.

Yoga Discipline of Freedom: The Yoga Sutra Attributed to Patanjali, Barbara Stoler Miller, Bantam Books, 1998.

How to Know God: The Yoga Aphorisms of Patanjali, Swami Prabhavananda and Christopher Isherwood, Vedanta Society of Southern California, Mentor Books, 1969.

Vivekananda: The Yogas and Other Works, published by the Ramakrishna-Vivekananda Center of New York, Copyright 1953 by Swami Nikhilananda, Trustee of the Estate of Swami Vivekananda.

Yoga Philosophy of Patanjali, Swami Hariharananda Aranya, State University of New York Press, 1983.

The I-dea of I, Swami Venkatesananda, The Chiltern Yoga Trust, 1973.

An Introduction to Yoga Philosophy: An annotated translation of the Yoga Sutras, Ashok Kumar Malhotra, Ashgate, 2001.

Patanjali's Vision of Oneness: an Interpretive Translation, Swami Venkatesananda., free internet download at dailyreadings.com/ys.

Other Texts Useful for Students of Yoga:

To Know Your Self: The Essential Teachings of Swami Satchidananda, Edited by Philip Mandelkorn, Integral Yoga Publications, 1988.

The Living Gita: The Complete Bhagavad Gita, Sri Swami Satchidananda, Integral Yoga Publications, 1988.

Concentration and Meditation, Swami Sivananda, The Divine Life Society, 1975.

All About Hinduism, Sri Swami Sivananda, Divine Life Society, 1977.

Bliss Divine, Swami Sivananda, The Divine Life Society, 1974.

The Yoga Tradition: Its History, Literature, Philosophy and Practice, Georg Feurstein, Hohm Press, 1998.

Tiruvalluvar: the Kural, P.S. Sundaram, Penguin Books 1990.

About Sri Swami Satchidananda
and Integral Yoga® Publications

His Holiness Sri Swami Satchidananda (Sri Gurudev) is a world-renowned spiritual teacher and Yoga Master. A much-loved teacher, well-known for his combination of practical wisdom and spiritual insight, he dedicated his life to the service of humanity, demonstrating by his own example the means of finding abiding peace.

Not limited to any one organization, religion or country, Sri Gurudev's message of peace, both individual and universal has been heard worldwide. He received many honors for his service, including the Martin Buber Award for Outstanding Service to Humanity, the B'nai Brith Anti-Defamation League's Humanitarian Award, the Albert Schweitzer Humanitarian Award, and the prestigious U Thant Peace Award.

In 1966, the Integral Yoga Institutes were founded under his direction and today there are Integral Yoga Institutes and Centers throughout the world offering classes and workshops in all facets of the yogic science including Hatha Yoga, meditation, nutrition, stress reduction, Teacher Training Certification Programs and retreats.

Sri Gurudev advocated the principle that "Truth is One, Paths Are Many." He sponsored innumerable interfaith symposiums, retreats, and worship services around the world. Witnessing the genuine peace and joy experienced by the participants, he was inspired to create a permanent place where all people could come to experience their essential oneness and the peace that is their True Nature. The Light Of Truth Universal Shrine (LOTUS), dedicated to the Light of all faiths and to world peace, was opened in 1986. It is located at Satchidananda Ashram-Yogaville in Buckingham, Virginia, a residential and teaching center that serves as the international headquarters for the Integral Yoga Institutes and Centers.

*For more information about **Sri Swami Satchidananda**, please visit: www.swamisatchidananda.org.*

*For wholesale orders, contact **Integral Yoga Distribution** at 1-800-232-1008, or at yogahealthbooks.com.*

*For retail orders, contact **Shakticom** at 1-800-476-1347.*

*To contact **Rev. Jaganath**: www.revjaganath.com.*

Books by Sri Swami Satchidananda:

To Know Your Self

The Living Gita

Integral Yoga Hatha

The Yoga Sutras of Patanjali

The Golden Present (Daily Readings)

Beyond Words

Enlightening Tales as Told by Sri Swami Satchidananda

Guru and Disciple

The Healthy Vegetarian

Kailash Journal

Satchidananda Sutras

Heaven on Earth: My Vision of Yogaville

Books about Swami Satchidananda:

Boundless Giving: The Life and Service of Sri Swami Satchidananda

Sri Swami Satchidananda: Apostle of Peace

Sri Swami Satchidananda: Portrait of a Modern Sage

The Master's Touch

Other books from Integral Yoga Publications:

Imagine That—A Child's Guide to Yoga

LOTUS Prayer Book

Meditating with Children

Dictionary of Sanskrit Names

Yoga for Kids—by Kids

Sparkling Together

Everybody's Vegan Cookbook